# Springer Series on PSYCHIATRY

## Carl Eisdorfer, Ph.D., M.D., Series Editor

**1**

## Stress and Human Health
Analysis and Implications of Research

Glen R. Elliott, Ph.D., M.D., and
Carl Eisdorfer, Ph.D., M.D.
**Editors**

**2**

## Treatment of Psychopathology
## in the Aging

Carl Eisdorfer, Ph.D., M.D., and
William E. Fann, M.D.
**Editors**

**Carl Eisdorfer, PH.D., M.D.,** is President of the Montefiore Medical Center and Professor of Psychiatry and Neuroscience, Albert Einstein College of Medicine and Montefiore Medical Center.

**William E. Fann, M.D.,** is Professor of Psychiatry and Associate Professor of Pharmacology at Baylor College of Medicine and Chief of the Psychiatry Service at the Veterans Administration Medical Center in Houston, Texas.

# TREATMENT OF PSYCHOPATHOLOGY IN THE AGING

Carl Eisdorfer, PH.D., M.D.
William E. Fann, M.D.

Editors

SPRINGER PUBLISHING COMPANY ▪ NEW YORK

Springer Publishing Company, Inc.
200 Park Avenue South
New York, New York 10003

82 83 84 85 86 / 10 9 8 7 6 5 4 3 2 1

*Library of Congress Cataloging in Publication Data*

Main entry under title:

Treatment of psychopathology in the aging.

  (The Springer series on psychiatry ; 2)
  Includes bibliographical references and index.
  1. Geriatric psychiatry.  2. Geriatric psychopharma-
cology.  I. Eisdorfer, Carl.  II. Fann, William E.
III. Series. [DNLM: 1. Aging. 2. Mental disorders—
In old age. Wl SP685SEM v.2 / WT 150 T784]
RC451.4.A5T73 1982     618.97'6891     82-10379
ISBN 0-8261-3810-1

Printed in the United States of America

# Contents

v

# Preface

The widespread emergence of programs and facilities to care for aged patients suffering from cognitive or emotional problems is long overdue. This development probably reflects the demographic changes in our population as well as the recognition that older persons are not merely in difficulty "because they are old," but rather at considerable risk for a number of specific disorders which are, in fact, diagnosable and treatable.

This book is designed to bring together many of the current concepts and practices in the psychiatric care of older patients. The collection of works by notable clinicians and investigators is oriented toward the recognition that older patients should not be treated in a cavalier fashion, as if age were of no consequence, or from the nihilistic posture that nothing much can be done for the aged. An optimistic view is appropriate, with realistic caveats.

Either or both biologic and psychosocial strategies may be of considerable value in the treatment of older patients. Recent observations about both the effectiveness and side effects of medication have made this a subject of significant interest, not only for the clinical psychiatrist or other physician, but for the nonmedical clinician as well. Nonpharmacologic therapies are also to be considered, and they add to the choice of appropriate approaches, which is a key to the management of the older patient.

The range of illnesses and strategies for dealing with them covered in this book is oriented to clinicians and clinical investigators who have an interest in the treatment of the aged, perhaps the most rapidly growing field among the mental health disciplines.

We have begun to recognize that the standard adult dosages of medication and their frequently recognized side effects, well-studied in middle-aged and younger adults, may be misleading in the clinical care of aged patients. There are problems in prescribing medications to older persons distinct enough to require an understanding of the factors involved, and on occasion, significant alterations in approach.

The pharmacodynamics and pharmacokinetics of the various medications used may differ in the older individual. The older patient is much more likely to have coexisting physical problems and need other medications, which can further complicate treatment. Many older patients are not open to psychology, and approaching them through psychotherapy can often be especially difficult if rigid formulations are adapted. Indeed, the setting in which older persons are treated and the nature of those treatments can be of serious consequence as factors in their care.

A recognition of the complex of biologic, psychological, and social factors in patient management should be a stimulus for more interest and involvement by clinicians. It is hoped that this book will help clarify some of the variables involved.

Grateful acknowledgment is made to the Upjohn Company of Kalamazoo, Michigan, which provided the funding and made all the arrangements for the conference where the material for this book was presented and refined.

C. E.
W. E. F.

# Contributors

MONICA D. BLUMENTHAL, M.D., PH.D., is late Professor of Psychiatry, University of Pittsburgh School of Medicine, and Director of Geriatric Services, Department of Psychiatry, Western Psychiatric Institute and Clinic, Pittsburgh, Pennsylvania.

DONNA COHEN, PH.D., is Associate Professor of Psychiatry and Neurosciences, Albert Einstein College of Medicine; Director of the Division of Geriatric Psychiatry, Albert Einstein College of Medicine and Montefiore Medical Center; and Director, Research and Evaluation, Beth Abraham Hospital, Bronx, New York.

THOMAS CUMMINGS, B.A., is Research Assistant, Psychiatry Service, Veterans Administration Medical Center, Bronx, New York.

BONNIE M. DAVIS, M.D., is Staff Physician, Bronx Veterans Administration Medical Center, and Assistant Professor of Medicine and Psychiatry, Mt. Sinai School of Medicine, New York City.

JOHN M. DAVIS, M.D., is Director of Research, Illinois State Psychiatric Institute, and Gilman Professor of Psychiatry, University of Illinois School of Medicine, Chicago, Illinois.

KENNETH L. DAVIS, M.D., is Chief of Psychiatry, Bronx Veterans Administration Medical Center, and Associate Professor of Psychiatry, Mt. Sinai School of Medicine, New York City.

YVONNE DE NIGRIS, M.A., is Mental Health Associate, Psychiatry Service, Veterans Administration Medical Center, Bronx, New York.

MARCIA DIVOLL, B.S., is Research Scientist, Division of Clinical Pharmacology, New England Medical Center Hospital, and Instructor in Psychiatry, Tufts University School of Medicine, Boston, Massachusetts.

DAVID L. DUNNER, M.D., is Chief of Psychiatry, Harborview Medical Center, and Professor of Psychiatry and Behavioral Sciences, University of Washington, Seattle, Washington.

IRWIN FEINBERG, M.D., is Director, Sleep Laboratory, San Francisco Veterans Administration Medical Center, and Professor of Psychiatry, University of California at San Francisco.

MAX FINK, M.D., is Professor of Psychiatry in the Department of Psychiatry and Behavioral Science, School of Medicine, State University of New York, Stony Brook, New York.

SANFORD FINKEL, M.D., is Medical Director, Barclay Hospital, Chicago; Chairman, American Psychiatric Association Task Force on the 1981 White House Conference on Aging; and Assistant Clinical Professor of Psychiatry, Northwestern University Medical Center, Chicago, Illinois.

WILLIAM J. FREED, PH.D., is Senior Staff Fellow, Adult Psychiatry Branch, Division of Special Mental Health Research, Intramural Research Program, National Institute of Mental Health, St. Elizabeth's Hospital, Washington, D.C.

ROBERT O. FRIEDEL, M.D., is Professor and Chairman, Department of Psychiatry, Medical College of Virginia, Virginia Commonwealth University, Richmond, Virginia.

CHARLES M. GAITZ, M.D., is Head, Gerontology Center, Texas Research Institute of Mental Sciences, and Clinical Professor of Psychiatry, Baylor College of Medicine, Houston, Texas.

DAVID J. GREENBLATT, M.D., is Chief, Division of Clinical Pharmacology, New England Medical Center Hospital, and Professor of Psychiatry and Associate Professor of Medicine, Tufts University School of Medicine, Boston, Massachusetts.

JEFFREY B. HALTER, M.D., is Associate Professor of Medicine, Department of Medicine, University of Washington, and Associate Director, Geriatric Research, Education, and Clinical Center, Veterans Administration Medical Center, Seattle, Washington.

BARRY J. HOFFER, M.D., is Professor of Pharmacology, University of Colorado Medical Center, Denver, Colorado.

THOMAS B. HORVATH, M.D., is Clinical Director, Psychiatry Service, Bronx Veterans Administration Medical Center, and Associate Professor of Psychiatry, Mt. Sinai School of Medicine, New York City.

A. KOEGLER, M.D., is Resident in Psychiatry, New York University Medical Center, New York City.

JARY M. LESSER, M.D., is Research Psychiatrist, Illinois State Psychiatric Institute, Chicago, Illinois.

MICHAEL LEVY, M.D., is Director, Special Treatment Unit, Psychiatry Service, Bronx Veterans Administration Medical Center, and Assistant Professor of Psychiatry, Mt. Sinai School of Medicine, New York City.

JOAN C. MARTIN, PH.D., is Professor of Psychiatry, Department of Psychiatry, and Professor of Psychology, Department of Psychology, University of Washington, Seattle, Washington.

RICHARD C. MOHS, PH.D., is Clinical Psychologist, Bronx Veterans Administration Medical Center, and Assistant Professor of Psychiatry, Mt. Sinai School of Medicine, New York City.

LARS OLSON, M.D., is Associate Professor of Histology, Karolinska Institute, Stockholm, Sweden.

PATRICIA N. PRINZ, PH.D., is Associate Professor of Psychiatry and Behavioral Sciences, University of Washington, and Director, Sleep and Aging Program, Geriatric Research, Education, and Clinical Center, Veterans Administration Medical Center, Seattle, Washington.

MURRAY RASKIND, M.D., is Associate Professor of Psychiatry and Behavioral Sciences, University of Washington, and Director, Geriatric Research, Education, and Clinical Center, Veterans Administration Medical Center, Seattle, Washington.

DONALD S. ROBINSON, M.D., is Professor and Chairman, Department of Pharmacology, Marshall University School of Medicine, Huntington, West Virginia.

GORDON S. ROSENBERG, B.A., is Research Assistant, Psychiatry Service, Veterans Administration Medical Center, Bronx, New York.

ALISON ROSS, B.A., is Research Assistant, Psychiatry Service, Veterans Administration Medical Center, Bronx, New York.

CARL SALZMAN, M.D., is Director of Psychopharmacology, Massachusetts Mental Health Center, Boston, and Associate Professor of Psychiatry, Harvard Medical School, Cambridge, Massachusetts.

NANCY L. SEGAL, M.A., is Research Psychologist, Department of Psychiatry, University of Chicago School of Medicine, Chicago, Illinois.

ANN P. STREISSGUTH, PH.D., is Professor of Psychiatry, Department of Psychiatry, University of Washington, Seattle, Washington.

RICHARD C. VEITH, M.D., is Clinical Investigator, Geriatric Research, Education, and Clinical Center, Veterans Administration Medical Center, and Assistant Professor of Psychiatry and Behavioral Sciences, University of Washington, Seattle, Washington.

RICHARD JED WYATT, M.D., is Chief, Adult Psychiatry Branch, Division of Special Mental Health Research, Intramural Research Program, National Institute of Mental Health, St. Elizabeth's Hospital, Washington, D.C.

JEROME A. YESAVAGE, M.D., is Assistant Professor, Department of Psychiatry and Behavioral Sciences, Stanford University School of Medicine, Stanford, California, and Chief, Psychiatric Intensive Care Unit, Veterans Administration Medical Center, Palo Alto, California.

# TREATMENT OF PSYCHOPATHOLOGY IN THE AGING

# CHAPTER 1

# Monoamine Oxidase Inhibitors in the Elderly

## Donald S. Robinson, M.D.

## INTRODUCTION

Various genetic, biologic, and environmental factors can influence drug metabolism. Although it has been appreciated for years that elderly patients tolerate drugs less well than younger ones (1, 2), the pharmacokinetic and pharmacodynamic explanations for this intolerance in the older patient have only recently been forthcoming. Age-related changes in drug response can be due either to altered kinetics or to receptor sensitivity (3). Decreased activity of microsomal drug-metabolizing enzymes with aging has now been documented in pharmacokinetic studies for a variety of drugs (4, 5).

Altered response to antidepressant drug therapy in the elderly is of particular interest and clinical concern. Impaired psychotropic drug metabolism with advancing age has been reported for the widely used and overused benzodiazepine agents (6–8) and the tricyclic antidepressants (9–11).

The resurgence of interest in the monoamine oxidase inhibitors (MAOIs) brings into question their potential therapeutic role in the older depressed patient as well as their potential for side effects and toxicity. The clinical role and therapeutic spectrum of MAOIs has only recently been subjected to intensive scrutiny and investigation (12). There has been little study or report of MAOI use in the geriatric population.

This work is supported in part by grant RO1 MH27836 from the National Institutes of Mental Health, and was carried out in collaboration with Alexander Nies, M.D., Veterans Administration Hospital, Coatesville, PA, and Thomas B. Cooper, Rockland Research Institute, Orangeburg, NY. The invaluable assistance of Diantha Howard, Derek Nicoll, Mary Varese, and Sally Roberts is gratefully acknowledged.

1

Although the tricyclic antidepressants have significant disadvantages in the aged patient, which are largely related to their anticholinergic actions (13), there has been reluctance on the part of many clinicians to consider MAOIs as an alternative antidepressant therapy since it has not been known previously whether these drugs are less well tolerated in the older adult. There is ample documentation that the more popular and widely used tricyclic antidepressant drugs can and often do present significant problems in the elderly, both because of predisposition to troublesome side effects (14) and the now well-documented impairment of drug metabolism and clearance (9, 11).

There is emerging evidence that MAOIs are well tolerated, with few side effects in the older patient, as discussed below. One can speculate that MAOIs might possess special efficacy and therapeutic advantage in the older patient, based on the observation that MAO activity increases with aging in a variety of tissues including brain and platelet (15–17). There is also evidence that depressed patients have higher mean platelet MAO activities than age-matched and sex-matched normal controls (18). This relationship of age and enzyme activity appears to be a generalized phenomenon observed in several human tissues. In two separate series of human brain studies there have been strong positive correlations of MAO activity with age in several brain regions, using as substrates both benzylamine and tryptamine (15, 16). Associated with this increased MAO activity, regional concentrations of norepinephrine show a trend for a gradual decline with age. Serotonin levels do not appear to change significantly with aging. These findings in human brains are consistent with the notion that MAOIs might represent a more specific therapy for elderly patients with primary depressive disorders and depressions associated with dementia.

## RESEARCH

We have been engaged in a double-blind comparison of phenelzine and amitriptyline in depressed outpatients (19). In this clinical trial, comparative efficacy and side effects have been studied. We have examined clinical and drug level data from this and our previous placebo-controlled trials (20, 21) to see whether age may be an important variable influencing drug pharmacokinetics or clinical response to either drug. Patients ranged in age from 19 to 74 years in these 3 outpatient trials. In the amitriptyline treatment group, there was no correlation of age and response rate to drug. However, in the patients treated with phenelzine 60 mg/day, the response to phenelzine improved significantly with aging

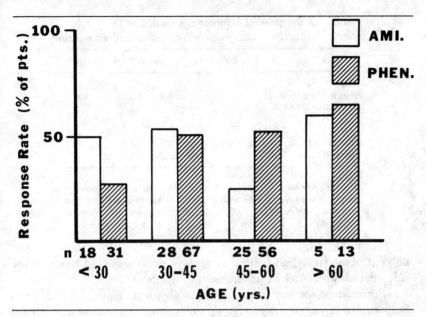

FIGURE 1.1.   Response rate by age strata to amitriptyline (AMI) 150 mg/day
(N=67) or phenelzine (PHEN) 60 mg/day (N=147) in depressed outpatients
treated for 6 weeks in double-blind, controlled clinical trials (19–21). Sample
sizes (N) are given for each group. Therapeutic response rate is the percent of
patients who exhibited pronounced symptomatic improvement or were symptom
free at the end of the 6-week drug treatment period. The trend for greater
clinical improvement with increasing age in the phenelzine treatment group is
statistically significant (p<.01, Wilcoxon rank order test). Amitriptyline response
rate is not related to age.

(Figure 1.1), being best in the group over 60 years of age. It is interesting that percent platelet MAO inhibition achieved during phenelzine
therapy did not relate to age, using either benzylamine or tryptamine as
substrates. Thus, while elderly patients tended to have higher pretreatment MAO activity than younger patients, they did not show more
marked percent inhibition during phenelzine treatment.

It is also interesting that the number of side effects reported by
patients during amitriptyline and phenelzine treatment were fewer for
phenelzine than for amitriptyline. Patients over the age of 50 years
treated with phenelzine reported the fewest drug side effects (Table
1.1). One side effect more common and troublesome to the older patient
treated with phenelzine was orthostatic dizziness. Eight of 12 older
patients (over 50 years of age) reported this symptom during phenelzine
treatment, whereas only 50% of younger patients did so. Thirty-one

TABLE 1.1 Number of Symptoms Reported as Drug Side
Effects during Treatment with Amitriptyline and Phenelzine

| Age and Drug | Number of Symptoms (Mean + SEM[a]) |
|---|---|
| **<50** | |
| Amitriptyline (N=42) | 3.4 + 0.3[b] |
| Phenelzine (N=46) | 2.5 + 0.2 |
| **>50** | |
| Amitriptyline (N = 13) | 2.8 + 0.6 |
| Phenelzine (N=12) | 2.2 + 0.3 |

[a]SEM=Standard Error of Mean
[b]The mean number of side effects reported per patient attributable to
drug treatment was significantly higher than for older patients treated
with amitriptyline (150 mg/day) or patients treated with phenelzine
(60 mg/day).

percent of amitriptyline-treated patients over 50 years old reported this
side effect, as did 43% of patients under age 50.

Fortunately, orthostatic dizziness with phenelzine, although more
frequent, was not troublesome to the point that treatment with the
antidepressant drug required interruption, except in a very few instances. However, patients who experienced this symptom did have
more prominent postural changes in blood pressure. As shown in Table
1.2, there is a significant decrease in both systolic and diastolic standing

TABLE 1.2 Change in Standing Blood Pressure with
Antidepressant Drug Treatment: Effects of
Phenelzine and Amitriptyline in Relation to Age

| Age and Drug | Pretreatment | Treatment |
|---|---|---|
| **<50** | | |
| Phenelzine (N=46) | 125 ± 15 | 118 ± 16 |
| | 82 ± 10 | 82 ± 10 |
| Amitriptyline (N=43) | 124 ± 15 | 121 ± 14 |
| | 85 ± 10 | 87 ± 12 |
| **>50** | | |
| Phenelzine (N=12) | 144 ± 20 | 116 ± 27[a] |
| | 89 ± 13 | 77 ± 17 |
| Amitriptyline (N=14) | 130 ± 17 | 130 ± 12 |
| | 88 ± 7 | 90 ± 8 |

[a]Changes in both systolic and diastolic blood pressure are
significant ($p<.01$, paired t-test) in patients over 50 years
treated with phenelzine 60 mg/day for 6 weeks. There was
no change in blood pressure in patients treated with amitriptyline (150 mg/day).

blood pressures in the age group over 50 years treated with phenelzine; this change does not occur with amitriptyline treatment.

    With the development of a sensitive assay for phenelzine in plasma (22), it is now possible to measure plasma drug levels as well as platelet MAO inhibition during phenelzine therapy. As shown in Figure 1.2, there is a trend for increasing plasma phenelzine concentrations with age as well as with duration of drug treatment. The age correlation is significant at 2 weeks; thereafter, the age correlation tends to disappear. Plasma phenelzine levels also correlate positively with the orthostatic change in blood pressure at 6 weeks of treatment (r=.46; p<.01).

## DISCUSSION

Our findings are in keeping with the recent preliminary report of Ashford and Ford (23), although our outpatient trials did not focus on a geriatric age group per se. In their report of 14 patients (mean age=70 years) treated with tranylcypromine or phenelzine, the MAOIs were generally well tolerated, except for 2 patients. One patient treated with

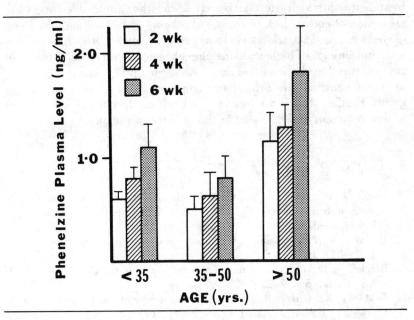

FIGURE 1.2. Mean plasma phenelzine concentrations by age strata during treatment with phenelzine 60 mg/day. Age correlated positively with phenelzine plasma levels (r=.32 [p<.05], .16, and .14 at 2, 4, and 6 weeks, respectively).

tranylcypromine and haloperidol demonstrated an exacerbation of parkinsonism. Another patient treated with phenelzine developed choreiform movements that subsided when the MAOI was discontinued. Patients in our clinical trials tolerated phenelzine better, with a lower overall incidence of side effects than with amitriptyline. We noted no unusual difficulties in the older age group that received phenelzine. Dropouts or early terminations were not overly represented in the older age group receiving phenelzine. Orthostatic dizziness was more commonly reported, but it was not particularly troublesome. This symptom was associated with documented orthostatic change in blood pressure of greater magnitude in the over-50-year age group, but again, it did not require dose reduction or discontinuance of drug therapy. Our patients are cautioned to arise and to change positions slowly, especially in the morning and during the night.

Preliminary experience suggests that MAOIs overall are equally or more efficacious than amitriptyline in treating outpatients with depressive disorders. Our experience with somewhat younger patients is consistent with Ashford and Ford (23), whose geriatric patients responded to MAOIs after they had failed previously on tricyclic antidepressants. Their treatment failures on tricyclics were due to either intolerable anticholinergic side effects or lack of therapeutic benefit. Ashford and Ford employed a reduced MAO dosage in their geriatric patients. This is in keeping with our findings of higher plasma phenelzine concentrations in the older patient. A reduced phenelzine dose also seems appropriate in view of the increased sensitivity to orthostatic change in blood pressure in this age group. Further studies are indicated to evaluate the clinical role of MAOIs in the treatment of depression in the geriatric population.

## REFERENCES

1. Smith, J. W., Seidl, L. G., Cluff, L. E.: Studies on the epidemiology of adverse drug reactions: V. Clinical factors influencing susceptibility. Ann. Intern. Med. 65:629–640, 1966.
2. Hurwitz, N.: Predisposing factors in adverse reactions to drugs. Br. Med. J. 1:536–539, 1960.
3. Bender, A. D.: Pharmacodynamic principles of drug therapy in the aged. J. Am. Geriat. Soc. 23:296–303, 1974.
4. O'Malley, K., Crooks, J., Duke, E., et al: Effect of age and sex in human drug metabolism. Br. Med. J. 3:607–609, 1971.
5. Vestal, R. E., Norris, A. H., et al: Antipyrine metabolism in man: Influence of age, alcohol, caffeine, and smoking. Clin. Pharmacol. Ther. 18:425–432, 1975.

6. Greenblatt, D. J., Harmatz, J. S., Shader, R. I.: Factors influencing diazepam pharmacokinetics: Age, sex, and liver disease. Int. J. Clin. Pharmacol. Biopharm. 16:177–179, 1978.
7. Greenblatt, D. J., Allen, M. D., Shader, R. I.: Toxicity of high dose flurazepam in the elderly. Clin. Pharmacol. Ther. 21:355–361, 1977.
8. Greenblatt, D. J., Harmatz, J. S., et al: Factors influencing blood concentrations of chlordiazepoxide: A case for multiple regression analyses. Psychopharmacology 54:277–282, 1977.
9. Nies, A., Robinson, D. S., et al: Relationship between age and tricyclic antidepressant plasma levels. Am. J. Psychiatry 134:790–793, 1977.
10. Gram, L. F., Sondergaard, I. B., et al: Steady-state kinetics of imipramine in patients. Psychopharmacology 54:255–261, 1977.
11. Dawling, S., Crome, P., Braithwaite, R.: Pharmacokinetics of single oral doses of nortriptyline in depressed elderly hospital patients and young health volunteers. Clinical Pharmacokinetics 5:394–401, 1980.
12. Robinson, D. S., Nies, A., Ravaris, L., et al: Clinical pharmacology of phenelzine. Arch. Gen. Psychiatry 35:629–635, 1978.
13. Fann, W. E.: Pharmacotherapy in older depressed patients. J. Gerontol. 31:304–310, 1976.
14. Davies, R. K., Tucker G. J., et al: Confusional episodes and antidepressant medication. Am. J. Psychiatry 181:127–131, 1971.
15. Robinson, D. S., Davis, J. M., et al: Ageing, monoamine, and monoamineoxidase levels. The Lancet 1:290–291, 1972.
16. Robinson, D. S.: Changes in monoamine oxidase and monoamines with human development and aging. Federation Proc. 34:103–107, 1975.
17. Robinson, D. S., Sourkes, T. L., et al: Monoamine metabolism in human brain. Arch. Gen. Psychiatry 34:89–92, 1977.
18. Nies, A., Robinson, D. S., Harris, L. S., Lamborn K. R.: Comparison of monoamine oxidase substrate activities in twins, schizophrenics, depressives, and controls, in: Neuropharmacology of Monoamines and Their Regulatory Enzyme, edited by Usdin E. New York, Raven Press, 1974.
19. Ravaris, C. L., Robinson, D. S., et al: A comparison of phenelzine and amitriptyline in the treatment of depression. Arch. Gen. Psychiatry, 37:1075, 1080, 1980.
20. Robinson, D. S., Nies, A., Ravaris, C. L., Lamborn K. R.: The monoamine oxidase inhibitor, phenelzine, in the treatment of depressive-anxiety states. Arch. Gen. Psychiatry 29:407–413, 1973.
21. Ravaris, C. L., Nies, A., et al: A multiple-dose control trial of phenelzine in depressive anxiety states. Arch. J. Psychiatry 33:347–350, 1976.
22. Cooper, T. B., Robinson, D. S., Nies, A.: Phenelzine measurement in human plasma: A sensitive GLC-ECD procedure. Communications in Psychopharmacology 2:502–519, 1978.
23. Ashford, J. W., Ford, C. V.: Use of MAO inhibitors in elderly patients. Am. J. Psychiatry 136:1466–1467, 1979.

CHAPTER 2

# Use of Antipsychotic Drugs in the Elderly

John M. Davis, M.D.
Nancy L. Segal, M.A.
Jary M. Lesser, M.D.

## INTRODUCTION

Psychosis is an all-too-common problem among the aged. It can affect patients who have experienced a schizophrenia-like illness for many years that is still acting past the age of 65. It also can occur in patients who have the onset of schizophrenic symptoms after the age of 65. Psychosis can also occur secondary to organic impairment. Excellent evidence from well-controlled studies showing that antipsychotic drugs produce a clinically substantial benefit in schizophrenic patients is reviewed by Klein and Davis (1). Fluphenazine enanthate has been found by Raskind and coworkers (2) to be effective in the treatment of late paraphrenia. Although there have been several well-controlled double-blind studies on the treatment of psychosis in the elderly (2–10), most of the studies were performed on patients under 65 years of age. The use of antipsychotic drugs in treating psychosis consequent to organic brain problems (such as senile Alzheimer's dementia) or in the treatment of psychosis with onset late in life has not received a great deal of investigation. The question arises whether the same clinical and/or pharmacologic factors that apply to the psychoses in patients under 65 years old also apply to the treatment of psychoses in the elderly. The present evidence indicates that in most situations the same clinical information applies. For example, haloperidol has been found to be superior to placebo in the well-controlled double-blind studies of Sugarman and coworkers and Tobin and coworkers (3, 4). In addition, thioridazine has been found to be useful in a variety of studies in treating psychosis in the elderly (5). Haloperidol or fluphenazine was found in a carefully done double-blind study to be as effective as thioridazine in a geriatric population by Tsuang et al. (6), Rosen (7), Smith et al. (8), and Branchley and coworkers (9). Acetophenazine has also been found in controlled studies to be an effective drug for treating psychosis in the aged in a study by Honigfeld and coworkers (10). There is no doubt that the antipsychotic compounds are very effective in treating psychoses in the elderly when compared to the improvement produced by placebo.

## Maintenance Medication

The next question that arises in considering drug treatment is the matter of maintenance therapy. Many elderly patients experience the onset of psychosis after age 65. Most of the evidence on maintenance medication is based on patients with recurrent schizophrenic illness that develops during their twenties. It is important to recognize that this information should not be uncritically generalized to psychotic episodes in the elderly. First, there is the problem of treating patients with recurrent episodes of schizophrenia before and after age 65, or with patients who have been continuously ill with schizophrenia over many years and are now over 65. If the patient becomes psychotic, is treated with an antipsychotic compound, and improves, should he be administered maintenance antipsychotics for several years or for the rest of his life? There are many controlled studies in the literature on this issue as it applies to nongeriatric schizophrenic patients. Every properly controlled study has found that a significantly fewer number of patients on maintenance antipsychotic drugs relapsed than comparable patients maintained on a placebo. This finding, however, may not always be true in the elderly. Many patients have chronic-remitting schizophrenia after 65, so maintenance medication is indicated. This generalization may not necessarily apply to all patients because, occasionally, it is observed clinically that there are patients whose schizophrenic illness appears to "burn out" with age (11). In our opinion, the decision of whether or how long to keep a patient on maintenance antipsychotics should be determined for each patient separately, on a clinical basis. We would be more likely to discontinue antipsychotics in an elderly patient who has been ill for many years, particularly if he has been treated with relatively low doses (11, 12). We would be more likely to maintain a patient on antipsychotic medication if a review of his medication history showed that he seemed clinically to require high doses of drugs, if he seemed to have active schizophrenic illness, or if he showed a history of relapses after discontinuation of drugs. In such patients, one uses maintenance medication because they have relapsed in the past without maintenance medication. Among the elderly, many patients have the onset of illness late in life, often after 55, and may not have an illness identical to schizophrenia. Since the basic indication for maintenance antipsychotics is past relapses, it is important not to put patients on maintenance antipsychotics automatically after their first episode. Many clinicians stabilize patients on antipsychotics for a period of several months after an episode so that they will not relapse into the same episode. In addition, we would not advocate maintenance antipsychotics for patients whose first episode of psychosis develops late in life.

The duration of treatment depends on the natural history of the underlying disorder. Some schizophrenic patients require treatment for many years. In the elderly, the psychosis often occurs as a single episode, and long-term treatment is not necessary. A few weeks of treatment may be sufficient for complete recovery, and even a few doses during a single day may have a substantial antipsychotic effect.

## Mode of Action

Although these drugs were initially referred to as tranquilizers, this term is an inaccurate conceptualization of how they work, as they do not benefit psychosis by producing a state of blissful sedation. Some antipsychotic drugs produce a modest degree of sedation, others produce essentially minimal or no sedation, whereas some may be slightly stimulatory at certain doses. If improvement was produced by sedation, the more sedative drugs should be more effective. Stimulatory, neutral, or minimally sedative antipsychotic drugs are equally effective. Sedative drugs per se produce no beneficial effect in schizophrenia. Sedative properties are not related to antipsychotic properties. If antipsychotics produced their beneficial effects through alleviation of anxiety, then the greatest drug-placebo difference would occur with anxiety, and substantially less difference would occur with other supposedly secondary symptoms. This is not the case. All the symptoms of psychosis are alleviated approximately equally by antipsychotic drugs. Retarded psychotic patients are speeded up. Excited patients are slowed to a more normal rate of activity. Delusions, hallucinations, catatonic posturing, and bizarre movements lessen with drug treatment. Schizophrenic thinking, as measured by psychological tests, dissipates along with the other symptoms of schizophrenia.

In our laboratory, in collaboration with Holzman, Ericksen, and Hurt, we have studied the effect of antipsychotic drugs in schizophrenic thought disorder. In this study, Holzman and Hurt quantified thought disorders through an instrument developed in Holzman's laboratory that essentially counted the number of thought distortions in a sample of schizophrenic speech. This is a direct quantification of disordered thoughts, which is conceptually distinct from the assumption that thought is disturbed if the patient has hallucinations or delusions. The schizophrenic thought disorder was evaluated blindly, with the rater not knowing whether the patient was a schizophrenic or control, on a drug or in a drug-free baseline period. The results, showing the improvement of schizophrenia in terms of symptomatology as measured by the Brief Psychiatric Rating Scale and in terms of the thought disorder as measured directly, are presented in Figure 2.1. It would seem that antipsychotic drugs turn off schizophrenia to the same extent and at the same rate as they turn off the symptoms of schizophrenia.

Therefore, the best label for these drugs is antipsychotic. To call them antischizophrenic would be too narrow because they benefit many different psychoses—mania, psychotic depression, certain drug-induced

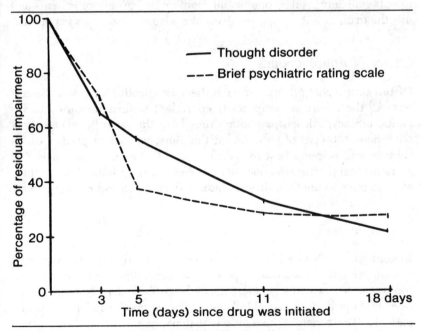

FIGURE 2.1. Effect of antipsychotic medication on disordered thought and BPRS scores of schizophrenics.

psychoses such as amphetamine type, and psychosis consequent to brain disorder. Among the elderly, antipsychotics are the indicated drugs in treating psychotic illness. Minor tranquilizers, such as the benzodiazepines and barbiturate or nonbarbiturate sedatives, have no antipsychotic properties. A wide variety of pharmacologic studies indicate that antipsychotic drugs benefit schizophrenia by blocking brain dopamine receptors. Exactly how the dopamine blockade relates to the underlying schizophrenia of the illness is unknown at present. It is also unknown whether the dopamine-receptor blockade is the mechanism of action in other psychoses, such as psychosis consequent to various organic brain disorders. Insofar as it is reasonable to generalize from data on schizophrenia to geriatric psychosis, the important concept is that dopamine-receptor blockade, or something akin to this, is probably responsible.

The conceptualization that antipsychotics directly correct the psychosis is slightly different than the conceptualization that the antipsychotic drugs have a suppressant effect on certain target symptoms, such as anxiety. The target-symptom theory is a derivative of the underlying notion that schizophrenia may be a defense against anxiety and that the antipsychotic agents are really tranquilizers or antianxiety agents. If one uses the anxiety model, one would monitor the anxiety of patients and use the drug as if it were a sedative. We advocate a different approach.

## Choice of Antipsychotics

Of the antipsychotics, promazine is the least effective and most dangerous. All the others are empirically equivalent in their measured therapeutic efficacy. All antipsychotic drugs have the same beneficial effect on various subtypes of patients. At this time, we cannot predict which subtype will respond best to specific drugs. Occasionally, one may find an individual patient who does better on one antipsychotic than another, so switching to another drug is indicated in a nonresponding patient.

## Dosage in the Elderly

In general, much lower doses are needed in elderly patients compared to younger ones. The relative potency of one antipsychotic in comparison to another can only be approximated (see Table 2.1). Note that some psychotic episodes in the elderly may require doses similar to a young patient's. The generality that elderly patients require lower dosages than younger schizophrenics should not be forgotten. However, like all rules it has exceptions.

TABLE 2.1 Antipsychotic Dose Ratios vs.
Chlorpromazine

| Drug | Dose Ratio |
| --- | --- |
| Chlorpromazine (Thorazine) | 100 |
| Triflupromazine (Vesprin) | 28.4 |
| Thioridazine (Mellaril) | 95.3 |
| Prochlorperazine (Compazine) | 14.3 |
| Perphenazine (Trilafon) | 8.9 |
| Fluphenazine (Prolixin) | 1.2 |
| Fluphenazine (Prolixin decanoate) | .67 |
| Trifluoperazine (Stelazine) | 2.8 |
| Acetophenazine (Tindal) | 23.5 |
| Carphenazine (Proketazine) | 24.3 |
| Butaperazine (Repoise) | 8.9 |
| Mesoridazine (Serentil) | 55.3 |
| Piperacetazine (Quide) | 10.5 |
| Haloperidol (Haldol) | 1.6 |

## AGE EFFECTS ON PHARMACOKINETICS

Aging causes a number of physiological changes that alter drug pharmacokinetics, which are summarized in the reviews of Triggs and Nation
(13) as well as Shader and Greenblatt (14) as follows:

1. Sugar, fats, and vitamins are less well absorbed by the G.I. tract, but
   in general, absorption is not markedly altered (15); the more important cause of such deficiencies is poor food preparation and/or intake.
2. Cardiac output decreases by 30–40%; renal and splanchnic flow also
   decrease.
3. Drug distribution is altered as fat replaces functional tissue in the
   aging process (16). For nonpolar lipid-soluble drugs such as antipsychotics, this may increase the volume of distribution. However, to
   our knowledge this possible alteration has not been investigated for
   the antipsychotics.
4. Hepatic-enzyme activity decreases, often resulting in a decrease in
   drug clearance.
5. The concentration of albumin relative to globulin decreases. If a drug
   is tightly bound in albumin, there may be an increase in the unbound fraction of the drug, which is free to distribute to tissue and
   thereby create higher relative concentration at the receptor site.
6. Glomerular filtration rate and creatinine clearance decrease, but the
   serum creatinine level may remain normal because of a decrease in
   skeletal muscle mass. There is often a decreased clearance of drugs,

such as lithium, that are normally eliminated in the kidney. Antipsychotics are almost completely metabolized, and hence are not excreted as unchanged drugs in clinically important amounts in the kidney.

## Drug-Drug Interactions

Elderly patients are more apt to have concomitant medical problems while receiving many medications. In addition, they are vulnerable to physiological alterations because of decreased reserve in various organ systems, and hence are under a greater risk from drug-drug interactions. Drug-drug interactions that may involve the antipsychotics follow.

## Absorption Interactions (17–19)

Following antacid therapy, Fann and his coworkers (18, 19) found a significant lowering of plasma chlorpromazine (CPZ), a finding consistent with urinary excretion studies. Neither study, however, investigated the rate of absorption as distinct from the completeness of absorption. The decreased absorption was assumed to be caused by the actual binding of chlorpromazine within the gut by the antacid-gel.

Rivera-Calimlim et al. (20) found that younger age, chronicity of illness, and prolonged drug treatment were associated with decreased CPZ plasma levels. The group believed that this possibly was the result of impaired gut absorption or accelerated metabolism of CPZ.

## METABOLIC INTERACTIONS

Curry et al. (1970) found that barbiturates increase the rate of chlorpromazine metabolism and consequently decrease its steady-state plasma levels by inducing liver-microsomal enzymes. The elderly brain may be more sensitive to the sedative effects of drugs at given brain levels. Due to impaired liver metabolism, elderly patients could have higher plasma levels and, consequently, higher brain levels of a drug. This would cause a greater drug effect. Similarly, patients with hepatic coma are very sensitive to CNS impairment by chlorpromazine. Is this because of impaired liver metabolizing capacity, or is it due to the greater sensitivity of the brain to sedative agents?

Maxwell's group (21) studied the plasma disappearance and cerebral effects of chlorpromazine (CPZ) in 24 patients with cirrhosis versus a matched control group. No pharmacokinetic differences were found between the two groups. Drowsiness and EEG slowing were present in all patients. Mild confusion and deterioration of visual-motor testing were observed in 3 of 4 patients who had a history of prior encephalopathy. These 3 also exhibited the greatest EEG slowing. The authors concluded that the susceptibility of some patients with cirrhosis to CPZ probably reflects increase CNS sensitivity rather than differences in hepatic drug metabolism.

Maxwell's study suggests that Bender's early conclusion (22) that the "central nervous system is perhaps the system most sensitive to alterations in drug activity with age" is still very relevant. It also supports Hamilton's (23) early conclusion that the neuronal loss due to aging is responsible for the altered reactivity and sensitivity of the aged to neurogenic agents. Both Bender and Hamilton were aware early of the importance of addressing age-related changes in receptor-site sensitivity.

## Age, Plasma Levels, and Clinical Efficacy

Martensson and Roos (24) and Axelsson and Martensson (25) report no marked relationship between age and plasma level of thioridazine. Forsman and Ohman (26) have also reported marked age-related changes in a study of serum haloperidol levels. If anything, there is a slight increase in plasma level with age, but this is small and certainly should not be considered well defined. This would be relevant if there were a relationship between plasma levels and clinical variables. However, the relationship between plasma levels of an antipsychotic drug and a therapeutic response has not been extensively investigated. Curry and his coworkers (27–29) did the first clinical open study on this topic. They postulated an inverted U-shaped relationship between therapeutic response and plasma CPZ level. Patients who showed a poor clinical response had plasma levels that were either too low or too high to be effective. These very high levels may produce CNS toxicity or other side effects that interfere with a therapeutic response. We emphasize that, to have a controlled study, a constant dose over time is required for definitive evidence. Either the one dose can be constant, or patients can be randomly assigned various doses. If dosage is adjusted clinically, nonresponders will receive a higher dose because the clinician is trying to help them. This will result in a high plasma level, thus confounding the relationship of plasma level to therapeutic response. In further research, our group found that most nonresponders to butaperazine and fluphenazine have low plasma levels (30–

34). With both butaperazine and fluphenazine, there is some suggestion that a few nonresponders have extremely high plasma levels, thus supporting the notion of the inverted U-shaped relationship originally suggested by Curry and his coworkers; but since this is based on a very limited number of patients, the Scotch verdict is "not proved" at this time.

Research on the relationship between clinical efficacy and drug plasma levels is in its beginning stages, and there are correlations between the two still to be defined. Present evidence suggests an inverted-U relationship. The finding that steady-state plasma levels may be slightly increased in the elderly should be interpreted within the context of the limited data on 3 studies of phenothiazines relating age to plasma levels. Plasma level studies show that antipsychotic drugs are metabolized at substantially different rates in different patients. A fast metabolizer will show very low plasma levels and need a higher-than-normal dose to achieve an adequate response. Slow metabolizers will have high plasma levels and may develop central nervous system or autonomic toxicity on a normal dose. This is one reason why it is necessary to adjust the dose for the individual patient. The limited amount of evidence on the half-life of antipsychotics in the elderly indicates that, on average, the drugs have slightly prolonged half-lives in older patients. Therefore, we would hypothesize that psychoses occurring in the elderly are more responsive to antipsychotic medication than those occurring in younger persons. Conversely, the elderly may be more susceptible to central nervous system toxicity as a consequence of pathological changes in the aging brain. In the absence of well-controlled studies, we can only conclude that although there is no precise evidence explaining the greater sensitivity to these medications in the aged, the evidence we have suggests that this is primarily caused at the end-organ, as opposed to the rate of metabolism (which does, nevertheless, contribute to a modest degree).

In determining the dosage, the clinician assesses the severity of the psychotic problem and the risk of side effects, as well as any relevant causative factors. For example, a patient with no previous psychotic illness who develops transient psychotic symptoms as a consequence of organic brain disease may require a very small dose of an antipsychotic drug. In addition, excess sedation may be particularly harmful in the case of an impaired brain.

On the other hand, a patient who required large doses in the recent past for treatment of manic or schizophrenic episodes and was able to tolerate such doses without undue side effects would initially be treated with a modest dose that would gradually be increased. Obviously, in an extremely disturbed patient, one would rapidly increase the dose to higher levels. Since there are substantial individual differences, each dose should be adjusted according to the patient, and all side effects should be monitored.

There is the usual sigmoid dose-response relationship. Patients on extremely low doses show less improvement than patients on moderately low doses, but after the point of diminishing returns, an extra-high dose will not provide more benefit than a high dose. Intramuscular drugs act quicker than oral drugs, and should be one-third to one-half the oral dose. After the first injection, oral doses generally suffice in a patient who voluntarily takes medication. In patients who are unreliable, a long-term depot form such as fluphenazine (Prolixin) can be administered intramuscularly every 1–4 weeks (2).

## SIDE EFFECTS

### Allergic and Miscellaneous Side Effects

Thioridazine can produce pigmentary retinopathy when given in high doses (e.g., 1,600 mg/day for a month). This often interferes with vision and may not be entirely reversible, so it is a serious side effect. For that reason, the maximum dose of thioridazine is generally considered to be 800 mg a day.

Chlorpromazine given in long-term high doses can produce skin discoloration as well as opacities of the lens and the cornea that do not interfere with vision.

The antipsychotics can produce a wide variety of rashes. In addition, chlorpromazine can cause a contact dermatitis in nurses and others who handle the drug and a photosensitive reaction from which sunburn results following relatively mild exposure to the sun.

Agranulocytosis has an incidence on the order of about 1 case per million. It appears most frequently in elderly women receiving chlorpromazine 3–8 weeks after the onset of phenothiazine treatment. Agranulocytosis has not been proven to be caused by the nonphenothiazine antipsychotics (haloperidol, molindone, or loxapine). The white blood cell count drops precipitously, essentially to zero, in a few days. The disorder generally presents as an infection with a sore throat and fever. Patients should not receive another phenothiazine, as a repeat episode might occur. Agranulocytosis should not be confused with a gradual decline of the white blood count to levels of 4,000 or so, which is probably a different side effect.

Phenothiazines can produce a cholestatic jaundice that occurs from 1 to 7 days after a prodrome of fever, nausea, abdominal pain, and malaise. This side effect generally occurs in the first few months of treatment, and dissipates within several weeks. The reaction is associated with eosinophils in the plasma and liver, and in a broad sense is an allergic reaction that can recur when the offending phenothiazine is readministered. There is no evidence that proves beyond a reasonable doubt that nonphenothiazine antipsychotics such as molindone, loxapine, and haloperidol cause jaundice.

## Central Nervous System

Drowsiness generally occurs in the first few weeks of treatment, but tends to disappear gradually as patients become tolerant to the drug's sedative side-effects. The antipsychotic drugs do not cause barbiturate-type or narcotic-type withdrawal symptoms and are, in this sense, non-addicting. The problem with self-medication is not that patients abuse these drugs with higher doses, but rather that patients often do not take their medication reliably. Occasional G.I. symptoms such as nausea or vomiting can occur with sudden cessation of high-dose phenothiazines.

In rare instances, antipsychotic drugs can produce a single, isolated seizure, which requires lower doses or anticonvulsants. Appropriate investigation should be conducted to determine whether the seizure was caused in part by a previously undiagnosed brain disease.

Acute extrapyramidal side effects, including pseudoparkinsonism, akathisia, and dystonic reactions, occur in 15–50% of patients. Pseudo-parkinsonism syndrome is identical to Parkinson's disease, characterized by akinesia, muscle rigidity, tremor, drooling, masklike faces, a shuffling gait, and loss of associated movements. Sometimes, when the parkinsonian symptoms are superimposed on psychotic flatness of affect or catatonic posturing, they are not entirely obvious. Patients appear apathetic and "zombie-like," and this can be falsely attributed to their age or psychosis. Patients with akathisia cannot remain still, as there is a compulsion to move. Constant pacing, repetitive leg movements, and restlessness are often difficult to distinguish from psychotic agitation. Dystonic reactions typically occur within the first week of treatment. They can occur as early as 2–25 hours after single dose of an antipsychotic drug such as prochlorperazine (Compazine) for nausea. Dystonic spasms of the face, neck, back, or other manifestations such as oculogyric crisis or torticollis opisthotonos occur. The patient often has hypersalivation associated with dystonic spasms of the neck and facial muscles. These muscle spasms are painful, and can be quite alarming to the patient.

Intramuscular or intravenous administration of anticholinergic drugs rapidly relieve dystonic reactions. Oral anticholinergic antiparkinsonian drugs such as benztropine (Cogentin) or procyclidine (Kemadren) are the standard treatment for less acute extrapyramidal side effects. Amantadine is also useful. Prophylactic antiparkinsonian drugs can reduce the incidence of extrapyramidal side effects by approximately 50% (e.g., from 30% to 15%). Furthermore, since patients can develop some tolerance to extrapyramidal producing properties with a few months of treatment, the antiparkinsonian drug should often be gradually discontinued.

Tardive dykinesia is a movement disorder that has its gradual onset after long-term, high-dose antipsychotic drug administration. The symptoms, essentially identical to Huntington's chorea, are choreiform movements in the oral region such as lip smacking, sucking, jaw movements, fly-catcher's tongue, and writhing tongue movements, as well as choreiform movements of the extremities, and sometimes of the entire body. There is a low spontaneous base rate of occurrence of such symptomatology in drug-free individuals. However, patients who have been treated on high doses of long-term antipsychotic medication have a substantial incidence of this movement disorder (35). On rare occasions, it can occur in patients who have had short-term or low-dose administration. There is a higher prevalence in the aged and a slightly higher occurrence in females over males, perhaps due to the increased longevity of females. The greater prevalence in the aged probably is a consequence of the fact that elderly schizophrenics have been taking neuroleptic medication for a longer period of time than younger schizophrenics. Since there is a significant incidence in the development of tardive dyskinesia after many years of antipsychotic drug treatment, the clinician should weigh these risks as well against the benefits of long-term maintenance. There is slightly less need to be concerned with patients whose life expectancy is limited, relative to that of a much younger person. It should be noted that many elderly patients show dissipation of psychosis in a few weeks of treatment with antipsychotics, and do not require long-term medication. Before tardive dyskinesia was recognized, antipsychotic drugs had been used for the treatment of nonpsychotic conditions, such as anxiety. Since minor tranquilizers are effective in simple anxiety, it is generally wise to avoid the use of antipsychotics in nonpsychotic conditions. However, since some nonpsychotic patients apparently do respond to an antipsychotic after doing poorly on minor tranquilizers, there is empirical justification for their use in this type of patient.

There is evidence from a variety of sources that elderly patients should be particularly sensitive to CNS toxicity produced by anticholinergic agents. For example, the central anticholinergic syndrome is frequently observed in patients with Parkinson's disease treated with anticholinergic agents. Furthermore, there is a definite age relationship. The older the patient, the greater the risk of central anticholinergic syndrome secondary to these anticholinergic agents. Autopsied brain studies show a decrease in acetylcholine transferase, an enzyme used as a marker for the central cholinergic system with the aged. It would follow that elderly patients may be particularly susceptible to anticholinergic toxicity, and for this reason we will closely consider anticholinergic toxicity. Cases of the central anticholinergic syndrome can occur in patients receiving a single anticholinergic compound, but since patients are often taking several different anticholinergics, it is possible that anticholinergic toxicity can accumulate. We have observed that, occasionally, the clinical symptoms of patients placed on a combination of anticholinergics (including tricyclics) have worsened. The hypothesis we chose to investigate was whether this apparent worsening of the clinical picture could be anticholinergic toxicity caused by the combined anticholinergic properties of all the drugs used (36).

Physostigmine has reversed experimentally induced anticholinergic delirium in normal volunteers and central anticholinergic poisoning in drug abusers, attempted suicides, and parkinsonian patients receiving anticholinergic antiparkinsonian agents. What had not been previously studied was whether the toxic confusional state observed in psychiatric patients during administration of antiparkinsonian drugs in combination with phenothiazines and/or tricyclic antidepressants is essentially an atropine psychosis and hence can be reversed by physostigmine. Our double-blind study was designed to investigate whether or not the apparent worsening after the administration of a polypharmacy of psychotropic agents was an atropine-like psychosis superimposed on the underlying schizophrenic illness, and whether this site could be alleviated by the administration of physostigmine.

Three schizophrenics who were receiving phenothiazines and benztropine mesylate for their parkinsonian side effects developed an intermittently occurring toxic confusional state that was clinically consistent with an "anticholinergic syndrome." All patients developed symptoms consistent with the "central anticholinergic syndrome," which is characterized by a marked disturbance of short-term memory, impaired attention, disorientation, and visual and auditory hallucinations associated with peripheral anticholinergic signs. Without an evaluation of mental status, these symptoms may not be obvious because of the original psychosis and the overlap of toxic and psychotic symptomatology. A 15-point rating scale (15 being the most severe) based on serial mental status exams was designed to evaluate the confusional state. It rated symptoms such as visual and auditory hallucinations, disorientation, and short-term memory loss. The patients were intramuscularly administered a placebo and physostigmine (4 mg) on a double-blind basis, and were evaluated for the alleviation of the confusional state by a rater who was unaware of whether a placebo or physostigmine was being given. In contrast to the placebo, which caused no significant change in the symptom complex, physostigmine dramatically reversed the toxic symptom complex for approximately 3 hours after injection. The 5 target symptoms were specific to the anticholinergic syndrome and were reversed with physostigmine, whereas the original functional (schizophrenic) symptoms were not reversed.

In contrast to the relatively easily diagnosed central anticholinergic toxicity seen in nonpsychotic patients, the "central anticholinergic syndrome" presents a difficult diagnostic problem in psychotics because many of these patients are already delusional, confused, and agitated. In addition, the anticholinergic toxic symptomatology is in the direction of the primary psychosis, with some overlap of symptoms. Diagnosis, therefore, becomes quite important. If some nonspecific diagnostic formulation is used, then the symptoms of schizophrenia can blur into the symptoms of an organic psychosis. If the worsening is in some nonspecific way attributed to the drugs being administered but the diagnosis is not made, then all drugs can be stopped in a sort of a nonspecific-avoidance reaction. This overlap may lead physicians to increase psychotropic medications, leading to a predictable worsening of the central anticholinergic symptoms. Consequently, the patients are left without the benefit of antipsychotic agents. The correct diagnosis can be made with consideration of the possibility of focusing on the presence of peripheral anticholinergic signs. Selective medication reduction or discontinuation can thereby relieve the central anticholinergic syndrome. The antiparkinsonian agents, which may be the chief offenders, are those that can most easily be dispensed with. It has recently been shown that many patients do not actually need their antiparkinsonian medication. On a mg/kg basis, the antiparkinsonian medications are more potent in producing anticholinergic changes than the phenothiazines or tricyclic antidepressants. It is important to remember, however, that phenothiazines and tricyclic antidepressants are given at a much higher absolute mg dosage. Most atropine confusional states will clear within a day if the drugs are discontinued. In rare cases in which the diagnosis remains uncertain or in which the rapid alleviation of the anticholinergic symptoms is needed, the use of physostigmine may prove a useful diagnostic and therapeutic tool.

It is necessary to use physostigmine with caution in patients who have no medical contraindications, starting with conservative, low test doses and carefully observing for signs of cholinergic toxicity. Atropine sulfate to reverse cholinergic toxicity should be readily available when physostigmine test doses are administered. The importance of our study is in proving that this picture is essentially atropine toxicity. Memory deficit is typical of atropine toxicity. A convenient test for immediate memory is to tell the patients to remember 3 numbers, then wait approximately a minute, and ask the patient to repeat the numbers. The second evidence that this is essentially atropine toxicity is provided by the fact that it can be dramatically reversed by physostigmine.

## Endocrine Effects

Antipsychotic drug treatment can cause weight gain; patients receiving the medication experience appetite increases and eat more than usual. The actual mechanism of appetite stimulation is not known. Molindone seems not to cause weight gain. The antipsychotic drugs produce changes on many endocrine parameters—for example, increases in prolactin. Gynecomastia is observed, generally in females but also in males.

## Autonomic Nervous System

The antipsychotics produce a variety of effects on the autonomic nervous system, such as alpha-receptor blockade and an atropine-like blockade of cholinergic receptors. Patients develop some degree of tolerance to these effects after several weeks of treatment. A particularly important autonomic effect in the aged is postural hypotension; elderly patients may faint and fall, causing broken limbs and hips, lacerations, and subdural hematomas. Most types of hypotensive episodes occur in the first few weeks of treatment, and are more prevalent after intramuscular medication. The antipsychotic drugs can produce a wide variety of atropine-like effects: dry mouth, blurred vision, nasal congestion, constipation, paralytic ileus (rarely), and bladder paralysis. Thioridazine has been noted to cause an inhibition of ejaculation, a side effect that can be alarming if the cause is not known.

## Differential Incidence of Side Effects

Thioridazine causes the least extrapyramidal side effects, but has a moderate degree of sedation and anticholinergic properties. Chlorpromazine is intermediate in relative prevalence of side effects. Most of the remaining antipsychotics, such as fluphenazine, perphenazine, haloperidol, thiothixene, loxitane, and molindone, fall in the high-extrapyramidal, low-sedation, low-autonomic relative-prevalence classification. There may be occasions when a drug would be chosen because it lacks a certain type of toxicity. For example, a patient who had a previous episode of the central anticholinergic syndrome should receive a low anticholinergic antipsychotic. Clinical studies indicate that there is a fairly even trade off between high-autonomic-sedative, but low-extrapyramidal vs. low-autonomic-sedative, high-extrapyramidal drugs, in terms of total significance of the toxicity.

## Cardiovascular Interactions

Antipsychotics can produce some T-wave changes, but as far as is known, these are benign and without medical import. Sudden death is common after age 40, and hence can occur coincidentally in a patient receiving drugs. Among elderly patients on drugs, sudden death can be falsely attributed to the medication.

Since hypertension is a common disorder in the elderly, it is important to consider in detail drug-drug interactions between antipsychotic drugs and drugs used to treat hypertension. Guanethidine is a potent antihypertensive agent. Both antipsychotic drugs and tricyclic-antidepressant drugs may interact with guanethidine. This effect is most prominent with tricyclic drugs, but can also occur with phenothiazines, and, by inference, other antipsychotics. Tricyclic antidepressants, such as amitriptyline, nortriptyline, doxepin, imipramine, desipramine, and protriptyline, administered in clinically efficacious doses, reverse the therapeutic effects of guanethidine in hypertensive patients. In our laboratory, Fann and his coworkers (37, 38) have shown that doxepin, in doses of 200–300 mg/day, reverses guanethidine's antihypertensive effects.

Since chlorpromazine and related antipsychotic agents are frequently used in the treatment of psychotic patients who coincidentally also are hypertensive, we believe that it is important to evaluate whether chlorpromazine blocks the action of guanethidine when administered in doses used clinically (38, 39). Four chronically hospitalized adult psychiatric inpatients with essential hypertension who had persistent hypertension of a moderate to severe degree were studied (38, 39). On admission, their standing blood pressures ranged from 230 to 172 mm Hg systolic and from 150 to 110 mm Hg diastolic. The patients were admitted to our research ward, and all drugs were discontinued. After a clinically effective dose of guanethidine was determined, each patient was maintained on that dose of guanethidine sulfate for a period of 7 days or more prior to the administration of the proposed "antagonist." Chlorpromazine, ranging in total daily dosage from 100 to 400 mg, was then added to the guanethidine regimen for a period of no less than 12 days. Chlorpromazine was then discontinued, and guanethidine treatment continued for a postantagonist phase of 9 days or longer. In 6 instances, chlorpromazine was administered. Haloperidol was used 3 times, and thiothixene once. After the patients were taken off all drugs and their blood pressure lowered with guanethidine, chlorpromazine was administered. Analysis of the data indicated that chlorpromazine in clinically utilized doses, ranging from 100 to 400 mg/day, significantly reversed the antihypertensive effects of guanethidine in all 6 instances in which it was used as an antagonist. Significant, but less dramatic, reversals occurred when haloperidol and thiothixene were added. The mechanism of action underlying the antagonism of guanethidine's hypotensive effects by antipsychotic agents is probably that these drugs antagonize guanethidine's access to the neuron, specifically by blockade of the norepinephrine uptake pump. Tricyclic antidepressants inhibit the neuronal uptake of norepinephrine and the hypertensive agents. Our studies, as well as other investigations, have shown that chlorpromazine is a potent inhibitor of norepinephrine uptake.

## RESEARCH QUESTIONS IN NEED OF INVESTIGATION

Since most of the double-blind studies on the use of antipsychotic agents involved typical schizophrenics whose illness had its onset in young adulthood, there may be some difficulty in generalizing the findings to late paraphrenia or psychosis secondary to a given type of brain disorder. It is reasonably safe to generalize from studies of younger schizophrenics to patients who have had chronic schizophrenic illness for their entire lives and who are now beyond age 65. However, some patients have a functional psychiatric illness that develops after age 55. Raskind and his associates (2) specifically investigated the use of antipsychotics in patients with late paraphrenia. All patients had paranoid delusions as well as an onset after age 55, in the absence of:

1. dementia,
2. acute medical illness, or
3. parkinsonism.

It would be helpful to have controlled studies verify the efficacy of antipsychotic drugs in late paraphrenia or in other functional diseases that have their onset late in life. In a similar sense, there is a need for information about the use of antipsychotic drugs in a variety of psychoses secondary to various types of organic brain disease, such as acute deliriums and chronic dementia.

There is a need for studies of different antipsychotic drugs in geriatric patients. For example, drug treatment of disorders specifically diagnosed as late paraphrenia by the criterion of Raskind and coworkers could be investigated, as could the use of antipsychotics in certain forms of chronic brain syndromes diagnosed by a specific set of diagnostic criteria. It is important that such studies exclude patients with preexisting schizophrenia since there is much less information on nonschizophrenic psychotic disorders in the elderly. Ideally, double-blind placebo controls should be used, but sometimes this is not practical, such as in treating acute deliria of various etiologies. The emergency situation may demand that patients immediately receive effective treatment and not undergo a placebo trial. In such a case, historical controls could be used. However, many of the psychoses secondary to brain disease are common, but psychoses secondary to one given brain disease may be relatively uncommon, which raises statistical problems for a group study. Obviously, the more stringent the exclusion and inclusion criteria used in a study of a subtype of psychoses, the more specific the information that will be achieved. In antipsychotic drugs for a miscellaneous group of elderly patients it is difficult to generalize to patients with a specific etiology. The most important exclusion criterion is preexisting schizophrenia. We already know that antipsychotic drugs help elderly schizophrenics. Now we must determine the effectiveness of antipsychotic drugs in other types of psychoses. Hence, the model used by Raskind and his coworkers can be extended to different types of psychoses found in geriatric patients to achieve a more exact specification of match between the disease studied, the presenting symptoms, and the use of antipsychotic medication.

# REFERENCES

1. Klein, D. F. and Davis, J. M.: Diagnosis and drug treatment of psychiatric disorders (Ed.: Kaplan), Williams and Wilkins, 1969.
2. Raskind, M., Alvarez, C., and Herlin, R. N.: Fluphenazine enanthate in the outpatient treatment of late paraphrenia. *J. Amer. Geriat. Soc.* 27:459–463, 1979.
3. Sugarman, A. A., Williams, B. H., and Aldersteing, A. M.: Haloperidol in the psychiatric disorders of old age. *Amer. J. Psychiat.* 120:1190, 1964.
4. Tobin, J., Brousseau, J. and Lorenz, A.: Clinical evaluation of haloperidol in geriatric patients. *Geriatrics* 25:119–122, 1970.
5. Lehmann, E. and Ban, T.: Comparative pharmacotherapy of the aging patient. *Laval Med.* 38:588–595, 1967.
6. Tsuang, M. M., Lo, L. M., Stotsky, B., and Cole, J. O.: Haloperidol versus thioridazine for hospitalized psychogeriatric patients. *J. Amer. Geriat. Soc.* 19:593–600, 1971.
7. Rosen, H. J.: Double blind comparison of haloperidol and thioridazine in geriatric outpatients. *J. Clin. Psychiatry* 40:17–20, 1979.
8. Smith, G. R., Taylor, C. G., and Linkous, P.: Haloperidol versus thioridazine for the treatment of psychogeriatric patients: A double-blind clinical trial. *Psychosomatics* 15:134–138, 1974.
9. Branchey, M., Lee, J., Amen, R., and Simpson, G.: High and low-potency neuroleptics in elderly psychiatric patients. *JAMA* 239:1860–1862, 1978.
10. Honigfeld, G., Rosebaum, M., Blumenthal, I., Lambert, H., and Roberts, A.: Behavioral improvement in the older schizophrenic patient. *J. Amer. Geriat. Soc.* 13:57–71, 1965.
11. Prien, R. F., Levine, J., Cole, J. O.: Indications for high dose chlorpromazine therapy in chronic schizophrenia. *Dis. Nerv. System* 31:739–745, 1970.
12. Prien, R. F., Levine, J., and Cole, J. O.: High dose trifluoperazine therapy in chronic schizophrenia. *Amer. J. Psychiat.* 126:305–313, 1969.
13. Triggs, E. J. and Nation, R. L.: Pharmacokinetics in the aged: A review. *J. Pharmacokinetics and Biopharmaceutics* 3:387–418, 1975.
14. Shader, R. I. and Greenblatt, D. J.: Pharmacokinetics and clinical drug effects in the elderly. *Psychopharmacology Bulletin* 15:8–14, 1979.
15. Crooks, J., O'Malley, K., and Stevenson, I. H.: Pharmacokinetics in the elderly. *Clinical Pharmacokinetics* 1:280–286, 1976.
16. Novak, L. P.: Aging, total body potassium, fat-free mass, and cell mass in males and females between ages 18 and 85 years. *J. Gerontology* 27:438–443, 1972.
17. Forrest, F. M., Forrest, I. S., and Serr, M. T.: Modification of chlorpromazine metabolism by some other drugs frequently administered to psychiatric patients. *Biological Psychiatry*, 2:53, 1970.
18. Fann, W. E., Davis, J. M., Janowsky, D. S., et al.: Chlorpromazine: effects of antacids on its gastrointestinal absorption. *J. Clin. Pharm.* 13:388–390, 1973.

19. Fann, W. E., Davis, J. M., Janowsky, D. S., And Schmidt, D.: The effect of antacids in the blood levels of chlorpromazine. *Clin. Pharm. & Ther.* 14: 135, 1973.
20. Rivera-Calimlim, L., Nasrallah, H., Gift, T., et al.: Plasma levels of chlorpromazine: Effect of age, chronicity of disease, and duration of treatment. *Clin. Pharm. & Ther.* 21:115–116, 1977.
21. Maxwell, J. D., Carella, M., Parkes, J. D., et al.: Plasma disappearance and cerebral effects of chlorpromazine in cirrhosis. *Clinical Science* 43:143–151, 1973.
22. Bender, A. D. Pharmacologic aspects of aging: A survey of the effect of increasing age on drug activity in adults. *J. Amer. Geriatric Soc.* 12:114–134, 1964.
23. Hamilton, I. D.: Aged brain and the phenothiazines. *Geriatrics* 21:131–138, 1966.
24. Martensson, R. and Roos, B. E.: Serum levels of thioridazine in psychiatric patients and healthy volunteers. *European J. Clin. Pharm.* 6:181–186, 1973.
25. Axelsson, R., and Martensson, E.: Serum concentration and elimination from serum of thioridazine in psychiatric patients. *Curr. Ther. Res.* 19:242–246, 1976.
26. Forsman, A., and Ohman, R.: Applied pharmacokinetics of haloperidol in man. *Curr. Ther. Res.* 21:396–411, 1977.
27. Curry, S. H., Davis, J. M., Janowsky, D., and Marshall, J. H. L.: Interpatient variation in physiological availability of chlorpromazine as a complication factor in correlation studies of drug metabolism and clinical effect (*Neuropsychopharm.* 5:72–76, 1976). In A. Cerletii and F. J. Bove (eds). *The Present Status of Psychotropic Drugs.* Excerpta Medica, Amsterdam, 72–76, 1969.
28. Curry, S. H., Janowsky, D. S., Davis, J. M. and Marshall, J. H. L.: Factors affecting chlorpromazine plasma levels in psychiatric patients. *Arch. Gen. Psychiat.* 22:209–215, 1970.
29. Curry, S. H., Marshall, J. H. L., Davis, J. M., and Janowsky, D. S.: Chlorpromazine plasma levels and effects. *Arch. Gen. Psychiat.* 22:289–296, 1970.
30. Smith, R. C., Dekirmenjian, H., Crayton, J., Klass, D., and Davis, J. M.: Blood levels of neuroleptic drugs in non-responding chronic schizophrenic patients. *Arch. Gen. Psychiat.* 36(5):579–584, 1979.
31. Smith, R. C., Dekirmenjian, H., Davis, M. M., Crayton, J., and Evans, H. Plasma butaperazine levels in long-term chronic non-responding schizophrenics. *Communications in Psychopharmacology* 1(1):319–324, 1977.
32. Hicks, R. and Davis, J. M. Pharmacokinetics in geriatric psychopharmacology. In *Psychopharmacology of Aging*, C. Eisdorfer and W. E. Fann (eds.), Spectrum, New York, 169–212, 1980.
33. Garver, D. L., Dekirmenjian, H., Davis, J. M., Casper, R., and Ericksen, S.: Neuroleptic drug levels and therapeutic response: Preliminary obser-

vations with red blood cell bound butaperazine. *Amer. J. Psychiat.* 134(3):304–307, 1977.

34. Davis, J. M., Ericksen, S. E., and Dekirmenjian, H.: Plasma levels of antipsychotic drugs and clinical response. In *Psychopharmacology: A Generation of Progress*, M. A. Lipton, A. DiMascio, and K. F. Killiam (eds.), Raven Press, New York, 905–915, 1978.

35. Fann, W. E., Davis, J. M., and Janowsky, D. S.: The prevalence of tardive dyskinesias in mental hospital patients. *Dis. Nerv. Syst.* 33:182–186, 1972.

36. El-Yousef, M. K., Janowsky, D. S., Davis, J. M. and Sekerke, H. J.: Reversal by physostigmine of antiparkinsonian drug toxicity: A controlled study. *Amer. J. Psychiat.* 130:141–145, 1973.

37. Fann, W. E., Cavanaugh, J. H., Kaufmann, J. S., Griffith, J. D., Davis, J. M., Janowsky, D. S., and Oates, J. A.: Doxepin: Effects on transport of biogenic amines. *Psychopharmacologia* 22:111–125, 1971.

38. Fann, W. E., Janowsky, D. S., Oates, J. A., and Davis, J. M.: Chlorpromazine reversal of the antihypertensive action of guanethidine. *Lancet* 2:436–437, 1971.

39. Janowsky, D. S., Fann, W. E., Davis, J. M., and Oates, J. A.: Chlorpromazine reversal of the antihypertensive action of guanethidine. *Am. J. Psychiat.* 133(4):808–812, 1973.

# CHAPTER 3

# Benzodiazepines in the Elderly

David J. Greenblatt, M.D.
Marcia Divoll, B.S.

## INTRODUCTION

Benzodiazepines are frequently administered to the elderly. The use of prescription drugs increases with age, and in the 60-and-over age group, the use of minor tranquilizers and sedatives is high (1). In one study, benzodiazepines were the psychoactive drugs most frequently prescribed to chronically ill elderly patients (2). In another study, prescriptions for diazepam represented 56% of all psychoactive drug prescriptions written for persons aged 55 years or older (3).

Epidemiological studies have demonstrated that the elderly may be more susceptible to central nervous system depression from this class of drugs. The frequency of drowsiness among recipients of diazepam and chlordiazepoxide was almost twice as high in patients over the age of 70 years as it was in patients 40 years old or younger (4). Adverse reactions attributed to flurazepam among 2,542 monitored hospitalized medical patients were infrequent and relatively minor, but the frequency of adverse reactions was considerably higher in the elderly than in the young (5). The frequency of toxicity among those 80 or over reached 7.1%, whereas only 1.9% of those younger than 60 experienced unwanted effects of flurazepam. The risk of toxicity increased substantially with larger doses. Unwanted effects were attributed to flurazepam in 39% of patients 70 years or older who received an average daily dose of 30 mg or more. Excessive central nervous system depression such as

We are grateful for the assistance and collaboration of Ann Locniskar, Lawrence J. Moschitto, Jerold S. Harmatz, and Dr. Richard I. Shader.

drowsiness, confusion, and ataxia were the most common side effects manifested. Oversedation and confusion were also experienced by 26% of elderly patients receiving flurazepam who were confined to long-term care facilities during a 1-year period (6).

Central nervous system depression from nitrazepam is also significantly more common in the elderly than the young (7). In the same hospital-based monitoring program, 11% of those aged 80 or older receiving nitrazepam experienced central nervous system depression. This increased to 55% in this group when the daily dose averaged 10 mg or more.

Two types of phenomena may explain the apparent susceptibility of the elderly to central nervous system depression—increased receptor site sensitivity and pharmacokinetic alterations caused by the aging process. If receptor site sensitivity increases with age, any given drug concentration at the receptor site of action may lead to a greater pharmacodynamic response in an elderly individual. Changes in pharmacokinetic variables such as prolonged elimination half-lives and decreased metabolic clearance may lead to higher steady-state plasma concentrations of drugs and may increase levels at the receptor site, thereby enhancing the pharmacological action.

Physiological changes caused by the aging process may play a role in altered metabolism of drugs. It is well documented that kidney function declines with age (8). A person's glomerular filtration rate and renal plasma flow may decrease by as much as 50% by the age of 80. Though serum creatinine levels may be normal and no active intrinsic renal disease may be present, creatinine clearance is diminished in the elderly individual (9). Alterations in kidney function caused by the aging process may alter the clearance of drugs eliminated totally or partially intact from the body via the kidneys.

However, the benzodiazepines available on the market today are biotransformed in the liver by either nitroreduction, oxidation, or conjugation. Therefore, hepatic function is critical for their elimination from the body. The usual clinical tests of liver function (serum bilirubin, transaminase, etc.) do not appear to differ significantly between elderly and young (10, 11), but changes in drug-metabolizing capacity are not necessarily reflected in conventional liver function tests.

## BENZODIAZEPINE KINETICS IN THE ELDERLY

The work in our laboratory has focused on pharmacokinetic alterations of benzodiazepines in the elderly. (See Table 3.1.) We have chosen this class of compounds for a number of reasons. Although the benzodiaze-

TABLE 3.1  Metabolic Biotransformation of Benzodiazepines

| Parent Compound | Metabolic Pathway | Metabolic Product |
|---|---|---|
| **Oxidative reactions** | | |
| Diazepam | Demethylation | Desmethyldiazepam[c] |
| Desmethyldiazepam[a] | Hydroxylation | Oxazepam |
| Chlordiazepoxide | Demethylation | Desmethylchlordiazepoxide[c] |
| Desalkylflurazepam[b] | Hydroxylation | 3-OH Desalkylflurazepam |
| Clobazam | Demethylation | Desmethylclobazam[c] |
| Alprazolam | Hydroxylation | Hydroxylated metabolites |
| Triazolam | Hydroxylation | Hydroxylated metabolites |
| | | |
| **Conjugative reactions** | | |
| Lorazepam | Glucuronidation | Lorazepam glucuronide |
| Oxazepam | Glucuronidation | Oxazepam glucuronide |
| Temazepam | Glucuronidation | Temazepam glucuronide |
| | | |
| **Nitroreduction reactions** | | |
| Clonazepam | Nitroreduction | 7-Aminoclonazepam |
| Nitrazepam | Nitroreduction | 7-Aminonitrazepam |

[a]Formed from its precursors clorazepate and prazepam.
[b]Formed from its precursor flurazepam.
[c]Pharmacologically active metabolites appearing in plasma in clinically important amounts.

pines are similar in structure, they are biotransformed in the liver by oxidation, conjugation, and nitroreduction. Thus, we are able to compare the drug-metabolizing capacity of elderly individuals to that of young controls for several different metabolic pathways. The benzodiazepines are also safe for study in this population, and many of the derivatives are available for intravenous administration. Finally, they are easily quantitated in body fluids following single doses. Most important, information derived from pharmacokinetic studies of the benzodiazepines in the elderly allows a better understanding of the effects of this class of drugs in this population.

Although age is an important factor in the ability to metabolize benzodiazepines, other determinants are also influential. The gender of the study population is an important determinant of pharmacokinetic variables. The aging process may have different effects on drug disposition depending on the sex of the population. Studies of age-related changes in drug metabolism must be stratified for gender.

Age-related alterations in the binding of drugs to plasma albumin may also influence pharmacokinetic findings. Plasma albumin concentrations decline with age. This, in turn, may lead to an increase of the free fraction of drugs that are extensively bound to albumin. Since only the unbound fraction is available for metabolic biotransformation and elimination, the volume of distribution and clearance of total (free plus bound) drug may not provide a clear picture of drug metabolism. Pharmacokinetic variables should be corrected for differences in the free fraction.

Environmental factors such as cigarette smoking may also alter pharmacokinetic findings. Cigarette smoking is known to induce the liver microsomal system increasing the metabolic clearance of drugs dependent on the same biotransformation system.

## OXIDATIVE PATHWAYS

Diazepam, desmethyldiazepam, chlordiazepoxide, and desalkylflurazepam undergo oxidative biotransformation.

### Diazepam

Diazepam is initially biotransformed by N-demethylation of the parent drug, to yield the pharmacologically active desmethyldiazepam. Desmethyldiazepam is then hydroxylated to a 3-hydroxy derivative, oxazepam.

Studies from our laboratory have shown that kinetic variables for total (free plus bound) diazepam are influenced by both age and sex (12). Volumes of distribution are larger in females than males of both age groups, and larger in the elderly than in the young of both sexes. Total clearance of diazepam is less in elderly males than in young males, but total diazepam clearance in the two female groups is nearly identical.

Protein binding of diazepam declines with age. After correction for protein binding, unbound volumes of distribution are larger in females than in males of both age groups, but the effect of age is small. Clearance of unbound diazepam is greater in females than in males of both age groups. Unbound clearance in elderly males is 50% less than in young males—a greater difference than for clearance of total diazepam. The age effect on unbound diazepam clearance in women is considerably less than in men.

Age was also associated with larger values of distribution volume and prolonged elimination half-lives of diazepam in a study by Klotz (13). Reduction in total clearance did not reach significance between young and old, but most of the subjects were male, and the study was not stratified for gender. In a study of 19 young and elderly subjects of both sexes, MacLeod et al. found that women had lower clearance of total diazepam than men (14). This finding was not influenced by age. However, the effects of cigarette smoking, protein binding, and underlying medical disease were not assessed.

## Clorazepate and Prazepam

Desmethyldiazepam is formed from two precursor compounds, clorazepate and prazepam. Regardless of the precursor, the disposition and elimination properties of desmethyldiazepam in the elderly are similar to those of diazepam (see Figure 3.1) (15, 16). Women have higher clearance of unbound desmethyldiazepam than men, regardless of age; unbound clearance declines with age in men but changes little with age in women. Protein binding of desmethyldiazepam also declines with age. Therefore, clearance values of the compound must be corrected for age-related changes in binding. As in the case of diazepam, distribution of desmethyldiazepam is more extensive in women and in the elderly (see Figure 3.2).

## Chlordiazepoxide

Chlordiazepoxide is transformed by N-demethylation yielding desmethylchlordiazepoxide. We have studied age-related changes of chlordiazepoxide only in males. The mean elimination half-life of oral chlordiazepoxide in elderly men is significantly longer than in young subjects, and chlordiazepoxide clearance is significantly less than in the young controls (17). Roberts et al. also found a decrease in plasma clearance and prolongation of the elimination half-life of intravenous chlordiazepoxide in elderly men (18). We are presently studying the disposition and elimination of chlordiazepoxide in elderly women.

## Flurazepam

Desalkylflurazepam, formed from its precursor flurazepam, appears to undergo 3-hydroxylation. Only trace concentrations of flurazepam appear in plasma following usual therapeutic doses in humans, but the extent of conversion of flurazepam to this active metabolite is not known. As in the case of diazepam and desmethyldiazepam, desalkylflurazepam half-life is prolonged in the elderly as opposed to the young, particularly among elderly men (see Figure 3.3) (19). The effect of age

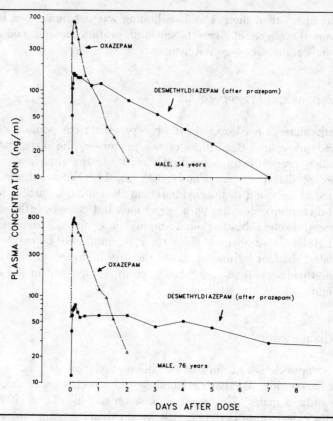

FIGURE 3.1. Example of the differential effect of age on the disposition of oxidized vs. conjugated benzodiazepines. Two healthy male volunteers, one aged 34 years (above) and one aged 76 years (below) ingested a single 30-mg dose of oxazepam and a single 20-mg dose of prazepam (a precursor of desmethyldiazepam) on two occasions separated by several months. Drug concentrations in plasma were measured by gas chromatography at multiple points in time after each dose. The pattern of elimination of oxazepam (transformed by glucuronide conjugation) is nearly identical for the two subjects. However, for desmethyldiazepam (transformed by aliphatic hydroxylation, a form of oxidation) the rate of elimination is greatly reduced in the elderly man as opposed to the young man.

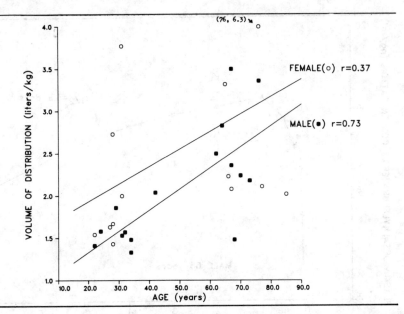

FIGURE 3.2.    Apparent volume of distribution of desmethyldiazepam (formed from its precursor prazepam) in relation to age and sex. Volume of distribution increases with age in both sexes, and is larger in women than in men (see reference 15 for study details).

on the accumulation of desalkylflurazepam during chronic therapy of 15 mg doses of flurazepam is consistent with the longer elimination half-life. Steady-state plasma concentrations are significantly higher in elderly as opposed to young males, whereas age-related differences among women are small. However, no increased sensitivity to flurazepam among elderly subjects was found at the plasma desmethylflurazepam concentrations achieved after 2 weeks of 15 mg doses. This was consistent with previous studies demonstrating the safety of 15-mg flurazepam doses among elderly individuals (5).

## Other Benzodiazepines Transformed by Oxidation

A number of other benzodiazepines currently under investigation are transformed by oxidative mechanisms. Clobazam, a 1,5-benzodiazepine, is metabolized by demethylation, yielding the active metabolite desmethylclobazam. Triazolam and alprazolam are relatively short-acting triaz-

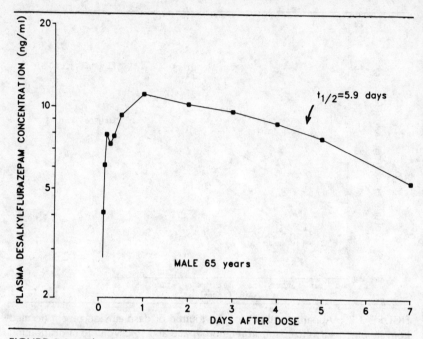

FIGURE 3.3.    Plasma concentrations of desalkylflurazepam in an elderly man who ingested a single 15-mg dose of flurazepam (Dalmane).

olo benzodiazepine derivatives metabolized by hydroxylation. Preliminary findings of kinetic studies of these drugs in elderly subjects are suggestive of age- and sex-related changes similar to those observed with other oxidized benzodiazepines (20).

## CONJUGATIVE PATHWAYS

Hydroxylated benzodiazepine derivatives such as oxazepam and lorazepam are biotransformed by glucuronide conjugation. Age-related findings with these derivatives contrast with results of studies of benzodiazepines metabolized by oxidative pathways. The glucuronide conjugation pathway appears to be minimally influenced by age or sex.

### Lorazepam

Studies from our laboratory comparing lorazepam pharmacokinetics between young and elderly subjects reveal no striking differences (21). Values of volume of distribution average about 9% less in the elderly

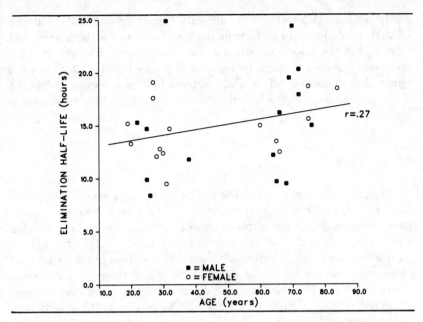

FIGURE 3.4. Relation of age to lorazepam elimination half-life. Solid line was determined by least squares regression analysis. The association (r=.27) is not significant.

than in the young group. Values of elimination half-life in the elderly are not significantly different from those in the young groups (see Figure 3.4). Total clearance averages 21% lower in the elderly than in young volunteers; the difference just reached statistical significance. Gender does not appear to influence the distribution or clearance of lorazepam in either age group. We are presently determining the free fraction of lorazepam in many of these same subjects. Preliminary findings show lorazepam to be 8–12% unbound. Since the compound is not tightly bound to plasma albumin, differences in protein binding between young and elderly subjects will probably not influence kinetic variables.

Kraus and associates also found that the disposition of lorazepam was not affected by the aging process in a group of 11 males aged 15–73 years (22). There was a trend toward decreased binding with increasing age, but this difference did not reach significance.

## Oxazepam

As in the case of lorazepam, neither age nor gender importantly influences the distribution, elimination half-life, or clearance of oxazepam (see Figure 3.1) (23). Protein binding of oxazepam declines with age, partly because of lower plasma albumin concentrations in the elderly. Clearance of unbound oxazepam declines with age in both men and women, but the association did not reach significance. The effects of sex are greater, with a reduced clearance and longer half-lives in females as opposed to males regardless of age. Others have also suggested that the aging process has relatively little effect on the disposition of oxazepam (24).

## Temazepam

Temazepam is a 3-hydroxy-1,4-benzodiazepine used extensively in the Eastern Hemisphere as a hypnotic agent. Like lorazepam and oxazepam, the major pathway of temazepam in humans involves conjugation with glucuronic acid. The clearance of total temazepam is higher in men than in women, and is essentially uninfluenced by age (25). Unbound clearance is reduced, but not significantly, in the elderly of both sexes. However, it is still higher in men than in women of corresponding age. Unbound volume of distribution tends to be smaller in the elderly than in the young of both sexes. The effect of age on temazepam kinetics has not been reported from other laboratories.

## NITROREDUCTION PATHWAYS

Nitrazepam and clonazepam are both biotransformed by nitroreduction. Kangas et al. reported that the elimination half-life of 5 mg of oral nitrazepam was prolonged in 12 elderly patients compared to 25 young volunteers (40.4 vs. 28.9 hrs) (26). However, clearance was approximately the same in both groups. The longer half-life may be partially explained by higher volumes of distribution in the elderly group. In a second study, no difference in nitrazepam disposition was found in the elderly (27). The findings of these two studies are not easily interpreted since the elderly population was ill or partially immobilized, and no stratification was made for gender.

## CONFIRMATION OF FINDINGS

Many of the same subjects have participated in a number of our pharmacokinetic studies with the benzodiazepines. This has enabled us to compare the ability of the same individual to oxidize or conjugate different

benzodiazepines. The elimination half-lives among oxidized benzodiazepines were highly intercorrelated (diazepam vs. desmethyldiazepam,
r=0.77, p<.001; diazepam vs. desalkylflurazepam, r=0.90, p<.001;
desmethyldiazepam vs. desalkylflurazepam, r=0.93, p<.001). The clear-
ances of conjugated benzodiazepines were also intercorrelated (oxazepam vs. lorazepam, r=0.60, p<.025; oxazepam vs. temazepam, r=0.80,
p<.001; lorazepam vs. temazepam, r=0.85, p<.001) (see Figure 3.5)
(28).

Antipyrine is often used as an indicator of drug oxidizing activity in
humans. Several studies have demonstrated an age-related decline in
antipyrine oxidation. A recent study from our laboratory revealed a high
degree of consistency within individuals in the ability to metabolize
antipyrine and oxidized benzodiazepines (28).

Acetaminophen is biotransformed by conjugation in the liver. We
are presently studying acetaminophen and the conjugated benzodiazepines in these individuals.

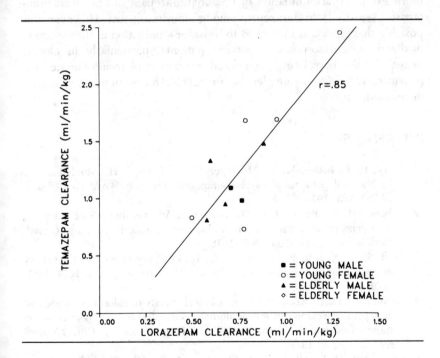

FIGURE 3.5. Relation of lorazepam clearance to temazepam clearance among
a series of subjects who received single doses of the two drugs on different
occasions. Solid line was determined by least squares regression analysis.

## SUMMARY

The benzodiazepines are frequently administered to the elderly population. Age-related changes in the disposition and elimination of this class of drugs have been demonstrated. However, these age-related changes appear to be dependent not only on the gender of the individual, but also on the metabolic pathway of the benzodiazepine in question.

The metabolic clearance of benzodiazepines initially biotransformed by oxidative pathways (diazepam, desmethyldiazepam, desalkylflurazepam) is reduced in the elderly, particularly in elderly men. However, the clearance of benzodiazepines transformed by glucuronide conjugation (oxazepam, lorazepam) is minimally affected by age or sex. Nitroreduction (e.g., of nitrazepam and clonazepam) may also be altered by age, but further study is needed to interpret these findings.

The clinical implications of these age- and sex-related changes have not been established. In the case of 15 mg doses of flurazepam, the more extensive accumulation of desalkylflurazepam did not lead to increased sensitivity to flurazepam among elderly subjects. However, it is possible that clinicians may need to consider a reduction in the dosage of oxidized benzodiazepines in elderly patients, particularly in elderly males. Studies correlating age-related changes in pharmacokinetics and pharmacodynamics are needed before specific recommendations can be developed.

## REFERENCES

1. Parry, H. J., Balter, M. B., Mellinger, G. D., Cisin, I. H., Manheimer D. I.: National patterns of psychotherapeutic drug use. *Arch. Gen. Psych.* 28:769–783, 1973.
2. Achong, M. R., Bayne, J. R. D., Gerson, L. W., Golshani, S.: Prescribing of psychoactive drugs for chronically anxious elderly patients. *Canad. Med. Assoc. J.* 118:1503–1508, 1978.
3. Skoll, S. L., August, R. J., Johnson, G. E.: Drug prescribing for the elderly in Saskatchewan during 1976. *Canad. Med. Assoc. J.* 121:1074–1081, 1979.
4. Greenblatt, D. J., Koch-Weser, J.: Clinical toxicity of chlordiazepoxide and diazepam in relation to serum albumin concentration: A report from the Boston Collaborative Drug Surveillance Program. *Eur. J. Clin. Pharmacol.* 7:259–262, 1974.
5. Greenblatt, D. J., Allen, M. D., Shader, R. I.: Toxicity of high-dose flurazepam in the elderly. *Clin. Pharmacol. Ther.* 21:355–361, 1977.
6. Marttilla, J. K., Hammel, R. J., Alexander, B., Zustiak, R.: Potential unto-

ward effects of long-term use of flurazepam in geriatric patients. *J. Amer. Pharmaceut. Assoc.* 17:692–695, 1977.

7. Greenblatt, D. J., Allen, M. D.: Toxicity of nitrazepam in the elderly: A report from the Boston Collaborative Drug Surveillance Program. *Br. J. Clin. Pharmacol.* 5:407–413, 1978.

8. Friedman, S. A., Raizner, A. E., Rosen, H., Solomon, N. A., Sy, W.: Functional defects in the aging kidney. *Ann. Intern. Med.* 76:41–45, 1972.

9. Rowe, J. W., Andres, R., Tobin, J. D., Norris, A. H., Shock, N.W.: Age-adjusted standards for creatinine clearance (letter). *Ann. Intern. Med.* 84:567–568, 1976.

10. Cohen, T., Gitman, L., Lipschutz, E.: Liver function studies in the aged. *Geriat.* 15:824–836, 1960.

11. Kampmann, J. P., Sinding, J., Moller-Jorgensen, I.: Effect of age on liver function. *Geriat.* 30:91–95 (August), 1975.

12. Greenblatt, D. J., Allen, M. D., Harmatz, J. S., Shader, R. I.: Diazepam disposition determinants. *Clin. Pharmacol. Ther.* 27:301–312, 1980.

13. Klotz, U., Avant, G. R., Hoyumpa, A., Schenker, S., Wilkinson, G. R.: The effects of age and liver disease on the disposition and elimination of diazepam in adult man. *J. Clin. Invest.* 55:347–359, 1975.

14. MacLeod, S. M., Giles, H. G., Bengert, B., Liu, F. F., Sellers, E. M.: Age- and gender-related differences in diazepam pharmacokinetics. *J. Clin. Pharmacol.* 19:15–19, 1979.

15. Allen, M. D., Greenblatt, D. J., Harmatz, J. S., Shader, R. I.: Desmethyldiazepam kinetics in the elderly after oral prazepam. *Clin. Pharmacol. Ther.* 28:196–202, 1980.

16. Shader, R. I., Greenblatt, D. J., Ciraulo, D. A., Divoll, M., Harmatz, J. S., Georgotas, A.: Effect of age and sex on disposition of desmethyldiazepam from its precursor clorazepate. *Psychopharmacol.* 75:193–197, 1981.

17. Shader, R. I., Greenblatt, D. J., Harmatz, J. S., Franke, K., Koch-Weser, J.: Absorption and disposition of chlordiazepoxide in young and elderly male volunteers. *J. Clin. Pharmacol.* 17:709–718, 1977.

18. Roberts, R. K., Wilkinson, G. R., Branch. R. A., Schenker, S.: Effect of age and parenchymal liver disease on the disposition and elimination of chlordiazepoxide (Librium). *Gastroenterol.* 75:479–485, 1978.

19. Greenblatt, D. J., Divoll, M., Harmatz, J. S., MacLaughlin, D. S., Shader, R. I.: Kinetics and clinical effects of flurazepam in young and elderly noninsomniac volunteers. *Clin. Pharmacol. Ther.* 30:475–486, 1981.

20. Greenblatt, D. J., Divoll, M., Puri, S. K., Ho, I., Zinny, M. A., Shader, R. I.: Clobazam kinetics in the elderly. *Brit. J. Clin. Pharmacol.* 12:631–636, 1981.

21. Greenblatt, D. J., Allen, M. D., Locniskar, A., Harmatz, J. S., Shader, R. I.: Lorazepam kinetics in the elderly. *Clin. Pharmacol. Ther.* 26:103–113, 1979.

22. Kraus, J. W., Desmond, P. V., Marshall, J. P., Johnson, R. F., Schenker,

42                                    Treatment of Psychopathology in the Aging

S., Wilkinson, G. R.: Effects of aging and liver disease on disposition of lorazepam. *Clin. Pharmacol. Ther.* 24:411–419, 1978.

23. Greenblatt, D. J., Divoll, M., Harmatz, J. S., Shader, R. I.: Oxazepam kinetics: Effects of age and sex. *J. Pharmacol. Exper. Ther.* 215:86–91, 1980.

24. Shull, H. J., Wilkinson, G. R., Johnson, R., Schenker, S. Normal disposition of oxazepam in acute viral hepatitis and cirrhosis. *Ann. Intern. Med.* 84:420–425, 1976.

25. Divoll, M., Greenblatt, D. J., Harmatz, J. S., Shader, R. I.: Effects of age and sex on the disposition of temazepam. *J. Pharm. Sci.* 70:1104–1107, 1981.

26. Kangas, L., Iisalo, E., Kanto, J., Lehtnen, V., Pynnonen, S., Ruikka, I., Salminen, J., Sallanpaa, M., Syvalahti, E.: Human pharmacokinetics of nitrazepam: Effects of age and diseases. *Eur. J. Clin. Pharmacol.* 15:163–170, 1979.

27. Casteleden, C. M., George, C. F., Marcer, D., Hallett, C.: Increased sensitivity to nitrazepam in old age. *Brit. Med. J.* 1:10–12, 1977.

28. Greenblatt, D. J., Divoll, M., Abernethy, D. R., Harmatz, J. S., Shader, R. I.: Antipyrine kinetics in the elderly: Prediction of age-related changes in benzodiazepine oxidizing capacity. *J. Pharm. and Exp. Ther.* 220:120–126, 1982.

# CHAPTER 4

# Sleep Disturbances in the Aged: Hormonal Correlates and Therapeutic Considerations

Patricia N. Prinz, PH.D.
Jeffrey B. Halter, M.D.

## INTRODUCTION

Sleep disturbances increase with advancing age. Sleeping pill use also increases markedly among older Americans. Although Americans over 60 represent only 11% of the population, they receive about 40% of all sleeping pill prescriptions (1). Impaired sleep in geriatric patients reflects not only the presence of health factors affecting sleep but also an age-change in sleep that can be observed in extremely healthy older individuals. This chapter reviews the sleep changes of healthy elderly people and discusses some of the hormonal correlates accompanying these sleep changes. Sleep pattern changes in cognitively impaired elderly are discussed, both for mildly and severely impaired old subjects. Some pharmacologic considerations for the treatment of impaired sleep in geriatric patients are also discussed, with an emphasis on the newer contributions to this field derived from recent sleep research efforts.

Support for this research was provided by the Veterans Administration and by PHS Grants AG 00667, MH 33688, RR 00037, and AG 01926.

## SLEEP CHANGES ACROSS THE LIFESPAN: CHANGES IN SLEEP PATTERN WITH AGE

Modern measures of sleep and wakefulness patterns are based on all-night polygraphic recordings of the electrical signals generated by various functions: brain (EEG), postural muscle (EMG), and eye movements (EOG). Although the brain's electrical activity undergoes changes as a function of age (2), this discussion is limited to the corresponding sleep stage changes.

Normal sleep is divided into two main categories, nonrapid eye movement (NREM) sleep and rapid eye movement (REM) sleep, which comprise a total of five stages (3). NREM sleep includes stages 1, 2, 3, and 4. REM sleep is the fifth stage (also called active or paradoxical or dreaming sleep). The patterning of the various sleep stages of NREM (stages 1–4), REM sleep, and the total amount of daily sleep change with normal aging. Roffwarg et al. (4), summarizing several studies, described the major changes across the lifespan: total sleep, percentage of REM sleep, and stage 4 sleep are all at maximum levels in early childhood and drop to more stable adult levels after puberty, followed by a further decline in senescence (4).

Human sleep stages are known to cycle in characteristic fashion. After sleep onset, the individual descends from stage 1 into 2, 3, and then 4, after which a REM period generally occurs. This sequence of sleep stages terminating in REM sleep is repeated 4–5 times across the night's sleep. Elderly individuals experience more frequent stage transitions and greater fragmentation of sleep with waking periods (see Figure 4.1). Additionally, stage 4 sleep is greatly reduced from childhood to adulthood and further reduced or absent in senescence. Time spent in REM has been observed to be consistently diminished in senescent sleep patterns as compared with young adult levels. At the same time, there is a significant increase in wakefulness, involving the number of awakenings and the length of time awake. Only minor, nonsignificant changes have been observed for NREM sleep stages 1, 2, and 3 in elderly subject groups as compared with young adult measurements (see Table 4.1) (4–9).

One of the more apparent age changes is the reduced amount of stage 4 sleep depicted in the comparison of polygraphic recordings of a young normal subject and an aged normal subject in Figure 4.2. The defining characteristic of stage 4 sleep is that high-voltage, slow-wave EEG activity occupies more than 50% of the total time in the epoch. Both amplitude and overall amount of stage 4 waves are decreased in the senescent sleep record (5, 10).

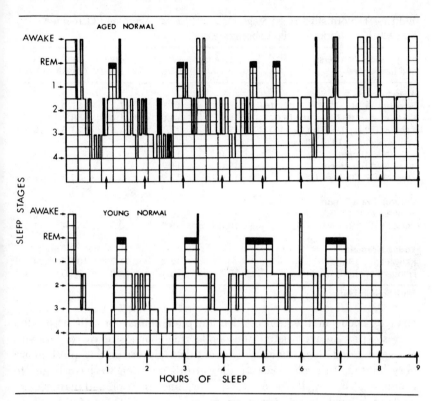

FIGURE 4.1.   Typical pattern of sleep and wakefulness across the night in an aged (90-year-old) and a young (22-year-old) subject. Compared to that of young adults, the senescent sleep recording contains little or no stage 4 sleep, reduced REM sleep, more frequent stage transitions, and more frequent—often longer—awakenings (2).

The biological significance of the decrease in stage 4 and REM sleep and increase in wakefulness is not well understood, although some hypotheses have been offered for these age-related changes in sleep patterns (11). Some useful information can be gained by examining correlative neurobiological changes with aging.

## HORMONAL CORRELATES

Since consistent changes in sleep accompany "normal" aging (reduced stage 4 and REM sleep together with increased nighttime wakefulness), corresponding physiological consequences may also be affected. Do age

TABLE 4.1 Normative Sleep Stage Data for Young, Aged, and Demented Subjects from Various Sleep Laboratories

| Subjects, Researchers, and References | Sleep Latency (mins.) | % Waking of TIB[a] | % Stage 4 of Sleep | REM (mins.) | % REM of Sleep |
|---|---|---|---|---|---|
| **Aged Normals** | | | | | |
| Feinberg et al., 1967 (5) (N=16) | 18.5 | 17.7 | 7.3 | 81.0 | 21.1 |
| Kales et al., 1967 (7) (N=10) | 18.0 | 18.0 | 1.4 | 68.2 | 19.7 |
| Kahn & Fisher, 1969 (6) (N=16) | 25.6 | 27.1 | 4.5 | 73.8 | 20.1 |
| Williams et al., 1974 (9) | | | | | |
| (N=10 men) | 32.0 | 16.0 | 0 | — | 21.3 |
| (N=10 women) | 15.0 | 11.7 | 4.0 | — | 22.2 |
| Prinz, 1977 (8) (N=11) | 12.6 | 12.9 | 6.1 | 75.8 | 18.4 |
| **Chronic Brain Syndrome** | | | | | |
| Feinberg et al., 1967 (5) | 31.0 | 30.8 | — | 53.1 | 16.9 |
| Prinz et al., 1981 SDAT (11) | 10.0 | 36.5 | 0 | 33.4 | 11.2 |
| **Young Normals** | | | | | |
| Kales et al., 1967 (7) | — | 2.2 | 11.2 | 109.7 | 24.0 |
| Feinberg et al., 1967 (5) | 10.4 | 6.1 | 13.0 | 90.0 | 22.7 |

[a]TIB=time in bed.

changes occur in the neuroendocrine phenomena normally associated with sleep? Can age-related neuroendocrine changes be correlated with the age-related sleep changes? Current data addressing this question are very limited. In preliminary studies of this question we have begun to examine 24-hour patterns of growth hormone, cortisol, and plasma catecholamine levels in relation to sleep.

## Growth Hormone

Growth hormone (GH), known to promote protein synthesis and tissue repair and growth in various somatic tissues and possibly brain tissues as well, is released from the neurohypophysis in response to various physiologic stimuli (12). Investigations of GH secretion in the elderly are of general value since GH may be involved in the altered energy metabolism in old age (13), and since GH is important as an anabolic factor in intermediary metabolism (14). Plasma GH level reflects the secretory rate of the hormone under normal physiological conditions. Studies of plasma levels can reveal age effects on GH secretory phenomena since the peripheral elimination of GH is not altered by age (15).

Physiologic stimuli that release GH include hypoglycemia, protein feeding, exercise, and stress (16). However, the largest consistent release of GH occurs in the first half of the night in association with

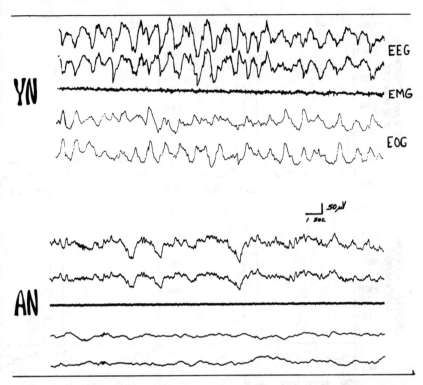

FIGURE 4.2. Age effect on slow-wave sleep. Shown in a epoch with maximum abundance of delta activity for a typical young normal (YN) and an aged normal (AN) subject. Large 100–200 microvolt waves occupy most of the epoch of the young normal but not aged normal subject.

slow-wave sleep onset (17–19). The pattern of plasma GH level as averaged across 24-hour observation periods of 7 young men is shown in Figure 4.3. When slow-wave sleep stages (3 and 4) predominate during the first half-night there is a consistent pulse of plasma GH (19). Since elderly adults experience diminished slow-wave sleep, it is also possible that they undergo a related reduction in nighttime GH release. Trends in this direction were indicated in earlier preliminary studies on small numbers of subjects (20, 21). In a more recent series of studies of nighttime GH release in 14 young and 16 aged men in excellent health (via physical examination), the GH peak associated with sleep onset was observed to be significantly suppressed in elderly males as compared to young men studied on the third of 3 consecutive nights in the sleep laboratory (11, 22, 23). Plasma GH levels were assayed at 20 minute intervals. Compared to young men, the aged men had nighttime peaks

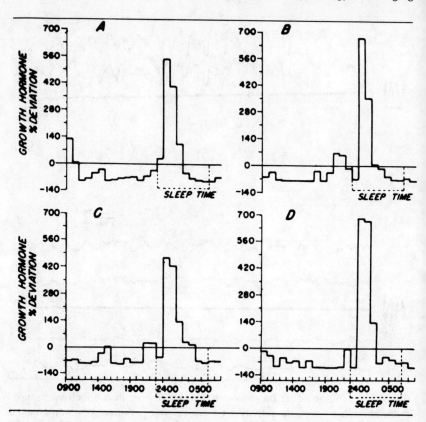

FIGURE 4.3. The 24-hour pattern of plasma growth hormone concentration expressed as percent deviation of the mean daily concentration. The average 24-hour curve of plasma growth hormone concentration in 7 young normal subjects is consistently higher during the first half of the time-in-bed period, irrespective of the 4 seasons of the year (19).

of GH that were small or absent and distributed more evenly across the night (see Figure 4.4 and 4.5 and Table 4.2). A significant reduction was observed in peak level (15.4 pg/ml vs. 4.3 pg/ml) and in integrated amount of GH in the first half-night (20.9 pg/ml vs. 5.0 pg/ml) for young normal and aged normal groups, respectively (see Table 4.2) Significant correlations were also observed between GH levels and quality of sleep (see Figure 4.6 and Table 4.2).

Twenty-four hour GH levels were examined to determine whether this age effect on GH pertained only to nighttime release. Age did not statistically alter GH levels during the daytime (out of bed) portion of the 24-hour period (see Figure 4.5 and Table 4.2). It appears that the age

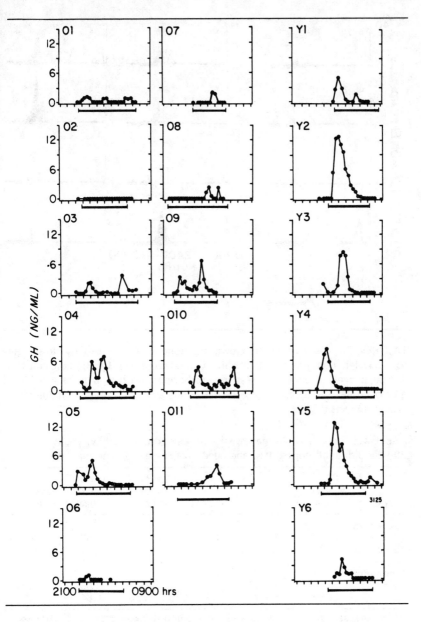

FIGURE 4.4.  Nighttime plasma growth hormone levels in 6 young (Y1–Y6) and 11 healthy aged (o1–o11) subjects. Note the high peaks of growth hormone release during the first half of the night in the young normals, and the more even distribution of smaller peaks in the aged subjects (22).

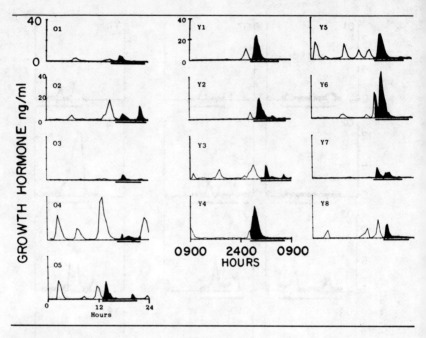

FIGURE 4.5. 24-hour plasma growth hormone levels in 5 healthy old subjects (o1–o5, left column) and 8 healthy young subjects (y1–y8, right column). Although aged subjects had less growth hormone in bed at night (blackened area of curve), GH release during the day (white area of curve) did not differ from young subjects (53).

TABLE 4.2 Sleep and plasma growth hormone (GH) in healthy, young (20–29-year-old) adult normal (YN) and aged (62–80-year-old) normal (AN) men[a]

| % Waking | % Stage 3 & 4 | % REM | First GH Peak | 1st Half-Night GH Integral | 2nd Half-Night GH Integral | ·Day GH Integral |
|---|---|---|---|---|---|---|
| **Young normal** | | | | | | |
| 11.13 | 22.85 | 23.76 | 15.42 | 20.93 | 3.37 | 26.75 |
| ±2.02 | ±2.30 | ±2.021 | ±3.05 | ±4.18 | ±.59 | ±6.25 |
| **Aged normal** | | | | | | |
| 27.83[b] | 9.95[b] | 16.35[b] | 4.28[b] | 4.96[b] | 3.06 | 48.06 |
| ±2.16 | ±1.89 | ±1.92 | ±.96 | ±1.22 | ±.84 | ±23.50 |

[a]Sleep data are expressed as percentage of time in bed. Mean ±SEM. GH is expressed as ng/ml (peak) ng/ml (integral). The Pearson correlation for percent stage 3 and 4 and the first GH peak level at night was nonsignificant within groups. For the combined AN + YN groups (N=30), the correlation coefficient was .463 (p<.01) (11,23).
[b]AN versus YN different, p<.05, t test.

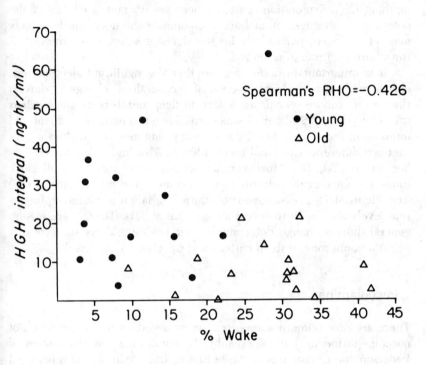

FIGURE 4.6.   All-night mean integrated growth hormone level for each young (•) or old (x) subject as plotted against his percent wakefulness of time in bed. These measures correlate significantly (r=.426, p<.05).

effect on spontaneous GH release pertains only to the first half of the nighttime hours spent in bed. The lack of a daytime age effect on spontaneous GH levels is in accord with clinical studies that employed various challenges (insulin hypoglycemia, arginine infusion) to elicit GH release in the elderly. These studies generally report minor or conflicting age effects (24–27).

The physiological significance of the nighttime reduction in GH with aging is not immediately apparent. Assuming that GH release at night has the same physiological effect as during the day, then daytime GH release would compensate for any nighttime reduction, and the observed age effect on GH would be inconsequential. However, this assumption may not be valid since varying dose levels of GH are reported to exert greater anabolic effects when given at night rather than in the morning (28). Exploration of GH's actions are warranted in view of the potential involvement of anabolic hormones in the declining lean body mass of the aged, particularly for the sleeping hours, when the organism's hormonal milieu is altered.

It is important to determine whether the significant sleep-pattern change with age is a consequence of a generalized change in diurnal rhythms or a more specific age effect on sleep and its correlates (such as GH). Our study of 24-hour plasma cortisol levels measured at 20 minute intervals in these same healthy aged and young men revealed no significant age differences in basal cortisol levels. This finding confirmed earlier studies (29, 30). Moreover, age effects were absent for all clock times and for diurnal patterns as well (as measured by cosinor analysis) (see Figure 4.7). Measurement of diurnal variation of plasma epinephrine levels also failed to reveal an age change (31). Thus, there was no general diurnal change detectable in our healthy elderly subjects that might account for the sleep pattern and GH changes observed.

## Catecholamines

There are now numerous reports of increased daytime plasma levels of norepinephrine (NE) in older subjects, confirming the observation of Pederson and Christensen (32) (see Figure 4.8). NE in plasma is believed to be derived mainly from NE released from peripheral postganglionic sympathetic nerve endings, which are particularly numerous in vascular walls (see Figure 4.9) (33, 34). Plasma NE is known to be increased in man at times when the sympathetic nervous system is activated, for example, during surgical stress, upright posture, or physical exercise (33–35), and to be decreased when the sympathetic nervous system is inhibited pharmacologically with clonidine (36) or when sympathetic efferents are blocked with high spinal anesthesia (37).

If higher plasma NE levels reflect a heightened sympathetic activation, and if older individuals have higher NE levels in the nighttime as well as the daytime, it is reasonable to hypothesize that this heightened sympathetic tonus could be interfering with sleep and promoting nighttime wakefulness, since physiologically or pharmacologically induced increases in sympathetic tonus are known to be accompanied by a more aroused state (as indicated by an EEG arousal pattern and behavioral attentiveness) (26, 38). It was observed in a preliminary study that healthy elderly males do indeed have significantly higher mean NE levels at night as well as during the day (see Figure 4.10) (31). Subsequent

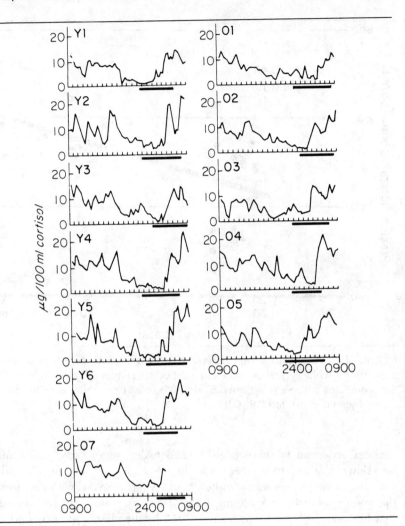

FIGURE 4.7. Twenty-four-hour plasma cortisol levels in young (Y1–Y7) and aged normal (O1–O5) subjects. Horizontal bar represents time in bed. Cortisol levels do not appear to be age-sensitive at any clock time, nor does integrated cortisol differ with age for these healthy subjects.

studies on larger numbers of subjects confirm this finding (see Figure 4.11). It can be inferred that these observations represent an age effect on the release of NE into the circulation rather than an age-related change of NE metabolism, since no age effect on the metabolic clearance rate of plasma NE has been demonstrated (39). The sleep pattern

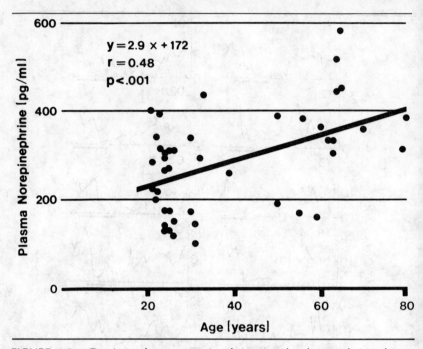

FIGURE 4.8.    Daytime plasma norepinephrine (NE) levels (pg/ml) in subjects aged 10–65 while supine (a), standing 5 (b) or 10 (c) minutes, or exercising (d). Age correlates with NE (r exceeds .5, p<. 05) in all cases. Similar results have been observed in our lab (59, 60).

changes observed in these healthy aged males (more wakefulness and less slow-wave and REM sleep) (see Figure 4.12) correlated significantly with the mean plasma NE for in-bed hours when analyzed with data from the young subjects (see Figure 4.13). This observation suggests either that high sympathetic tonus (as measured by the plasma NE) may underlie the fragmentation and deterioration of sleep in the elderly or that impaired sleep leads to increased sympathetic activity. This interesting possibility deserves further study, as a role for increased sympathetic activity in sleep abnormalities of the elderly would provide a rationale for the development of new pharmacological interventions that counteract nighttime sympathetic hyperactivity as potential sleep aids.

Interestingly, irrespective of whether the ongoing sleep stage is REM or NREM, plasma NE levels remain at stable low levels during sleeping hours (31). However, during periods of spontaneous nighttime wakefulness, small and inconsistent increases are observed. During the longer

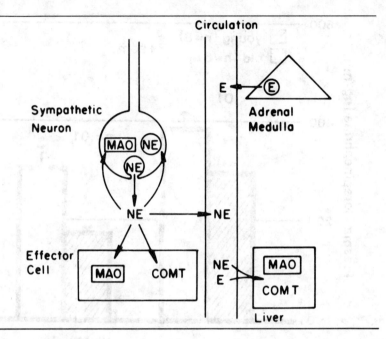

FIGURE 4.9.   Diagram of a postganglionic sympathetic nerve terminal releasing norepinephrine (NE), which is normally taken up again by the nerve ending or degraded locally by the enzymes catechol-o-methytransferase (COMT) or monoamine oxidase (MAO). However, some of the released NE spills over into the circulation before it is taken up again by the synaptic ending or degraded. In contrast, epinephrine (E) is secreted directly into the circulation.

awakenings induced by a tone stimulus as it approaches auditory threshold levels, more pronounced and consistent surges in plasma NE occurred (see Figures 4.14 and 4.15). The pulses of NE induced in this way are brief (1–10 minutes) and superimposed upon the preexisting basal level that is higher in the aged than in the young subject. This indicates that longer awakenings due to environmental factors such as noise might induce a temporary sympathetic discharge that is additive to an existing high level of sympathetic tonus in the elderly. Previous studies, based on hormonal and on psychophysiological evidence, indicated that the elderly are more responsive to sympathetic activation (40, 41). Further studies are needed to determine whether a heightened sympathetic responsivity at night may contribute to the greater susceptibility to noise-induced wakenings described in elderly subjects (42).

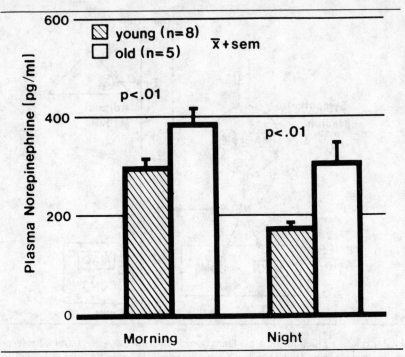

FIGURE 4.10.    Mean daytime (11:00 A.M.) and mean all-night plasma norepinephrine (NE) levels ± SEM for young and old subjects, showing higher NE
levels both at night and during the day in older subjects (31).

## New Areas for Study

There is a growing literature that implicates respiratory disturbances
during sleep as factors underlying impaired sleep (43). Additionally,
there is a growing awareness that these respiratory disturbances are
more pervasive and severe in older individuals. More severe snoring
(44), apnea, and hypopnea (45–47) have been reported in older subjects.
Nighttime respiration and oxygen saturation levels were monitored to
determine whether apnea or hypopnea might account for the sleep and
hormonal changes we observed in our healthy elderly subjects. It was
observed that oxygen saturation remained well above 90% across the
night in all our subjects. Four subjects had evidence of mild apnea (5 or
fewer episodes/hour lasting 10 seconds or more) and the remaining subjects were nonapneic. Thus, the milder age-related sleep-pattern
changes observed here for healthy elderly subjects (see Figure 4.12)

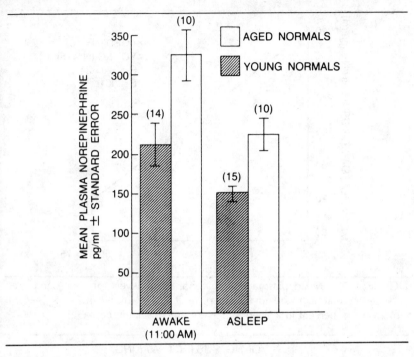

FIGURE 4.11. Mean plasma norepinephrine (NE) levels ± SEM for 14 young and 10 aged normal subjects at 11:00 A.M. and as averaged across bedtime hours (p<.01) or at 11:00 A. M. (p<.01) (52).

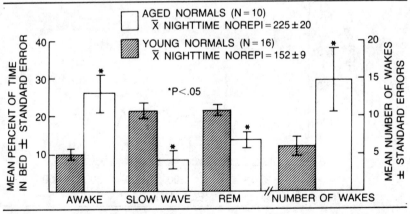

FIGURE 4.12. Sleep stages expressed as mean percent of time in bed ± SEM for healthy young (21–29-year-old) and aged (62–80-year-old) subjects. Aged men spend more time awake, awaken more frequently, and experience less slow-wave (stages 3 and 4) and REM sleep (52).

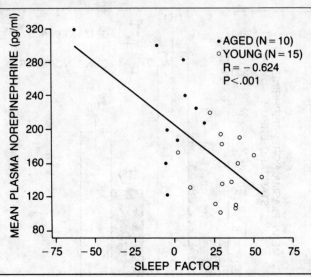

FIGURE 4.13. Mean plasma norepinephrine (NE) levels for young and aged subjects in relation to quality of sleep, as indicated by Sleep Factor (percent slow-wave + percent REM sleep − percent time awake in bed) (52).

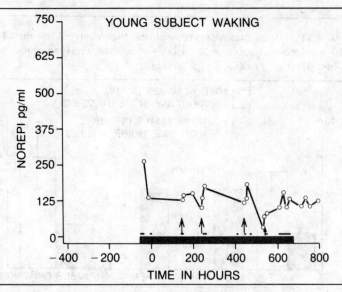

FIGURE 4.14. Plasma norepinephrine (NE) levels in a young normal subject during bedtime hours (dark bar). NE levels are low and consistent during the night with very little response to spontaneous awakenings (indicated by dashes) or experimentally induced awakenings ( ↑ ) to a tone stimulus approaching arousal threshold level.

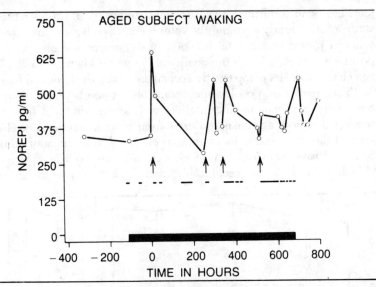

FIGURE 4.15.    Plasma norepinephrine (NE) levels in an aged normal subject across the night. All-night basal levels are higher than in the young subject. Surges in NE can be observed at time of induced awakening ( ↑ ), but are not as apparent during waking time generally across the night (dashes).

occurred in the absence of appreciable apnea. Nevertheless, these mild age-changes in sleep patterns correlated significantly with changes in certain neurohormonal phenomena. It seems reasonable to assume that as the health status of the aged individual becomes more impaired, and as apnea, myoclonus, or other sleep disturbing factors become pronounced, sleep patterns will become even more disturbed and be accompanied by even greater associated hormonal changes. The task ahead of us is to understand not only the multiple underlying factors contributing to impaired sleep in the elderly, but also the impact of the poor sleep per se on the overall health of the aged individual.

## PSYCHOMETRIC CORRELATES

It has been observed that sleep-pattern variables in elderly subject groups parallel mental function test scores. Feinberg et al. (5) observed that time spent in REM sleep was correlated positively with Wechsler Adult Intelligence Scale (WAIS) scores and Wechsler Memory Scores in a study of elderly men living in the community. The finding that amount of REM sleep and psychometric scores are correlated in typical elderly subjects has been confirmed by subsequent studies (6, 8). In a longitudinal study of 12 elderly community volunteers, the change throughout 18 years in preexisting mental function (WAIS) scores was observed to be positively correlated with the quality of sleep (see Figure 4.16) (8). Thus, age changes in sleep apparently accompany changes in mental function.

This relationship could reflect some (as yet poorly understood) function of sleep in maintaining intellectual function (48), or it may reflect the fact that both age changes derive from another common age change, such as the structural brain alterations observed to accompany aging (49, 50). Extensive neuroanatomical changes are observed in elderly individuals with clinically recognizable memory loss who are diagnosed as

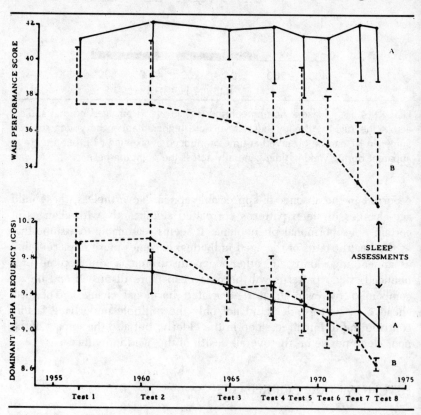

FIGURE 4.16.   Longitudinal change in intellectual function for an aged subject group with greater (Group A) or lesser (Group B) amount of REM sleep. Mean ages for these groups were similar. Group mean ± SD for WAIS performance scores are shown at periodic intervals over an 18-year period preceding the sleep pattern assessments (8).

having senile dementia. The most common form, senile dementia of the Alzheimer's type (SDAT), is a disorder involving primary neuronal degeneration of unknown etiology (51).

## Sleep Patterns in Senile Dementia of the Alzheimer's Type

Sleep pattern deterioration, increased waking, and decreased REM (measured as percent of time in bed) together with increased sleep-stage fragmentation have been reported to accompany dementing disorders of varying etiologies (5). Similar effects were observed in a recent study focusing on 24-hour spontaneous sleep/waking patterns in nondemented and SDAT patients (see Table 4.3) (52). Twenty-four-hour sleep/waking patterns of dementia patients were fragmented: patients slept more during the day and were awake more at night compared to age-matched-nondemented or young-adult controls. Additionally, dementia patients had significantly reduced amounts of stage 3 and 4 sleep and REM sleep (as percent of time in bed) (see Figure 4.17). Fragmentation of sleep, defined as the number of awakenings lasting a minute or longer in a given sleep period, was significantly greater in the dementia patients than age-matched controls (see Table 4.3).

It is often suggested that older individuals may have reduced demands on their time in retirement and thus sleep more during the day. Does the additional sleep from daytime naps compensate for the decreased nighttime REM sleep in either the normal elderly or the dementia patient groups (see Table 4.3)? Slow-wave sleep and REM sleep did not occur in sufficient amounts to compensate for the age-change at night, although they were present during the daytime naps of aged normals. Slow-wave and REM sleep were even more curtailed in the nap sleep of dementia patients (see Table 4.3). Thus, it appears that daytime napping only partially compensates for age changes in nighttime sleep (53).

## NEWER PHARMACOLOGIC CONSIDERATIONS

As pointed out by Kripke (47), there is now impressive evidence based on mortality data to suggest that sleep impairment (as measured by self-reports of excessive or extremely short nighttime sleep) is associated with excessive mortality in elderly subjects living in the community. Moreover, sleeping-pill use in the elderly is associated with a mortality

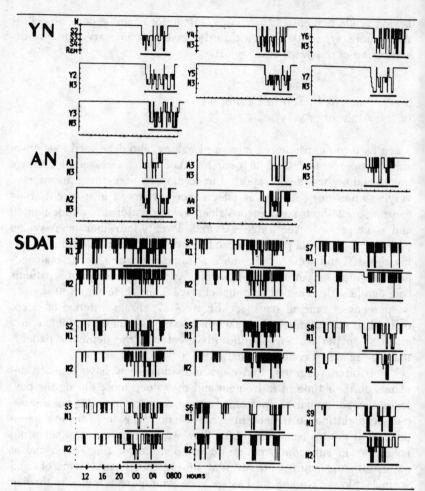

FIGURE 4.17. Twenty-four-hour sleep-stage plots for young normals (YN), aged normals (AN), and senile dementia patients of the Alzheimer's type (SDAT) on the last one or two of three consecutive 24-hour recording periods. The horizontal bar under each plot indicates time spent in bed. Increased fragmentation of the diurnal sleep/wake pattern can be seen in the SDAT records.

rate 50% higher than that of elderly persons who do not take sleeping pills (47). Mortality figures also indicate that more deaths occur during the last half-night of sleep than at any other time. Taken together, these observations suggest that the more extensive sleep disturbances and sleeping-pill use carry an associated health risk in the aged.

A growing number of sleep researchers have expressed concern that

TABLE 4.3 Nighttime and daytime sleep measures for 11 male aged normals and 10 male dementia patients (SDAT)[a]

| | Aged Normals | | SDAT Group—1979 | |
|---|---|---|---|---|
| | Mean | SD | Mean | SD |
| **Nighttime Sleep** | | | | |
| Total Time in Bed (TIB) | 449.73 ± | 50.62 | 475.29 ± | 75.21 |
| % Waking of TIB | 18.81 ± | 7.02 | 36.47 ± | 15.78 |
| % Stage 3 + 4 of TIB | 14.05 ± | 3.37 | 1.75 ± | 3.58 |
| % REM of TIB | 15.67 ± | 3.63 | 7.31 ± | 4.70 |
| Sleep Latency | 15.33 ± | 13.59 | 9.97 ± | 5.18 |
| REM Latency | 97.41 ± | 18.13 | 104.25 ± | 76.06 |
| Number of Awakenings from Sleep | 9.96 ± | 3.90 | 20.65 ± | 12.10 |
| **Daytime Sleep** | | | | |
| Minutes of Sleep | 6.55 ± | 19.50 | 78.67 ± | 57.82 |
| % Stage 3 + 4 of Sleep | 2.73 ± | 6.56 | 1.14 ± | 3.04 |
| % REM of Sleep | 0 ± | 0 | 0.97 ± | 2.10 |
| Number of Awakenings from Sleep | 0.55 ± | 1.29 | 12.60 ± | 6.53 |

[a]Mean ± SD for the last one or two of three consecutive 24-hour recording periods (53).

sleeping-pill use should be contraindicated in cases where the sleep disorder is related to underlying respiratory disturbances, since hypnotics generally depress central respiratory drive mechanisms. It is now recognized that respiratory impairment during sleep (predominantly apnea and hypopnea) induces hypoxia and frequent arousal from sleep. Deleterious effects on cardiovascular function may also occur (43). There is a growing awareness that sleep-related respiratory dysfunction is more pervasive and severe in older individuals. More severe snoring (44) and apnea and hypopnea (45–47) have been reported in older subjects. Approximately 40% of the elderly volunteers living in the community studied by Kripke (27) and by Carskadon and colleagues (4) were found to experience apneic and hypopneic episodes 30–70 or more times per night. Apnea of this degree is associated with frequent arousals, as often as 30–700 times per night, enough to result in nighttime insomnia or daytime sleepiness (47). Thus, elderly patients complaining of poor sleep and daytime sleepiness may have an underlying apnea problem in almost half of the cases. The use of hypnotic sleep aids in such patients could lead to even more severe respiratory impairment during sleep. Caution is therefore advisable in prescribing hypnotics for geriatric patients, particularly for those with the symptomatology indicative of apnea: snoring, obesity, hypertension, and notable irregular breathing sounds at night.

Another major area of concern in prescribing sleeping medications for elderly patients arises from the undesirable lingering hangover effects the following day. Barbiturates and benzodiazepines are known to impair psychomotor and cognitive function during the day following normal bedtime usage in young adults (54, 55). For those elderly subjects who are already slightly to moderately impaired in motor and mental functioning, this additional hangover effect could mean the difference between adequate and impaired ability to cope with the activities of daily living. For this reason, careful monitoring of dose levels so as to avert daytime impaired functioning is important in treating geriatric patients. This precaution must be doubly emphasized in view of the fact that many geriatric patients experience an age- or health-related alteration in drug metabolism, absorption, distribution, or elimination (56, 57).

It has been suggested that development of new sleep aids might profitably focus on hypnotic compounds whose pharmacokinetics are such that an adequate nighttime drug level is achieved followed by a more rapid clearance of the drug from the body, as is possible using hypnotics with single rather than multicompartment-model kinetics (54). Triazolam has been suggested as an example of a hypnotic with a body distribution approaching a single compartment model, with a more rapid clearance rate (54).

Future pharmacologic development of this sort may provide improved therapeutic options for the physician treating geriatric sleep disorders. In addition, the recent development of a nosology of sleep disorders will promote the development of more specific therapeutic approaches that more adequately address the underlying disorder causing the sleep impairment. For example, a list of the major factors currently recognized as impairing sleep would include situational states, affective disorders, various medical conditions, drug abuse, circadian rhythm disturbances, respiratory inadequacies during sleep, nocturnal myoclonus, neurological disorders such as narcolepsy, etc. (58). Other conditions may also contribute, such as a sympathetic hyperarousal state at night. As our sophistication in identifying the various sleep disorders improves, we can look forward to the development of more effective and specific therapeutic approaches for the treatment of sleep disorders.

## SUMMARY AND CONCLUSIONS

Age changes in sleep/waking patterns include decreased stages 4 and REM sleep, together with increased wakefulness while in bed at night. These age changes are more pronounced in mildly intellectually impaired elderly subjects, and are most extreme in senile dementia patients. Daytime napping does not appear to restore sleep stages 4 and REM to normative young adult levels.

The sleep changes of healthy elderly persons are accompanied by changes in certain hormonal measures. For example, growth hormone release at sleep onset is significantly reduced in older men compared with young men. This age effect correlates with the age sleep-change. In additional hormonal studies of these same subjects, significant age differences were observed in plasma norepinephrine level, both in the daytime and at night. Mean nighttime plasma norepinephrine levels were correlated with quality of sleep. Since plasma norepinephrine generally reflects the activity level of the sympathetic nervous system, these data raise the possibility that sympathetic hyperactivity may contribute to age-related sleep impairment. Further study will be required to determine if drugs that suppress this sympathetic hyperactivity may prove to be useful sleep aids for the elderly.

Not all hormonal measures studied revealed an age effect. Diurnal cortisol and epinephrine plasma levels were similar for this same young (21–29) and old (62–80) male subject group. Thus, a significant sleep-pattern change occurred in the absence of an age-related diurnal cortisol rhythm change and in the absence of appreciable apnea. Thus, age sleep-changes can be detected in extremely healthy individuals who have little or no evidence of circadian-rhythm or nighttime respiratory disturbance. For geriatric patients with impaired health, we can expect even greater deleterious effects on sleep. It is likely that several factors contribute to produce the impaired sleep pattern of the elderly, and further work is needed to evaluate potential factors such as apnea, myoclonus, and possibly sympathetic hyperactivity affecting sleep in the aged. For the sizable proportion of geriatric patients suffering from sleep apnea, therapeutic approaches employing hypnotics should be avoided. For cognitively impaired elderly persons, hypnotic usage should be carefully monitored to minimize daytime hangover effects impairing psychomotor and mental functions. Future research into the etiologies underlying the sleep disorders will foster the development of more effective and specific therapeutic approaches for the treatment of sleep disorders.

## REFERENCES

1. Mendelson, W. B.: *The Use and Misuse of Sleeping Pills*, New York: Plenum, 1980.
2. Prinz, P. N.: EEG during sleep and waking states, in: *Spec Annual Rev. of*

*Exper. Aging Res.* B. Eleftheriou and M. Elias (eds.), Bar Harbor: EAR, 1976, pp. 135–164.

3. Rechtschaffen, A., and Kales, A.: *A Manual of Standardized Terminology, Techniques and Scoring Systems for Sleep Stages of Human Subjects,* USPHS Publication 204, Washington: US GPO, 1968.

4. Roffwarg, H. P., Munzio, J. N., and Dement, W. C.: Ontogenic development of the human sleep-dream cycle, *Science* 152:604–619, 1966.

5. Feinberg, I., Koresko, R., and Heller, N.: EEG sleep patterns as a function of normal and pathological aging in man, *J. Psychiat. Res.* 5:1107–1144, 1967.

6. Kahn, E., and Fisher, C.: The sleep characteristics of the normal aged male, *J. Nerv. Ment. Dis.* 148:477–505, 1969.

7. Kales, A., Wilson, T., Kales, J., Jacobson, A., Paulson, M., Kollar, E., and Walter, R.: Measurements of all-night sleep in normal elderly persons: effects of aging. *J. Amer. Geriat. Soc.* 15:405–414, 1967.

8. Prinz, P. N.: Sleep and intellectual function in the aged, *J. Gerontol.* 32:179–186, 1977.

9. Williams, R. L., Karacan, I., and Hursch, C. J.: *Electroencephalog. (EEG) of Human Sleep: Clinical Applications* New York: Wiley & Sons, 1974.

10. Smith, J. R., Karacan. I., and Yang, M.: Ontogeny of delta activity during human sleep, *Electroencephalog. and Clin. Neurophysiol.* 43:229–237, 1977.

11. Prinz, P. N., Halter, J., Raskind, M., Cunningham, G., and Karacan, I.: Diurnal variation of plasma catecholamines and sleep-related hormones in man: relation to age and sleep patterns, in: *Proceed. of Conf. on Neuroendocrine Theories of Aging,* C. E. Finch (ed.), Bethesda: Raven Press, 1981.

12. Takahashi, S., Penn. N. W., Lajtha, A., and Reiss, M.: Influence of growth hormone on phenylalanine incorporation into rat-brain protein, in: *Protein Metab. of the Nervous System,* A. Latjha (ed.), New York: Plenum Press, 1970, pp. 355–361.

13. Dilman, V. M.: Age-associated elevation of hypothalamic threshold to feedback control, and its role in development, aging and disease, *Lancet* 1:1211–1219, 1971.

14. Snipes, C. A.: Effects of growth hormone and insulin on amino acid and protein metabolism, *Quart. Rev. Biol.* 43:127–147, 1968.

15. Taylor, A. L., Finster, J. L., and Mintz, D. H.: Metabolic clearance and production rates of human growth hormone, *J. Clin. Invest.* 38:2349–2358, 1969.

16. Ganong, W. F.: *Review of Medical Physiology,* 9th Ed., Los Altos: Lange Medical Publications, 1979.

17. Sassin, J. F., Parker, D. C., Mace, J. W., Gotlin, R. W., Johnson L. C., Rossman, L. G.: Human growth hormone release: relationship to slow-wave sleep and sleep-waking cycles, *Science* 165:513–515, 1969.

18. Takahashi, Y., Kipnis, D. M., and Daughaday, W. H.: Growth hormone secretion during sleep, *J. Clin. Invest.* 47:2079–2090, 1968.
19. Weitzman, E. D., de Graaf, A. S., Sassin, J. F., Hansen, T., Godtlibsen, O. B., Perlow, M., and Hellman, L.: Seasonal patterns of sleep stages and secretion of cortisol and growth hormone during 24-hour periods in northern Norway, *Acta Endocrinol.* 78:65–76, 1975.
20. Carlson, H. D., Gillin, J. C., Gordon, P., and Snyder, F.: Absence of sleep-related growth hormone peaks in aged normal subjects and in acromegaly, *J. Clin. Endocrinol. Metab.* 34:1102, 1972.
21. Finkelstein, J. W., Roffwarg, H. P., Boyar, R. M., Kream, J., and Hellman, L.: Age-related change in the twenty-four-hour spontaneous secretion of growth hormone, *J. Clin. Endocrinol. Metab.* 35:660–665, 1972.
22. Prinz, P., Blenkarn, D., Linnoila, M., and Wietzman, E.: Growth hormone levels during sleep in elderly males, *Sleep Res.* 5:187, 1976.
23. Prinz, P., Weitzman, E., Karacan, I., and Cunningham, G.: Spontaneous plasma levels of growth hormone in healthy young and aged men: relation to sleep. Submitted for publication, 1981.
24. Cartlidge, H. E. F., Black, H. M., Hall, M. R. P., and Hall, R.: Pituitary function in the elderly, *Gerontol. Clin.* (Basel), 12:65–70, 1970.
25. Dudl, R. J., Ensinck, J. W., Palmer, H. E., and Williams, R. H.: Effect of age on growth hormone secretion in man, *J. Clin. Endocrinol. Metab.* 37:11, 1973.
26. Laron, Z., Doron, M., and Amilkam, B.: Plasma growth hormone in men and women over 70 years of age, *Med. Sport* 4:126, 1970.
27. Sacher, E. J., Finkelstein, J., and Hellman, L.: Growth hormone responses in depressive illness, *Arch. Gen. Psychiat.* 25:263–269, 1971.
28. Rudman, D., Freides, D., Patterson, J. H., and Gibbas, D. L.: Diurnal variation in the responsiveness of human subjects to human growth hormone, *J. Clin. Invest.* 52:912–918, 1973.
29. Blichert-Toft, M.: Secretion of corticotrophin and somatotrophin by the senescent adenohypophysis in man, *Acta Endocrinol. Sup.* 195, 1975.
30. Green, M., and Friedman, M.: Hypothalamic-pituitary-adrenal function in the elderly, *Gerontologia Clin.* 10:334, 1968.
31. Prinz, P. N., Halter, J., Benedetti, C., and Raskind, M.: Circadian variation of plasma catecholamines in young and old men: relation to rapid eye movement and slow wave sleep, *J. Clin. Endocrinol. Metab.* 49:300–304, 1979.
32. Pederson, E. B., and Christensen, N. J.: Catecholamines in plasma urine in patients with essential hypertension determined by double-isotope derivative techniques, *Acta Med. Scand.* 198:373–1975.
33. Cryer, P.: Isotope-derivative measurements of plasma norepinephrine and epinephrine in man, *Diabetes* 25:1971, 1972.
34. Kopin, I. J., Lake, R. C., and Ziegler, M.: Plasma levels in norepinephrine, *Ann. Intern. Med.* 88:671, 1978.

35. Halter, J. B., Pfluge, A. E., and Porte, D., Jr.: Mechanisms of plasma catecholamines increase during surgical stress in man. *J. Clin. Endocrinol. Metab*. 34:936–946, 1977.
36. Metz, S. A., Halter, J. B., Porte, D., Jr., and Robertson, R. P.: Suppression of plasma catecholamines and flushing by clonidine in man, *J. Clin. Endocrinol. Metab*. 46:83, 1978.
37. Pfluge, A. E., and Halter, J. B.: Effect of spinal anesthesia on adrenergic tone and the neuroendocrine responses to surgical stress in man. *Anesthesiol*. 55:170, 1981.
38. Gellhorn, E.: *Autonomic Imbalance and the Hypothalamus*, New York: Univ. Minnesota Press, 1957.
39. Young, J. B., Rowe, J. P., Pallotta, J. A., Farrow, D., and Landsberg, L.: Enhanced plasma norepinephrine response to upright posture and oral glucose administration in elderly human subjects, *Metab*. 29:532–539, 1980.
40. Eisdorfer, C., Nowlin, J., and Wilkie, F.: Improvement of learning in the aged by modification of the autonomic nervous system, *Science* 170:1327–1329, 1970.
41. Eisdorfer, C.: Autonomic changes in aging, in: *Aging and the Brain*, C. Gaitz (ed.), New York: Plenum, 1974, pp. 145–151.
42. Zepelin, H., McDonald, C., Wanzie, F., and Zammit, G.: Age differences in auditory awakening thresholds, *Sleep Res*. 9:109, 1980.
43. Guilleminault, C., and Dement, W. C.: *Sleep Apnea Syndromes*, New York: Alan R. Liss, 1978.
44. Lugaresi, E., Coccagna, G., and Cirignotta, F: Snoring and its implications in sleep apnea syndrome, in: *Sleep Apnea Syndrome*, C. Guilleminault and W. C. Dement (eds.), New York: Alan R. Liss, 1978, pp. 13–22.
45. Ancoli-Israel, S., Kripke, D. F., Menn, S. J., and Messin, S.: Prevalence sleep apnea in a Veterans Administration sleep disorders clinic, *Sleep Res*. 9:185, 1980.
46. Carskadon, M. A., Van Den Hoed, J., and Dement, W. C.: Sleep and daytime sleepiness in the elderly, *J. Geriatric Psychiat*. in press.
47. Kripke, D.: Sleep related mortality and morbidity in the aged, in: *New Perspectives in Sleep Research*, E. D. Weitzman (ed.), New York, in press.
48. Feinberg, I., Braun, M., and Koresko, R.: Vertical eye-movement during REM sleep: effects of age and electrode placement, *Psychophysiol*. 5:556–561, 1969.
49. Brody, H.: An examination of cerebral cortex and brainstem aging, in: *Neurobiol. of Aging* 3, R. D. Terry and S. Gershon (eds.), New York: Raven Press, 1976, pp. 177–183.
50. Shiebel, M., and Scheibel, A.: Structural changes in the aging brain, in: *Aging*, Vol. 1. D. Harman and J. M. Ordy (eds.), New York: Raven Press, 1975.

51. Katzman, R., Terry, R. D., Bick, K. L. (eds.): *Alzheimer's Disease: Senile Dementia and Related Disorders*, New York: Raven Press, 1978.

52. Prinz, P. N., Vitiello, M. V., and Halter, J. B.: Sleep/waking patterns and plasma norepinephrine in young and aged normal men, abstract submitted, *Sleep Res.* 1981.

53. Prinz, P. N., Peskind, E. R., Raskind, M. A., Eisdorfer, C., Zemcuznikov, N., and Gerber, C. J.: Changes in the sleep and waking EEG in demented and nondemented elderly adults, *J. Amer. Geriat. Soc.* 30:2, 88–93, 1982.

54. Nicholson, A., Borland, R., Spencer, M., and Stone, B.: Hypnotics with single and multi-compartment model kinetics: sleep and behavioral studies in man, in: *New Advances in Sleep Research*, E. Weitzman (ed.), New York: Spectrum, in press.

55. Oswald, I., Adam, K., Borrow, S., Idzikowski, C.: The effects of two hypnotics on sleep, subjective feelings and skilled performance, in: *Pharmacology of the States of Alertness*, P. Passouant and I. Oswald (eds.), New York: Pergamon, 1979, pp. 51–63.

56. Friedel, R. O., and Raskind, M. A.: Psychophysiology of aging, in: *Spec. Rev. of Expt. Aging Res.*: Progress in Biology, B. Eleftheriou, and M. Elias (eds.), Palo Alto: [Pub]. 1977.

57. Vestal, R. E.: Aging and pharmacokinetics: impact of altered physiology in the elderly, in: *Physiol. and Cell Biol. of Aging*, Aging Vol. 8, A. Cherkin et al. (eds.), New York: Raven Press, 1979.

58. Sleep Disorders Classification Committee, H. P. Roffwarg, Chmn.: Diagnostic classification of sleep and arousal disorders, *Sleep* 2:1–137, 1979.

# CHAPTER 5

# A Novel Method for Local Administration of Neurally Active Agents

Richard Jed Wyatt, M.D.
William J. Freed, PH.D.
Barry J. Hoffer, M.D.
Lars Olson, M.D.

A major issue in pharmacology is how to target an active agent to a specific end-organ without that agent impinging on sites where it might cause untoward side effects. This was the theory behind Paul Ehrlich's magic bullet. Few, if any, drugs have been designed so well that they achieve this goal. Even aspirin, a relatively innocuous agent, can produce stomach ulcers and tinnitus when given in doses that are maximally effective for rheumatoid arthritis.

Since Parkinson's disease is associated with and very likely caused by a defect in brain dopamine, clinicians have tried to treat Parkinson's disease with the dopamine precursor, levodopa (L-dopa); dopamine itself does not cross the blood-brain barrier. L-dopa treatment, however, is capable of producing numerous side effects. The use of the peripheral decarboxylase inhibitor, carbidopa, with L-dopa has greatly decreased L-dopa's peripheral side effects because L-dopa is not converted to dopamine outside the brain; but many undesirable central effects of L-dopa treatment remain. If dopamine could be delivered to its target regions in the brain—at least one of which is the caudate—without being applied to other brain sites, it might provide a more effective and less toxic treatment than those currently available. Evidence that this might be possible is provided by a series of experiments described here.

One potential method of delivering dopamine specifically to the caudate nucleus would be to transplant live, functioning dopamine-containing tissues to areas close to the caudate. Our first indication that functional grafting of brain tissue might be possible came from experiments in the anterior chamber of the eye. Studies over many years had shown that a number of tissues could survive and grow in the anterior eye chamber when homologously transplanted (1). Substantia nigra and caudate, when sequentially grafted into the anterior chamber of the eye, grow and become interconnected (2). We then wondered if the same thing might happen if an embryonic substantia nigra was placed adjacent to the in situ caudate of an animal whose substantia nigra was previously destroyed. (Loss of substantia nigra neurons, of course, produces parkinsonian symptoms in humans.)

A good paradigm to test the functional properties of such brain grafts would be to use rats with unilateral substantia nigra lesions. These rats typically develop contralateral rotations when given apomorphine, probably as a consequence of dopamine receptor supersensitivity in the caudate nucleus on the lesioned side (3).

## METHODS

Briefly (4, 5), 150 gm Sprague-Dawley rats were lesioned with 6-hydroxydopamine injected into the right substantia nigra. One month following the lesions, the animals were tested for 40 minutes twice each week for at least 5 sessions in a rotometer that measured 360° turns following 0.1 or 0.25 mg per kg subcutaneous apomorphine. Substantia nigra grafts obtained from 17–18-day-gestation rat embryos were stereotaxically implanted into the right lateral vertical adjacent to the caudate. Adult rat sciatic nerve was implanted in other rats as a control.

## RESULTS

One to two months after grafting, the rats were again tested for turning (see Figure 5.1). Rats with substantia nigra grafts had significantly decreased turning compared with the controls (between groups $F(1,76)=7.43$, $p=0.008$, two-way analysis of variance), with the greatest difference appearing during the first 5 minutes after apomorphine injection. The rotation reductions found at 2 months were maintained at 4 and 6 months (see Figure 5.2).

The rats were examined by Falck-Hillarp fluorescence histochemistry at 2 months and 8–10 months following grafting. Multiple, partly fused grafts were found in all grafted animals. These were, for the most

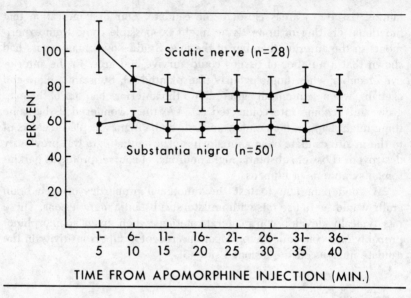

TIME FROM APOMORPHINE INJECTION (MIN.)

FIGURE 5.1.    Substantia nigra grafts: Turning after grafting as a percentage of turning before grafting for each of the eight 5-minute segments of the 40-minute testing sessions. The main effect of treatment was found to be statistically significant (F [1, 76]=7.43, p=0.008, two-way analysis of variance).

part, located along the medial surface of the caudate and partly fused with it. All but 1 graft contained visible catecholamine-containing (fluorescent) neurons. Extending from the cell bodies were numerous catecholamine-containing fibers, some of which ran into the caudate.

To confirm biochemically that the grafts were producing dopamine, circular punches were made of the grafts and the surrounding brain tissues. Dopamine was measured by a gas-chromatographic mass-spectrometric assay with an internal deuterated standard (6). The concentration of dopamine was highest in the graft, with a sharp gradient as distance increased between the graft and sampled tissue (see Table 5.1).

## DISCUSSION

The data generated by our experiments and similar work by Bjorklund's group (7) substantiate the hypothesis that grafts into the brain of adult animals can be functional. If these findings are extended to higher animals, it might be possible to provide patients having Parkinson's disease with a functional replacement for their lost dopamine-containing neu-

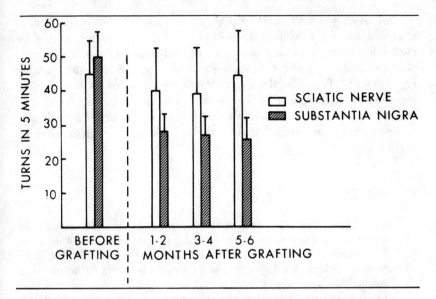

FIGURE 5.2. Mean rate of contralateral turning for animals that received substantia nigra grafts (N=15) or sciatic nerve grafts (N=7) for the 2 months prior to grafting and the first, second, and third 2-month periods following grafting. The bars represent the mean turning rate during the first 5 minutes following apomorphine injections; vertical lines indicate SEM.

rons. Furthermore, other catecholamine tissues, such as the adrenal, might be used; the latter could resolve many problems since the transplant could then be an autograft rather than having to come from embryonic brain.

Preliminary data comparing 13 rats with adult adrenal medulla grafts with 15 rats with sciatic nerve grafts indicate that the adrenal medulla is capable of reducing apomorphine-induced turning in animals with substantia nigra. Catecholamine-containing chromaffin cells were found in grafts of 5 of 6 animals examined histochemically. The axons of these neurons, however, did not project into the caudate, as did axons of neurons taken from embryonic substantia nigras.

TABLE 5.1 Dopamine Concentration in Graft and Host Brain as a Percentage of Normal Caudate

| | Graft | Caudate Adjacent to Graft | Caudate Remote from Graft |
|---|---|---|---|
| Substantia Nigra Graft | 265 | 127 | 19.8 |
| Sciatic Nerve Graft | | 11.9 | 24.2 |

Although we have used substantia nigra dopamine-containing neurons and adrenal medulla catecholamine cells as replacements in a rat model for Parkinson's disease, other central nervous system disorders characterized by discrete lesions might also be treated with suitable replacements. For example, hypothalamic neurons that contain regulating substances for growth hormone secretion might be capable of correcting the deficiency in animals that produce little or no growth hormone. A similar approach has recently been successful with antidiuretic hormone (8).

## REFERENCES

1. Olson, L. and Seiger, A.: Brain tissue transplanted to the anterior chamber of the eye. I. Fluorescence histochemistry of immature catecholamine and 5-HT neurons reinnervating the rat iris. Z. Zellforsch. 135:175–194, 1972.
2. Olson, L., Seiger, A., Hoffer, B. and Taylor, D.: Isolated catecholaminergic projections from substantia nigra and locus coeruleus to caudate, hippocampus, and cerebral cortex formed by intraocular sequential double brain grafts. Exp. Brain Res. 35:47–67, 1979.
3. Marshall, J. F. and Ungerstedt, U.: Supersensitivity to apomorphine following destruction of the ascending dopamine neurons: Quantification using the rotational model. Eur. J. Pharmacol. 41:361–367,1977.
4. Perlow, M. J., Freed, W. J., Hoffer, B. J., Seiger, A., Olson, L. and Wyatt, R. J.: Brain grafts reduce motor abnormalities produced by destruction of nigrostriatal dopamine system. Science 204:643–647, 1979.
5. Freed W. J., Perlow, M., Karoum, F., Seiger, A., Olson, L., Hoffer, B. and Wyatt, R. J.: Restoration of dopaminergic function by grafting of fetal rat substantia nigra to the caudate nucleus: Long-term behavior, biochemical and histochemical studies. Ann. Neurol. 8:5, 510–519, 1980.
6. Karoum, F., Gillin, J. C., Wyatt, R. J. and Costa, E.: Mass-fragmentography of nanogram quantities of biogenic amine metabolites in human cerebrospinal fluid and whole rat brain. Biomed. Mass Spectrometry 2:183–189, 1975.
7. Bjorklund, A. and Stenevi, V.: Reconstruction of the nigrostriatal dopamine pathway by intracerebral nigral transplants. Brain Res. 177:555–560, 1979.
8. Gash, D. and Sladek, J. R.: Vasopressin neurons grafted into Brattleboro rats: Viability and activity. Peptides 1:11–14, 1980.

# CHAPTER 6

# Hypnotics and the Elderly: Clinical and Basic Science Issues

Irwin Feinberg, M.D.
A. Koegler, M.D.

## INTRODUCTION

It might be useful to begin this discussion by defining "hypnotic." In the first Brook Lodge volume *Hypnotics* (1), some of the contributors used this term broadly, in the literal sense of any sleep-promoting substance. In their discussions, these authors included drug classes as diverse as barbiturates, antidepressants, neuroleptics, and antihistamines. Although drugs from each of these groups can be used appropriately to induce or encourage sleep, their pharmacologic properties are so different that it seems certain that their effects on sleep are produced by quite different mechanisms.

Our discussion in this chapter is limited to the classic group of sedative-hypnotics (SHs), which includes barbiturates, meprobamate, methyprylon, chloral hydrate, the entire class of benzodiazepines, and some other agents. Although benzodiazepines have a therapeutic ratio markedly superior to that of barbiturates, they nevertheless produce the same syndromes of intoxication and withdrawal. These syndromes were summarized for barbiturates by Essig (2), who based his descriptions on the classic studies of Fraser, Wikler, Isbell, and associates (3–5). Intoxication with sedative-hypnotics produces " . . . drowsiness, poor judgement, intellectual impairment, emotional instability, slurred speech, incoordination and a staggering gait, irritability, aggressive behavior, fighting, paranoid ideation."

*Overdose* produces coma, which is usually (except for benzodiazepines) life-threatening. *Withdrawal* from the addicted state produces
". . . an abstinence syndrome which is sometimes threatening to life.
Withdrawal manifestations include apprehension, weakness, tremulous-
ness, muscle twitches, anorexia, nausea, vomiting, insomnia, postural
hypotension and fever." In addition to these so-called "minor" withdrawal symptoms, the two major features of the syndrome are generalized convulsions, a delirium, or both. The delirium is characterized by
"disorientation in time and place, delusions, and the occurrence of auditory or visual hallucinations."

This chapter discusses certain clinical and basic science implications
of three sets of data regarding hypnotics as defined above. First, we
review in some detail their effects on the sleep EEG. Second, we comment briefly on the uncertain relations between sleep EEG patterns and
the complaint of insomnia. Third, we reemphasize what has been already remarked in an authoritative review by the Institute of Medicine
(6, 7): that there is little scientific knowledge of the nature and prevalence of insomnia in the elderly, or of its treatment.

In general, we believe that undue weight has been placed on sleep
EEG findings in both the clinical evaluation of hypnotics and the diagnosis
of insomnia. In contrast, the basic science implications of changes
wrought by SHs on EEG sleep patterns have received scant attention,
although their pursuit might yield insights into the mechanisms of hypnotic action. Such understanding, of course, often proves of clinical value.

## EFFECTS OF SEDATIVE-HYPNOTICS
## ON THE SLEEP EEG

The first question that arises is whether this chemically diverse pharmacologic group produces a common set of effects on sleep. In an early
paper describing the effects of phenobarbital and chlorpromazine on
sleep EEG patterns (8), we proposed that drugs in the SH class would
suppress stage 4 sleep and diminish the density of eye movement (EM)
during REM. We proposed also that these two effects would have different time courses: EM density would be suppressed promptly on administration and would recover quickly on withdrawal, whereas the suppression of stage 4 sleep (characterized by dense, high-voltage slow waves)
would occur gradually when the drug was given and would recover
slowly after withdrawal. This hypothesis received little notice. This was
unfortunate, because it predicted with remarkable accuracy the effects
that were to be found for benzodiazepines.

In this discussion, we shall consider in special detail the data on flurazepam, since this benzodiazepine is the most widely used hypnotic in the United States. Figure 6.1 shows the effects on eye-movement activity and stage 4 EEG of flurazepam (FZP), 30 mg administered before sleep, in four noninsomniac young adults (9, 10). The degree of suppression produced by 30 mg of FZP on EM density was about equal to that we found (8) for 200 mg of phenobarbital. In common with other benzodiazepines, FZP profoundly suppressed stage 4 EEG, an effect first described by Kales and coworkers (11).

A more systematic view of the sleep data available for sedative-hypnotics might have prevented some quite mistaken ideas regarding FZP effects. As mentioned above, it had been predicted that EM density would be suppressed by SH drugs. However, since EM activity was not reported in the first studies of FZP and for several years thereafter, it was concluded that this drug did not affect REM sleep and this apparent advantage was heavily emphasized in the early commercial promotion of FZP. Although later studies demonstrated that FZP produces the same

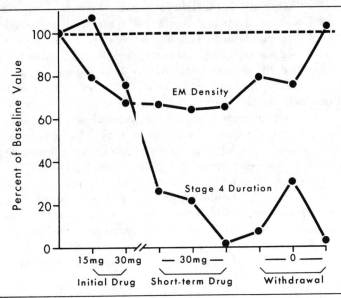

FIGURE 6.1.    Effects of administration and withdrawal of flurazepam on density of eye movements during REM sleep and on stage 4 EEG. Results are plotted as a percentage of the baseline value (which is 100%). EM density declined immediately on drug administration, and returned to baseline by the third night of withdrawal. Stage 4 showed an initial rise, and then declined to low levels in short-term drug with no significant recovery during the first 3 nights of withdrawal.

effects on EM density and REM duration as barbiturates and other SHs, the misapprehension that FZP does not affect REM sleep remains widespread in the medical community.

A second advantage that has been claimed for FZP was that it does not produce REM rebound on withdrawal. This indeed is the case, but this characteristic is equally true for barbiturates. We have found in the literature no adequate evidence that demonstrates that barbiturates produce REM rebound under ordinary conditions of clinical administration; moreover, we failed to observe REM rebound in a study of 3 different barbiturates (12). Thus, with respect to REM rebound, no differences have yet been demonstrated between FZP and barbiturates. (The strongest experimentally produced REM rebound in man that has been documented statistically was found after withdrawal of high doses of tetrahydrocannabinol or marijuana extract (13, 14). The highest levels of REM sleep observed in a clinical abstinence syndrome were those observed in delirium tremens (15, 16).

More recently, FZP has been recommended for its ability to increase sleep without habituation or a need for increased dosage. However, this claim was based on sleep EEG findings of quite small magnitude and uncertain clinical significance. The samples used were small, as is inevitable in most EEG sleep studies. These facts led the Institute of Medicine to conclude that the evidence was too weak to support the sweeping claims of superiority for FZP* (6, 7). Moreover, as we will discuss below, the relation between the sleep EEG itself and the subjective complaint of insomnia is so inconsistent that, for the vast majority of patients with this symptom, the sleep EEG cannot be used to define *either* the existence of insomnia or the adequacy of its treatment. (An interesting point in this regard was made recently by Church and Johnson (17). They noted a temporal dissociation between subjective response and sleep EEG changes after FZP. Subjective ratings of sleep improved promptly after drug administration and showed no further improvement over the week. In contrast, the EEG "improvement" was quite small initially, and increased over the 1-week drug period.)

There are no clinical studies that demonstrate a superiority of flu-

---

*Even those EEG studies that have been interpreted as demonstrating superiority of flurazepam over other hypnotics when used for a period of several weeks have not carried out the statistical tests required to demonstrate that one drug is *superior* to another, i.e., these studies have not demonstrated significantly more sleep time and significantly less waking with flurazepam as compared to other drugs. Instead, the studies have shown that flurazepam more frequently yields significantly increased amounts of sleep over baseline in longer-term use than do other agents. This is *not* the same as demonstrating that flurazepam produces significantly more sleep than other drugs in an appropriately randomized trial.

razepam over other sedative-hypnotics in long-term use. The sleep laboratory study (18) most frequently cited as demonstrating the ineffectiveness of chronic use of traditional (i.e., nonbenzodiazepine) hypnotics compared sleep patterns in middle-aged insomniacs who were taking multiple hypnotic doses with insomniac subjects who were not taking any medications. However, these samples must have come from vastly different populations. One group had insomnia that was so severe (or so unresponsive to hypnotics) as to require, for 8 of the 10 subjects, more than 1 hypnotic dose each night. The control group of insomniacs were so untroubled that they (apparently) were not taking any hypnotics on an ongoing basis. The finding that the group using drugs manifested as much awakening during the night as the control group could therefore be interpreted as the result of increased severity of insomnia in the drug users, or of the refractoriness of this special population to hypnotics. The sampling methods used in this study make it difficult to draw any conclusions regarding response to prolonged hypnotic use in the general population.

Kales and coworkers recently described what they regarded as a new syndrome—a worsening of sleep after withdrawal of short-acting benzodiazepine hypnotics (19, 20). Actually, a similar observation had been made earlier by Linnoila and coworkers (21) in studies of nitrazepam in geriatric patients. It seems quite likely that the phenomenon described is a real one; certainly, it is consistent with clinical experience that patients usually have difficulty sleeping for a few nights when a course of hypnotic treatment is terminated. However, the implications of this phenomenon for treatment practices require some thought. One may be able to prevent rebound insomnia by using, instead of short-acting hypnotics, drugs with long-lived metabolites, such as flurazepam or diazepam.* But this benefit would presumably be obtained at the cost of greater daytime sedation and psychomotor impairment as compared with shorter-acting agents. It would seem to us preferable to employ hypnotics with the shortest possible half-lives consistent with therapeutic effectiveness. Rebound insomnia at the end of a course of treatment could, in all probability, be prevented or substantially mitigated by tapering the dose for the last 2 or 3 nights.

Our review of the available literature leads us to conclude that

---

*It is by no means certain that long-acting benzodiazepines such as flurazepam do not produce rebound insomnia at some point after withdrawal. Sleep laboratory studies are usually carried out only during the first three nights of withdrawal. The rebound insomnia with flurazepam, because of its extremely long half-life and the build-up of its N-desalkyl metabolite (22), may not become apparent until the fourth or fifth night after withdrawal.

sedative-hypnotics in the two main chemical classes (barbiturates and benzodiazepines) produce the following effects on the sleep EEG:

1. Suppression of REM sleep with marked reduction of EM density, modest suppression of REM duration, and an increase in the duration of the amount of NREM sleep that precedes the first REM period (NREMP 1 or "REM latency")* The suppression of REM occurs promptly on drug administration and dissipates quickly on withdrawal, so that baseline levels are reached in a few days.

2. Suppression of stage 4 sleep with repeated administration.** As noted above, the stage 4 suppression requires several nights of drug administration, and recovery of stage 4 after withdrawal can be markedly delayed. For example, after 1 week of FZP treatment, stage 4 may not return to baseline levels for up to 2 weeks (25).

3. Increase in fast (beta) EEG frequencies. This effect has long been known to occur in the waking EEG (26). It is also prominent during sleep in REM periods.

4. An increase in sigma spindle activity. This effect has been documented by Gaillard and associates (27) and by Johnson et al. (28) and others for benzodiazepines. Other sedative-hypnotics, such as barbiturates, have not been evaluated with regard to the capacity to stimulate spindle production.

The clinical (behavioral) implications of each of these effects is unknown. It is not clear whether any of these EEG changes is correlated with the degree to which sleep is refreshing or satisfying, or with the amount of "hangover" and psychomotor impairment produced during waking. In addition to these potentially important clinical correlates, the effects of SH drugs on the sleep EEG pose a number of interesting basic science issues:

1. One important question is whether the combination of EM and stage 4 suppressions, with their differing time courses, is in fact unique to the sedative-hypnotic class. Thus far, this seems to be the case, although the question has not been systematically investigated.

2. Whether or not the effects are unique to the general class of seda-

---

*"NREMP 1" is used interchangeably with "REM latency." We have long maintained (23, 10) that it is not at all clear whether a change in NREMP 1 duration implies an effect on NREM or on REM sleep, although the latter is almost invariably assumed to be the case.
**There may be an increase in stage 4, especially early in the night, with a suppression in later cycles, on the first night of administration. This pattern has been reported for both secobarbital (24) and FZP (10) (see below).

tive-hypnotics, how can one account for the differing time courses of the EM density and the stage 4 effects that are so prominent with benzodiazepines? The prompt recovery of EM after FZP withdrawal is somewhat surprising in view of the long half-life of its N-desalkyl metabolite (22). Equally puzzling is the long depression of stage 4 after withdrawal, which persists after all of the drug has been eliminated from the plasma. A number of possible ad hoc hypotheses could be advanced, ranging from different receptors with different affinities to disuse atrophy. In any event, the remarkably different time course of these two effects on brainwave activity would seem worthy of further investigation.

3. Another question related to these effects is how the suppression of stage 4 is mediated. EEG waves are believed to result from slow, synchronous potential changes in cortical neurons and dendrites in response to subcortical pacemakers. (See review by Elul (29).) A reduction in amount of high-voltage activity could result from *either* a reduction in the average change in membrane potential or in the size of the pool of neurons changing potential synchronously. It seems likely, because of their depressing effect on neuronal metabolism, that sedative-hypnotics suppress delta wave amplitude by reducing the average membrane potential change. However, it remains possible that these effects are produced by a reduction in the size of the neuronal pools responding to their unknown pacemaker as a result of the interruption of certain critical synapses.

4. Is the increased brain excitability (lowered seizure threshold) that follows withdrawal of sedative-hypnotics from addicted individuals correlated with either the degree of REM or stage 4 suppression? Does its time course follow either effect? This question, of course, is of clinical importance as well as basic science interest.

5. Is the reduction in EM density produced by sedative-hypnotics a specific effect on sleep mechanisms or is it, instead, a direct effect on oculomotor excitability. There is considerable evidence that barbiturates and benzodiazepines affect the oculomotor system in the waking state. (See discussion in reference 12.) One cannot simply assume that the effects during sleep are on REM control mechanisms.

6. What discrete EEG changes underlie the reduction in stage 4? An epoch of EEG (typically 20–90 sec) is classified as stage 4 if the time occupied by high-voltage (over 75 microvolts) delta (.5–3 Hz) waves exceeds half the duration of the epoch. A reduction in visually scored stage 4 could, therefore, result from a reduction in the amplitude, density, or average period of delta waves. An analysis that distinguishes the changes in EEG waveforms that result in the suppression

of visually scored stage 4 could help shed light on the neurophysiological mechanisms underlying the drug effects. Such an analysis
might also provide clues as to why stage 4 EEG can be eliminated for
prolonged periods by benzodiazepines without an enormous increase
in hangover or other side-effects.

These questions are by no means comprehensive, but they do represent
interesting basic science issues that are often ignored because of preoc-
cupation with the clinical implications of the sleep EEG effects of sedative-hypnotics. It is clear, however, that with respect to the most striking difference between barbiturates and benzodiazepines—the difference in lethality—sleep EEG effects are thus far uninformative. Benzodiazepines distort EEG sleep stages far more than barbiturates, and yet
they are far less lethal.

## OBSERVATIONS ON THE EFFECTS
## OF FLURAZEPAM ON DELTA (.5–3 Hz)
## WAVEFORMS

Some data do exist with respect to one of the basic issues raised above.
Computer analysis of EEG waveforms permits one to distinguish among
the possible factors underlying the reduction in visually scored stage 4
EEG. We investigated this problem using a period and amplitude analysis carried out on a minicomputer (30). The program employed (PANV35)
measures the number, density, period, and amplitude of delta waves (as
well as those in the other main EEG frequency bands). The absolute
amounts of delta and the rates of decline of delta across sleep cycles
proved highly replicable in independent groups (31). The delta measures also showed extremely low within-subject variability with night-to-
night correlations ranging from .86 to .91 for measures of delta activity
in the average 20-second epoch of NREM sleep (30, 31).

Other investigators had already employed computer measurement
to show that delta-wave amplitude is reduced by benzodiazepines (27,
32). However, none had simultaneously measured the individual delta
characteristics described above, nor had tabulation of the computer
measures of delta been carried out for the physiological units of NREM
sleep—the NREM periods. Inclusion of these data in our analyses led to
several interesting new observations.

We administered 15 mg of FZP on the first night, then 30 mg for 7
consecutive nights to 4 noninsomniac medical students with a mean age
of 23.7 years. Recording was carried out on the first 2 and the last 3 drug

nights and on the first 3 withdrawal nights. Five consecutive nights of baseline recording for each subject had been obtained 2 months earlier as part of a previous study (9, 10).

Both visual scoring and computer measurement of EEG waveforms were carried out. Figure 6.1 (p. 77) presents the data for visually scored EM activity and for stage 4 EEG scored according to the Rechtschaffen and Kales (33) criteria. Figure 6.2 shows in detail the effects of FZP on visually scored sleep variables analyzed by successive periods of NREM and REM sleep. For the first 4 NREM sleep cycles, the breakdown of each NREMP into stages 2, 3, or 4 is shown as are the proportions of 4-second epochs of REM sleep with eye movement. On the initial drug nights (N1=15 mg, N2=30 mg) there was a marked increase in the duration of the first NREMP associated with a significant increase in the amount of stage 4. The suppression of eye movement was also apparent on this initial drug night. On the fifth through eighth nights of FZP administration (short-term drug condition), NREMP 1 remained elevated, although almost all its stage 4 had been replaced by stage 2. The level of EM activity was reduced by FZP, but its trend across the night was not affected. During the first 3 nights of withdrawal, NREMP 1 remained increased in duration, although, on average, REM duration and EM density did not differ significantly from baseline.

Figure 6.3 illustrates the biphasic response to FZP of visually scored stage 4. On the first nights of administration, stage 4 increased in NREMP 1 and decreased in NREMP 2. This change is of interest in two respects. First, this resembles that demonstrated by Lester et al. (24) for secobarbital, revealing yet another similarity between benzodiazepine and barbiturate effects on sleep EEG. Second, this change demonstrates extremely quick penetration of the blood-brain barrier by flurazepam, and indicates that its effects on stage 4 sleep (previously thought to require repeated administration) can be observed with a single 15-mg dose. Many psychoactive drugs produce effects on the sleep EEG that are much larger than those produced in waking brainwaves. The onset of these effects may prove useful in estimating the time of penetration of the blood-brain barrier.

Computer analysis of the FZP data yielded several interesting additional findings. First, as expected from the work of others, the amplitude of delta waves was reduced. In the short-term drug condition (sixth through eighth night of drugs), we found a 28% reduction in integrated amplitude in the .5–3 Hz band, summed across all delta activity in NREM ($p < .001$). There was no significant recovery of delta wave amplitude during the 3-day withdrawal period.

The findings for the number and for the time occupied by delta

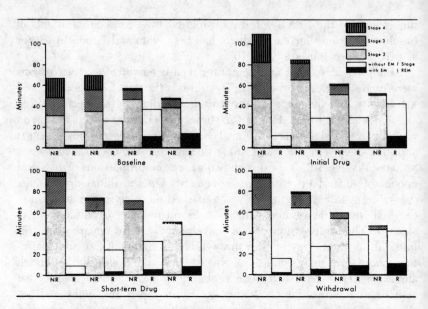

FIGURE 6.2.   Effects of flurazepam administration and withdrawal on NREM and REM patterns in the first four non-REM sleep cycles. Initial drug administration increased the length of the first NREMP (REM latency) and increased the amount of stage 3–4 EEG. Stage 4 EEG was virtually eliminated during both the short-term drug and withdrawal conditions. The first NREMP remained elevated during drug withdrawal, although REM measures did not differ significantly from baseline. This result suggests that the increased length of the first NREMP with flurazepam reflected an effect on NREM rather than on REM systems.

waves were quite different from those for amplitude. In spite of a reduction of 82% in the amount of visually scored stage 4, there was no reduction in either the total number of delta waves or in the total time they occupied in NREM sleep. This apparent paradox can be resolved when one considers that FZP significantly increased the total duration of NREM sleep (see Figure 6.4). This increase was in stage 2 EEG, which, while made up of delta waves with a relatively low density and amplitude, nevertheless contributes appreciably to the .5–3 Hz band (34). We found it interesting that the increase in stage 2 sleep contributed precisely the amount of delta activity required to maintain at baseline levels both the total number of delta waves and the total time they occupied. Of course, since this number of waves was spread out over a larger number of epochs of NREM sleep, the average number and duration of delta waves *per* NREM *epoch* were significantly reduced by the drug. It was of further interest to us that the increase in stage 2 EEG (and in total

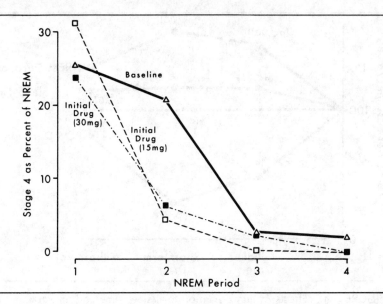

FIGURE 6.3.    The biphasic effect of flurazepam on stage 4 sleep. The first night of administration increased stage 4 EEG in the first NREMP, but decreased it in the second. This effect was less marked on the second night of administration. This result, which was statistically significant, demonstrates that flurazepam affects stage 4 EEG even on the first night of administration.

sleep) occurred largely in the first NREMP, which normally contains over 50% of the visually scored stage 4 of the entire night.

Thus, although FZP profoundly reduced visually scored stage 4, an apparently compensatory increase in stage 2 EEG maintained the number and time occupied by delta activity at baseline levels, although the total amplitude in the delta band was significantly and substantially reduced. Perhaps this compensatory process, if such it is, explains the relatively minor daytime effects produced by flurazepam in the face of almost total elimination of stage 4 sleep.

Neither the computer measures of delta activity nor visually scored stage 4 EEG showed any recovery during the 3 nights following withdrawal of flurazepam (Figure 6.5). This finding may shed some light on the rather vexing question posed above: whether the latency to the first REM period (NREMP 1 duration) reflects the state (sometimes described as "pressure") of NREM or REM systems. In considering this issue in light of the present data, we take note that REM duration and EM density recovered during withdrawal so that, on the third withdrawal night, they were at baseline levels. In contrast, NREMP 1 duration remained signifi-

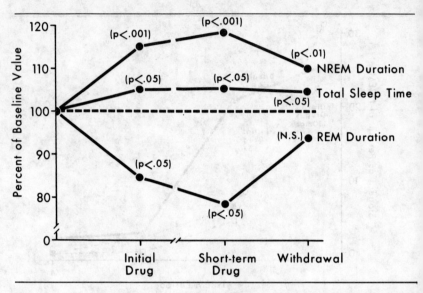

FIGURE 6.4.    Effects of flurazepam on total sleep time and on NREM and REM sleep. Although the amount of REM sleep was reduced, NREM sleep was increased by a greater amount so that the total sleep time was mildly increased.

cantly elevated during withdrawal, suggesting that under these experimental conditions the increase in NREMP 1 reflected a change in NREM rather than in REM systems. (See further discussion in reference 10.)

These findings indicate the value and feasibility of computer measurement of the sleep EEG in the study of sedative-hypnotic effects. They also illustrate the value of separate analyses by physiological units of sleep (the alternating NREMPs and REMPs) rather than by arbitrary units such as hours or thirds of the night.

The finding that flurazepam increased total sleep time by an amount of stage 2 sleep that acted to maintain the number of delta waves at baseline levels suggested (9, 10) an hypothesis regarding the mechanism of action of hypnotics: that hypnotics, at least in part, increase sleep by slowing down its metabolic processes so that a longer total sleep time is required to achieve the same amount of metabolic change. Whether or not this hypothesis is plausible, special consideration is merited by the question of how drugs that depress neuronal metabolism increase an active neuronal process such as sleep.

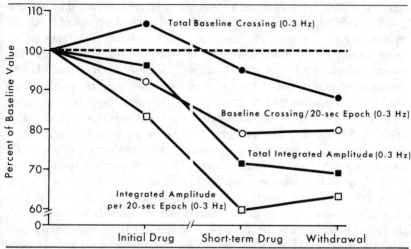

FIGURE 6.5.    Effects of flurazepam administration and withdrawal on the integrated amplitude and the number of half-waves in the .5–3 Hz frequency band. For each variable, both the total amount for all of NREM sleep and the amount in the average 20-second epoch of NREM sleep are shown. In the short-term drug condition, there was a significant (p<.001) reduction in total integrated amplitude but not in the total number of half-waves. However, since the same number of half-waves were distributed over a greater number of NREM epochs (increased total NREM sleep—see Figure 4) the number of half-waves per epoch of non-REM sleep was significantly (p<.001) reduced. During drug withdrawal, the amount of REM sleep increased and the amount of NREM sleep decreased. Since the rate of production of .5–3 Hz waves remained unchanged, the reduction in NREM sleep duration led to a significant (p<.01) reduction in total number of delta waves.

## RELATION OF SLEEP EEG
## TO THE COMPLAINT OF INSOMNIA

In the remainder of this chapter, we comment briefly on the relation of the sleep EEG to the complaint (symptom) of insomnia and on the related question of insomnia in the elderly. The brevity of our comments in these areas reflects the paucity of available information, and should not be construed as a reflection of our view of the importance of these questions.

It is now widely accepted that many patients who complain bitterly and continuously of insomnia—by which they usually mean sleepless-

ness—manifest total sleep times and sleep stage amounts that are normal for their age (see the technical appendix of the Institute of Medicine
report (6) for a summary of these data). This probably is the case for the
great majority of middle-aged patients with idiopathic insomnia. The
interpretation of this fact is controversial. Some claim that patients who
complain of insomnia but have normal EEG sleep patterns suffer from a
kind of "pseudoinsomnia." However, it is not clear what this term
means. Does it imply that the sleep of these patients is in fact normal in
spite of the fact that they perceive it to be highly unsatisfactory? There
would seem to be two main possibilities: either patients with idiopathic
insomnia really have nothing wrong with their sleep but suffer instead
from a psychiatric disorder (somatization or hypochondriasis) or else the
sleep EEG as conventionally analyzed simply does not reflect the physiologic abnormality that causes unrefreshing or unsatisfactory sleep. We
think the latter is more likely to be true. Of course, a more microscopic
analysis of sleep EEG data taking into account the amounts and temporal
distribution of EEG waveforms might reveal abnormalities not apparent
in visual sleep-stage scores. However, it is equally possible that the
sleep EEG does not contain the information that reflects the pathophysiology of insomnia. This pathology may depend upon subtle alterations of
memory processes that cause some persons to recall what appears to be
almost continuous low-level mentation during both NREM and REM sleep
(35). Such changes may involve small groups of neurons whose activity is
not reflected in the scalp EEG. Alternatively, idiopathic insomnia may
involve abnormalities of the neuroendocrine rhythms rather than the
EEG patterns of sleep. Still other probabilities exist for the frequent
discrepancies between objective and subjective complaints of insomnia
(6). At the present time, the comments of Kagan (36) and of Morgan (37)
remain true. Kagan noted that an important challenge for sleep research
was to "determine the relationship between objective data determined
in the sleep laboratory and the way a subject feels and acts on awakening." This challenge has yet to be met, and Morgan's statement that "it
is depressingly clear that we have little knowledge of the causes of poor
sleep and of what constitutes insomnia" remains valid.

## SLEEP EEG PATTERNS
## IN THE NORMAL ELDERLY

We have often emphasized that the changes in the sleep EEG with age
represent the most marked age-related changes in brain physiology
demonstrated thus far in man. It is our view that an understanding of

the etiology and functional significance of these changes will shed light on two basic problems of human neurobiology: the nature of aging in the central nervous system and the biological function of sleep. There have been no recent advances in our understanding of these profound questions. We restate them here in light of our concern that underlying basic science issues not be neglected.

While sleep EEG changes in the normal elderly are quite marked, their *clinical* significance has not yet been firmly established. The main sleep EEG changes in the normal elderly as compared to young adults include a reduction of 40% in the amount of visually scored stage 4 and of about 60% in the number of sleep spindles. The fragmentation of sleep is even more marked in old age. The number of EEG-defined awakenings is increased by about 75%, and the percentage of time in bed spent awake doubles. In contrast, changes in REM duration and eye-movement activity are minimal until extreme old age.

This description, based on initial studies of 15 normal elderly persons (mean age 72 years) (23), has been confirmed in all essential details in a recent study of 50 normal elderly subjects (Feinberg, Floyd, and Fein, unpublished observations). In view of the modest reliability of visual sleep-stage scoring, it is also remarkably consistent with the data in the literature (38). Elsewhere (23), we proposed that the changes in sleep in old age are correlated with the degree of cognitive impairment. Although there is some evidence consistent with this hypothesis, it has not yet been proved.

One might expect that the great increase in awakening and the decrease in the deep (stage 4) sleep in the elderly would be associated with a marked increase in the frequency of complaints of insomnia. In our experience, such complaints are quite uncommon. In a sample of over 50 elderly subjects, only one complained of insomnia, although the group as a whole showed all of the changes in EEG sleep patterns described above. In a sense, the situation with the elderly is the converse of that found in middle-aged and young insomniacs. The latter show near normal EEG sleep patterns, but have severe complaints: elderly normal subjects show severe fragmentation of sleep and loss of deep sleep and spindles, but voice relatively few complaints.

The elderly, however, do consume a disproportionate amount of the prescription hypnotics. Although persons over 65 years of age make up 15% of the population, they account for 39% of the prescribed hypnotics (6). A survey of national psychotherapeutic drug use by Parry and co-workers reported in 1973 (39) also found a relatively high use of hypnotics by the elderly.

It is not clear what the increased use of hypnotics signifies for the question of insomnia in geriatric populations. Elderly persons often have chronic illnesses and frequent contact with physicians. They may receive prescriptions for hypnotics because of pain associated with other illnesses such as arthritis. In addition, elderly persons may mention sleep disturbance in the course of the medical interview although they would not have consulted physicians for this complaint alone. They may, therefore, be prescribed hypnotics as part of the thorough workup of the conscientious physician.

We do not yet know whether the elderly would in any way be benefited by treatment for what might be termed the physiologic insomnia of old age for which no complaints have been voiced. For elderly patients who do complain of insomnia, rather limited data are available to guide us in their treatment. Frost and DeLucchi (40), in an EEG study of 6 women aged 67–82 years, found that 15 mg of FZP increased total sleep time and decreased total time awake significantly; the number of awakenings per night was not affected. Also unaffected was the amount of stage 3 and 4 sleep, which were at the extremely low levels expected for this age group. It would be of interest to measure, using waveform analyses of the sort described above, the frequency and amplitude characteristics of the increased non-REM sleep produced by the drug in the elderly. Two of the 6 subjects in Frost and DeLucchi's study showed significant side effects.

## CLINICAL COMPARISONS OF HYPNOTICS

Clinical studies of hypnotics in geriatric populations fail to substantiate any objective (EEG) or subjective advantage for either major class of hypnotics or for any individual drug. Linnoila and Viukari (21) found that nitrazepam, 10 mg, produced a marked rebound insomnia upon withdrawal from geriatric patients. This drug also caused quite pronounced side effects, including impaired memory, incontinence, and inability to conduct daily activities. In this study, thioridazine, a neuroleptic, produced a greater increase in sleep with fewer side effects than did nitrazepam. In another investigation, Viukari, Linnoila, and Aalto (41) compared the efficacy and side effects of 15 mg of FZP, 60 mg of fosazepam and 5 mg of nitrazepam in a cross-over study with 17 psychogeriatric patients. The drugs were equal in sleep-promoting effects. However, there was some evidence of tolerance to each by the end of the first week. In this study, nitrazepam again produced severe side effects that appeared to be more closely correlated with the existence of cerebrovascular disease than with chronological age. Two patients with vascular disease of the brain became amnesic after each of the hypnotics was administered.

Although there exists a widespread impression that flurazepam is superior to other benzodiazepines as a hypnotic, the available literature does not support this view. FZP was not more effective in the studies of Linnoila and coworkers described above. Fabre and colleagues (42) found .5 mg of triazolam superior to 30 mg of flurazepam in a 1-week double-blind study of 61 (triazolam) and 57 (FZP) outpatients. In a second study (43), Fabre, McLenden, and Harris, using the preference method of Jick et al. (44), found .5 mg of triazolam preferred to 30 mg of FZP and 500 mg of chloral hydrate in a double-blind 2-night crossover study. Reeves (45) found .25 mg of triazolam superior to 15 mg of FZP in a 28-day, double-blind study of 41 geriatric outpatients. Rather surprisingly, no tolerance was observed in this study over a 4-week treatment period. Reeves found triazolam was significantly superior ($p < .05$) to FZP in increasing the estimated sleep duration. Triazolam also led FZP in other ratings of sleep quality, but these differences were not statistically significant. Goldstein and coworkers (46) carried out a 4-week study of 15 mg of oxazepam, 15 mg of FZP, and 500 mg of chloral hydrate in 17 geriatric nursing home patients (mean age 82 years). The patients were treated for 6 days; sleep effects were measured by nurse observations and self-ratings. Oxazepam was found equal in efficacy to FZP on most measures and superior on a few.

In reviewing the literature on hypnotic efficacy, one cannot avoid the impression that superior results are obtained more frequently for drugs being evaluated for the first time. This seems to occur even though appropriate precautions have been taken to eliminate bias. Perhaps this phenomenon results from a preference for investigators to submit, and for editors to accept, studies in which positive results have been obtained for new pharmacologic agents.

## "HANGOVER" EFFECTS

We shall not review here the rapidly developing literature on psychomotor and cognitive impairment produced during the day by hypnotics administered prior to sleep. An excellent summary of these data was included in the Institute of Medicine report (6). We emphasize, however, the abundant evidence (47–51), that such impairment is much greater in the elderly than in young adults and can be life-threatening. The effects are probably more marked in the elderly because of diminished rates of clearance due to slower excretion and metabolism. The

changes produced are further exaggerated in the normal elderly by sub-
clinical brain impairment (diminished "cerebral reserve"), which is probably present in most if not all elderly persons. Even hypnotics usually
viewed as being quite mild, such as chloral hydrate, can cause severe
symptoms in susceptible elderly patients (52). For these reasons, we
would agree with the comments of Blumenthal elsewhere in this volume
(Chap. 12) that, where at all practical, hypnotics ought not be prescribed
to the elderly.

One of the more frequent indications for treatment is repeated episodes of nocturnal delirium or "Sundowner's syndrome." This behavior
pattern is fairly common in demented patients, and often urgently requires intervention. The causes of this interesting condition are unknown, although it has been suggested that an intrusion of REM processes into waking or an inability to distinguish dreams from reality may
be involved (23). Further research on this syndrome and its treatment
are needed, since it is frequently the cause of institutionalization for
patients who could otherwise be maintained with their families.

## IDEAL HYPNOTICS—
## WHERE SHOULD WE LOOK?

The classic sedative-hypnotics have many unsatisfactory characteristics.
The features of an "ideal" hypnotic, recently described by the Institute
of Medicine (6), are opposite to the effects of traditional drugs:

> The "ideal hypnotic" would be safe and effective. Evaluation of
> this drug would demonstrate that it would cause neither coma nor
> death when taken in overdose; it would not be attractive for abuse;
> it would not interact adversely with other medications; it would be
> free from such side effects as allergic reactions, respiratory depres-
> sion, and cardiovascular complications; it would be free of hangover
> effects, such as daytime drowsiness, memory and cognitive impair-
> ment, incoordination, and adverse mood changes; it would be safe
> for such special population groups as pregnant women, the elderly,
> and patients with pulmonary, renal, or liver insufficiency; it would
> not disrupt the order of natural sleep, including waveform charac-
> teristics; its onset and duration of action would be consistent with
> clinical use and need—that is, it would enable patients to fall asleep
> quickly, to sleep through the night, and to wake at the desired time;
> although it would promote sleep, it would not anesthetize the pa-
> tient so as to render him unresponsive to a full bladder, pain, tele-
> phone calls, fire alarms, a crying baby, or the smell of smoke; if

needed for prolonged use, neither tolerance nor dependence would develop, and upon cessation of treatment rebound insomnia would not occur; it would be inexpensive; it would not disrupt the normal physiological process associated with sleep or with circadian rhythms, such as changes in temperature and neuroendocrine responses; and it would effectively treat the problems of a wide variety of patients. (p. 156)

It seems unlikely that *any* new drug could prove such a paragon, but we emphasize that virtues such as these are probably forever unattainable within the traditional pharmacologic class of sedative-hypnotics. The two main chemical groups, benzodiazepines and barbiturates, seriously depress brain function and drastically distort the normal architecture of the sleep EEG. They impair daytime functioning, and may have other serious consequences. Thus, Kripke and coworkers (53) reported an intriguing and unexplained association between hypnotic use and earlier mortality in a large elderly population. A fundamentally improved hypnotic will probably come from an entirely different class of compounds. Such a development might occur serendipitously, but is more likely to result from advances in knowledge of the basic neurochemistry and neuroendocrinology of human sleep.

# REFERENCES

1. Kagan, F., Harwood, T., Rickels, K., et al. (eds): *Hypnotics: Methods of development and evaluation*. New York, Spectrum, 1975.
2. Essig, C. F.: Addiction to barbiturate and nonbarbiturate sedative drugs. In: *The Addictive States: Proceedings of the Association for Research in Nervous and Mental Disease*. Ed. by Wikler, A. Baltimore, Williams and Wilkins, 1968.
3. Fraser, H. F., Isbell, H., Eisenman, A. J., Wikler, A. Pescor, F. T.: Chronic barbiturate intoxication. *Arch. Int. Med.* 94:34–41, 1954.
4. Isbell, H.: Addiction to barbiturates and the barbiturate abstinence syndrome. *Ann. Int. Med.* 33:108–121, 1950.
5. Isbell, H., Altschul, S., Kornetsky, C. H., Eisenmen, A. J., Flanary, H. G., Frazer, H. F.: Chronic barbiturate intoxication: an experimental study. *Arch. Neurol.* 64:1–28, 1950.
6. Institute of Medicine: *Report of a Study: Sleeping Pills, Insomnia, and Medical Practice*. Nat. Acad. Sciences, Washington, D. C. 1979.
7. Solomon, F., White, C. C., Parron, D. L., Mendelson, W. B.: Sleeping pills, insomnia and medical practice. *New Eng. J. Med.* 300(14):803–808, 1979.
8. Feinberg, I., Wander, P. H., Koresko, R. L., Gottlieb, F., Piehuta, J. A.:

Differential effects of chlorpromazine and phenobarbital on EEG sleep patterns. *J. Psychiat. Res.* 7:101–109, 1969.

9. Feinberg, I., Fein, G., Walker, J. M., Price, L. J., Floyd, T. C., March, J. D.: Flurazepam effects on slow-wave sleep: Stage 4 suppressed but number of delta waves constant. *Science* 198:847–848, 1977.

10. Feinberg, I., Fein, G., Walker, J. M., Price, L. J., Floyd, T. C., March, J. D.: Flurazepam effects on sleep EEG: visual, computer and cycle analysis. *Arch. Gen. Psychiat.* 36:95–102, 1979.

11. Kales, A., Allen, C., Scharf, M. B., Kales, J. D.: Hypnotic drugs and their effectiveness: all-night EEG studies of insomniac subjects. *Arch. Gen. Psychiat.* 23:227–232, 1970.

12. Feinberg, I., Hibi, S., Cavness, C. March, J: Absence of REM rebound after barbiturate withdrawal. *Science* 185:534–535, 1974.

13. Feinberg, I., Jones, R., Walker, J. M., Cavness, C. March, J.: Effects of high dosage delta-9-tetrahydrocannabinol on sleep patterns in man. *Clin. Pharm. & Ther.* 17(4): 458–466, 1975.

14. Feinberg, I., Jones, R., Walker, J., Cavness, C., Floyd, T: Effects of marijuana extract and tetrahydrocannabinol on electroencephalographic sleep patterns. *Clin. Pharm. & Ther.* 19(6):782–794, 1976.

15. Gross, M. M., Goodenough, D., Tobin, M., Halpert, E., Lepore, D., Pearlstein, A., Sirota, M., Dibianco, J., Fuller, M., Kishner, L.: Sleep disturbances and hallucinations in the acute alcoholic psychoses. *J. Nerv. Ment. Dis.* 142:493–514, 1966.

16. Greenberg, R., Pearlman, C.: Delirium tremens and dreaming. *Am. J. Psychiat.* 124:133–142, 1967.

17. Church, M. W., Johnson, L. C.: Mood and performance of poor sleepers during repeated use of flurazepam. *Psychopharm.* 61:309–316, 1979.

18. Kales, A., Bixler, E. O., Tan, T.-L., Scharf, M. B., Kales, J. D.: Chronic hypnotic-drug use: ineffectiveness, drug-withdrawal insomnia, and dependence. *JAMA* 227(5): 513–517, 1974.

19. Kales, A., Scharf, M. B., Kales, J. D.: Rebound insomnia: a new clinical syndrome. *Science* 201:1039–1041, 1978.

20. Kales, A., Scharf, M. B., Kales, J. D., Soldatos, C. R.: Rebound insomnia: a potential hazard following withdrawal of certain benzodiazepines. *JAMA* 241(16):1692–1695, 1979.

21. Linnoila, M., Viukari, M: Efficacy and side effects of nitrazepam and thioridazine as sleeping aids in psychogeriatric inpatients. *Br. J. Psychiat.* 128:566–569, 1976.

22. Greenblatt, D. J., Shader, R. I., Koch-Weser, J.: Flurazepam hydrochloride. *Clin. Pharm. & Ther* 17(1):1–14, 1975.

23. Feinberg, I., Koresko, R. L., Heller, N.: EEG sleep patterns as a function of normal and pathological aging in man. *J. Psychiat. Res.* 5:107–144, 1967.

24. Lester, B. K., Coulter, J. D., Dowden, L. C., et al.: Secobarbital and nocturnal physiological patterns. *Psychopharmacologia* 13:275–286, 1968.

25. Kales, A., Bixler, E. O., Scharf, M., Kales, J. D.: Sleep laboratory studies of flurazepam: a model for evaluating hypnotic drugs. *Clin. Phar. & Ther.* 19(5):576–583, 1976.

26. Brazier, M. A., Finesinger, J. E.: Action of barbiturates on the cerebral cortex: electroencephalographic studies. *Archs. Neurol. Psychiat.* 53: 51–58, 1945.

27. Galliard, J. M., Aubert, C.: Specificity of benzodiazepine action on human sleep confirmed: another contribution of automatic analysis of polygraph records. *Biol. Psychiat.* 10:185–197, 1975.

28. Johnson, L. C., Hanson, K., Bickford, R. G.: Effect of flurazepam on sleep spindles and K complexes. *Electroencephalogr. Clin. Neurophysiol.* 40:67–72, 1976.

29. Elul, R.: The genesis of the EEG. In: *International Review of Neurobiology*, Vol. 15. Ed. by Pfeiffer, C. C., Smythies, J. R. New York: Academic, 1972, 227–272.

30. Feinberg, I., March, J. D., Fein, G., Floyd, T. C., Walker, J. M., Price, L. Period and amplitude analysis of 0.5–3 c/sec activity in NREM sleep of young adults. *Electroencephalogr. Clin. Neurophysiol.* 44:202–213, 1978.

31. Feinberg, I., Fein, G., Floyd, T. C.: Period and amplitude analysis of NREM EEG in sleep: repeatability of results in young adults. *Electroencephalogr. Clin. Neurophysiol.* 48:212–221, 1980.

32. Smith, J. R., Karacan, I., Keane, B. P., et al.: Automated sleep EEG analysis applied to the evaluation of drugs: illustration by study of chlorazepate dipotassium. *Electroencephalogr. Clin. Neurophysiol.* 41:587–594, 1976.

33. Rechtschaffen, A., Kales, A. (Eds.): *A Manual of Standardized Terminology, Techniques and Scoring System for Sleep Stages of Human Subjects.* National Institutes of Health Publication No. 204, U. S. Government Printing Office, Washington, D. C., 1968.

34. Johnson, L., Lubin, A., Naitoh, P., et al.: Spectral analysis of the EEG of dominant and nondominant alpha subjects during waking and sleeping. *Electroencephalogr. Clin. Neurophysiol.* 26:361–370, 1969.

35. Foulkes, W. D. Dream reports from different stages of sleep. *J. Abnorm. Soc. Psychol.* 65:14–25, 1962.

36. Kagan, F.: Introduction to Brook Lodge symposium on hypnotics. In: *Hypnotics: Methods of development and evaluation.* Ed. by Kagan, F. Harwood, T., Rickels, K., et al. New York: Spectrum, 1975.

37. Morgan, J. P.: Inpatient evaluation of hypnotic drugs. In: *Hypnotics: Methods of Development and Evaluation.* Ed. by Kagan, F., Harwood, T., Rickels, K., et al. New York, Spectrum, 1975.

38. Feinberg, I.: Functional implications of changes in sleep physiology with age. In: *Neurobiology of Aging.* Ed. by Terry, R. D., Gershon, S. New York, Raven Press, 1976.

39. Parry, H. J., Balter, M. B., Mellinger, G. D., Cisin, I. H., Manheimer, D.

I.: National patterns of psychotherapeutic drug use. *Arch. Gen. Psychiat.* 28:769–783, 1973.

40. Frost, J. D., DeLucchi, M. R.: Insomnia in the elderly: treatment with flurazepam hydrochloride. *J. Amer. Ger. Soc.* 27(12):541–546, 1979.
41. Viukari, M., Linnoila, M., Aalto, U: Efficacy and side effects of flurazepam, fosazepam, and nitrazepam as sleeping aids in psychogeriatric patients. *Acta Psychiat. Scand.* 57:27–35, 1978.
42. Fabre, L. F., Gross, L., Pasigajen, V., Metzler, C.: Multiclinic double-blind comparison of triazolam and flurazepam for seven nights in outpatients with insomnia. *J. Clin. Pharm.* 17(7):402–409, 1977.
43. Fabre, L. F., McLendon, D. M., Harris, R. T.: Preference studies of triazolam with standard hypnotics in outpatients with insomnia. *J. Int. Med. Res.* 4:247–254, 1976.
44. Jick, H., Slone, D., Dinan, B., Muench, H.: Evaluation of drug efficacy by a preference technique. *N. Eng. J. Med.* 275:1399–1403, 1966.
45. Reeves, R. L.: Comparison of triazolam, flurazepam and placebo as hypnotics in geriatric patients with insomnia. *J. Clin. Pharm.* 17(5 & 6):319–323, 1977.
46. Goldstein, S. E., Birnbom, F., Lancee, W. J., Darke, A. C.: Comparison of oxazepam, flurazepam and chloral hydrate as hypnotic sedatives in geriatric patients. *J. Amer. Ger. Soc.* 26(8):366–371, 1978.
47. Greenblatt, D. J., Allen, M. D., Shader, R. I.: Toxicity of high-dose flurazepam in the elderly. *Clin. Pharm. & Ther.* 21(3):355–361, 1977.
48. Greenblatt, D. J., Allen, M. D.: Toxicity of nitrazepam in the elderly: a report from the Boston collaborative drug surveillance program. *Br. J. Clin. Phar.* 5:407–413, 1978.
49. Castleden, C. M., George, C. F., Marcer, D., Challet, C.: Increased sensitivity to nitrazepam in old age. *Br. Med. J.*, 1:10–12, 1977.
50. Marttila, J. K., Hammel, R. J., Alexander, B., and Zustiak, R.: Potential untoward effects of long-term use of flurazepam in geriatric patients. *J. Amer. Pharm. Assoc.* 17(11):692–695, 1977.
51. MacDonald, J. B., MacDonald, E. T.: Nocturnal femoral fracture and continuing widespread use of barbiturate hypnotics. *Br. Med. J.* 2:483–485, 1977.
52. Miller, R. R., Greenblatt, D. J.: Clinical effects of chloral hydrate in hospitalized medical patients. *J. Clin. Pharm.* 19(10):669–674, 1979.
53. Kripke, D. F., Simons, R. N., Garfinkel, L., Hammond, E. C.: Short and long sleep and sleeping pills: in increased mortality associated? *Arch. Gen. Psychiat.* 36:103–116, 1979.

CHAPTER 7

# ECT in the Elderly

Max Fink, M.D.

Depressive disorders are common among the elderly. Loss of significant members of the family and friends, loss of a job, deterioration of physical state and illness, economic dependence, and the loss of self-esteem associated with these experiences lead to depressive reactions. Endogenous depression (including depression in the elderly and involutional melancholia) are also sufficiently frequent to be major factors in geriatric medicine. In addition, difficulties with memory, recall, concentration, cognition, reduced sleeping time, increased sleep awakenings, reduced libido, and anorexia increase with aging and the physical changes that accompany that process. Among the many physiologic changes are decreased secretion of testosterone and estrogen and increased monoamine oxidase activity in plasma and platelets (1).

Although most patients respond to reassurance, social casework, environmental change, and proper medical care for physical disability, a significant number require more intensive psychiatric care (2–4). The principal therapies of the depressive states in the elderly are reassurance, psychotherapy, and antidepressant drugs. Hypnotics, anxiolytics, hormonal replacements, tricyclic antidepressants, and monoamine oxidase inhibitors are widely used, but electroconvulsive therapy is recommended with sufficient frequency to be a principal treatment in these populations. It is recommended for those patients who fail to respond to antidepressant drugs or who develop complications of the treatment. Some patients may have medical illnesses for which the anticholinergic, autonomic, and sedative actions of the antidepressant drugs may be harmful, and ECT is preferred. In the severely ill, particularly those with

97

severe suicidal intent, cachexia, refusal of food, and hyperpyrexia, for whom a delay in therapeutic effect may be intolerable, convulsive therapy may be life-saving. And patients with severe depression with delusions of guilt or somatic disease, for whom the tricyclic drugs are not usually useful alone, may also be helped by ECT.

This review focuses on the use of convulsive therapy in the elderly. Other sources of information may be sought in Fink (1979), APA (1978), Kalinowsky and Hippius (1972), and Sargant and Slater (1963) (5–8).


## INDICATIONS

The decision to use convulsive therapy in the elderly is based on a complex calculus—on the severity of illness, the efficacy of ECT and of the alternate treatments, the risks of amnesia and problems of anesthesia with ECT, the cardiovascular and autonomic risks of antidepressant drugs, the need for special facilities and expense of ECT, the ease of drug administration, and the social stigma of having had ECT. In each instance, the experience of the physician will determine whether a patient is suitable for a course of ECT .

Convulsive therapy is particularly effective in patients with severe depressive mood disorders, accompanied by symptoms of vegetative dysfunction. In such conditions, ECT is more effective than the available drug therapies. It is most useful in patients with endogenous depression and involutional depression, when accompanied by insomnia, anorexia, weight loss, decreased libido, constipation, and dry mouth. In such patients, 4–8 seizures, given twice or three times a week, will relieve the depression and the accompanying vegetative symptoms. It is also effective in severely ill patients with refusal of food, inanition, and weight loss; severe agitation and restlessness; and those who are so depressed that they seek death. In such instances, ECT may be lifesaving.

Some severely depressed patients exhibit delusions of worthlessness, guilt, and somatic concern. Several authors report that the response of such patients to antidepressant drugs is poor, even when plasma levels are monitored, but that such patients respond well to ECT, suggesting that ECT may be considered a primary treatment in such cases (9–12). Recently, others have suggested that combined antidepressant and antipsychotic drug therapies may be effective in such delusional and depressed cases, but these reports do not consider the special risks of the combined treatment in the elderly (13–16).

Patients with evidence of brain dysfunction may respond to ECT. Among parkinsonism patients, there are those who do not respond to chemotherapies or in whom the usual regimen is no longer helpful. Although the first parkinsonism patients treated with ECT were those with manifest depressive disorders (17–23), recent reports find parkinsonism to be relieved in hospitalized, incapacitated patients in whom depressive illness is not a prominent feature, suggesting that ECT may have a special place in the management of these patients (24). ECT is also useful in patients exhibiting excitement and confusion in senile dementia (25), general paresis (17, 26–29), pseudodementia, and senile agitation (25, 30–33). Intoxications, particularly with delirium, have been reduced (25, 31 34–36), although a recent note found a case of bromide psychosis not to respond to ECT (37). A patient exhibiting an organic stupor after head injury is also described as responding to ECT (32).

Psychotic patients with renal, cardiac, and hepatic decompensation, or recent coronary occlusion, may be poor candidates for antidepressant drugs, particularly those drugs with autonomic and cardiovascular effects. Although there is some hope that the newer tetracyclic drugs, such as mianserin, may be devoid of these secondary effects, convulsive therapy is still to be considered in such cases. Although each seizure in ECT is physically demanding, stimulating elevations in blood pressure, arrhythmia, and tachycardia, the incidence of these effects leading to complications is low, even in patients with recent myocardial infarction. Recent reports cite the successful ECT treatment of patients with cardiac pacemakers (38–41). ECT has also been used successfully in a patient with severe diabetes (42), and in a patient with a shunt in place for normal hydrocephalus (43). On balance, for patients with severe medical conditions, ECT may be safer and more secure than present antidepressant drug therapy.

Convulsive therapy is to be considered in the severely ill, and is ordinarily reserved for patients who require hospitalization. Although outpatient treatments are still being done, it has become clear—particularly with the elderly in whom the risks of the treatment may be considerable—that the treatments should be given in settings where the means to prevent and treat the complications are at hand.

## COMPLICATIONS

The risks of induced seizures are considerable, but modern techniques, which are well described and generally available, are sufficient to reduce the risks so that ECT may be considered even in the most elderly of patients.

## Fracture

Fracture was common in the initial years of convulsive therapy, but the present methods of anesthesia with short-acting barbiturates, such as methohexital, and muscle relaxation with succinylcholine, have made fracture a rare event.

## Organic Psychosis and Amnesia

An organic psychosis, manifest as either amnesia alone or amnesia accompanied by confusion, confabulation, and disorientation, is still a risk of ECT (44–49). The incidence was higher in the early decades of ECT use, particularly when it was believed that amnesia was part of the therapeutic process, and the importance of oxygenation during the seizure was not recognized. But with the demonstration that the efficacy of ECT was not related to the degree of amnesia, three modifications of the treatment process were developed that reduced the incidence of organic psychosis: hyperoxygenation, unilateral nondominant placement of electrodes, and brief, low-voltage induction currents. When forced oxygenation was used during the treatment, particularly in patients in whom succinycholine muscle relaxation was used, amnesia was reduced (50). The demonstration by Blachly and Gowing (51) that multiple seizures could be given in a single session without significant amnesia, provided that oxygenation was well maintained, emphasized the importance of oxygenation.

Unilateral electrode placement for the induction of seizures was used occasionally, until the demonstration by Cannicott (52) that the therapeutic response of patients receiving ECT through unilateral electrodes was equal to those receiving treatments through bilateral electrodes and that the effects on memory functions were much less for the unilateral electrode inductions. Since then, many studies have replicated this observation. The reviews summarizing the findings agree that the effects on amnesia for unilateral ECT are less and that the therapeutic effects are equivalent (5, 48, 53, 54). Two recent reports highlight the significance of these observations for elderly patients. Seizures were induced in 9 elderly patients using unilateral and bilateral electrodes alternately. The recovery times, the time from the end of the seizure until the patient first breathed spontaneously, opened his eyes on command, and gave correct answers to questions of orientation, were measured (55). The recovery times were significantly longer with bilateral electrode placement than with unilateral, and the effects after bilateral placement were cumulative, while after unilateral placement they were not.

But this study did not assess the relative clinical efficacy of the two treatments. In a second report, Fraser and Glass (56) carried out a randomized trial of unilateral and bilateral ECT in 29 elderly depressed patients (64–86 years of age; mean=73±6). Behavioral and memory tests were repeated after the fifth treatment and 3 weeks after the last treatment. All patients but 1 showed full recovery at 3 weeks, and there was no difference between the groups in outcome. Memory performance was impaired before treatment and improved with treatment, reaching normal values at 3 weeks. Again, postictal recovery times were longer in the bilateral than the unilateral group after the first treatment; after the fifth treatments they were three times as long. Recovery times decreased during courses of unilateral treatment. These authors concluded " . . . that unilateral ECT is a safe and highly effective treatment for selected elderly patients suffering from depression, but that there is nothing to be said for the continued use of bilateral ECT."

Although the data are not as well developed for the merits of brief, low-threshold stimuli to induce seizures, there is evidence that higher-current intensities increase EEG abnormalities (5). The merit of these induction methods are being determined.

## Brain Damage

Much has been written about brain damage induced by ECT, but the facts are obscured by the failure of reviewers to take into account the progressive developments in the ECT process. Thus, in the first decades of ECT use, when amnesia was considered a factor in the improvement process and oxygenation was not used, pathological studies of brains taken from patients who died during a course of ECT exhibited structural damage. This was also true for experimental studies in animals. But more recent animal studies implicate hypoxia as the central factor in seizure-related brain damage, and as modern ECT methods have improved, death has become so rare that autopsies in patients dying during a course of modified ECT have not been reported. In almost all patients subjected to ECT, the recovery from the organic mental syndrome that may occur is well defined, as occurring within 2–4 weeks of the end of treatment. In many patients, cognitive tests are performed better after a course of ECT than during their pretreatment testing. From these experiences, we believe that the incidence of brain damage is so low that these risks are not a significant part of the present practice of ECT.

## Spontaneous (Tardive) Seizures

The appearance of spontaneous seizures outside the treatment room was reported more frequently in the first decades of ECT use, but is rare today. There has been some recent concern that ECT will kindle a seizure focus (57), but the present practice of ECT, in which seizures are spaced over 48–72 hours and are given under barbiturate anesthesia, serves to prevent the induction of seizure foci. (For seizure foci to develop in animals, seizures must be given by direct stimulation of the brain, without barbiturates, and with spacings defined in minutes and hours rather than days.)

## Other Complications

Death is rare in ECT today, with an incidence of less than 3.4 deaths in 10,000 patients treated. Again, death seems less frequent with modern induction methods and with the prophylaxis and treatments that are presently available. Most deaths have been associated with cardiovascular symptoms, with the increase in blood pressure or the development of an intractable arrhythmia. Some recent suggestions for treatment include the use of propranolol to modify arrhythmia (58) and sodium nitroprusside to modify hypertension (59).

Missed or incomplete seizures have always been a feature of the ECT process. With the more common usage of unilateral electrode placement and brief stimulus currents for induction, the frequency of missed seizures seems to be increasing. Following the suggestions of d'Elia and Raotma (54)—that the efficacy of seizures induced through unilateral electrode placement could be improved—and the observations of Blachly and Gowing (51) on multiple seizures, most treatments today are being done under monitored conditions, thereby assuring a full grand mal seizure in each induction. Although EEG and EMG monitoring may be more elegant, a practical and inexpensive method is that introduced by Addersley and Hamilton (60), in which a blood pressure cuff is inflated over the systolic pressure in one arm before succinylcholine is introduced into the other. This allows one limb to express the tonic and clonic phases of the seizure. If the total time is greater than 25 seconds, the induction is accepted. If it is shorter, the seizure induction is repeated.

## DRUGS AND ECT

The few studies that examined the effects of antidepressant drugs combined with ECT have not identified any benefits for the combination (61–66). On the contrary, the anticholinergic and autonomic effects of the antidepressant drugs increase the risks of complications in ECT. One example is cited in the report by Summers, Robins, and Reich (49), which associated the use of psychotropic drugs with an increased incidence of organic psychoses. In patients receiving lithium, ECT is associated with a similar increase (67–70). It is a reasonable conclusion that such combined therapy should not ordinarily be attempted, particularly in the elderly.

What of ECT in patients with medical illnesses requiring maintenance treatments? In such instances, attention should be paid to the potential interactions of the drugs with the effects of the seizure and with the anesthetic agents. This is particularly true for cardiovascular drugs that may interact with succinylcholine to produce a prolonged respiratory paralysis, arrhythmia, or cardiac arrest (71). It is also true for lithium (72) and magnesium (71), where the combination with succinylcholine may lead to prolongation of respiratory effects. There are few studies of these interactions, and it is prudent for the psychiatrist who is administering ECT and who is considering the continuation of medications for physical disabilities to consult the clinicians involved prior to undertaking a course of ECT.

Although the combined use of antidepressant drugs and ECT shows little benefit for the combination, the sequential use may sustain improvement better than sedative drugs (64) or no maintenance drugs (61, 63).

## RISK-BENEFIT ANALYSIS

Although the risks of ECT induction are defined, modern methods of induction reduce the risks significantly and seem to make the use of ECT secure in the severely depressed patient. ECT in the elderly is not to be taken lightly, and it is incumbent upon the therapist to use all means now available to provide the patient with a safe course of treatment—including the proper use of anesthesia and means of seizure induction to minimize the hazards of the development of an organic psychosis. In a recent careful study, the incidence of an acute organic mental syndrome after bilateral ECT was estimated at 48%, with an average duration of 20 days.

These patients differed from those who did not exhibit an organic psychosis only in their exposure to psychoactive drugs during the course of ECT and in the prior presence of significant medical illness (49). Age was not a factor in the difference between the groups. These findings parallel the studies of the interseizure EEG and neuropsychological tests during a course of convulsive therapy, where the degree of EEG slowing and dysfunction in cognitive tests is related not to age but to the presence of other illnesses, drugs, or prior abnormalities in the measures (5).

Thus, in the treatment of depressed patients, particularly the elderly, consideration must be given to the use of barbiturate anesthesia, unilateral electrode placement, hyperoxygenation, seizure monitoring, and the restriction of concomitant drugs to minimize the risks of treatment. Treatments should be given by therapists with experience with these methods, and in settings in which the facilities are available to treat the complications of the treatment. Combined treatments should be avoided, and where the continuation of medication for a patient's medical condition may be required, the collaboration of medical consultants (and their presence during treatment) should be considered. With these caveats, ECT should not be denied the elderly, as it may provide relief from a severely debilitating, and often fatal, illness.

## USE OF ECT

In our economic system, the elderly are likely to be impoverished and to seek their medical care in the hands of the state. Surveys of the use of ECT, undertaken in the past decade, find that ECT is used in about 5% of the mentally ill admitted to university hospitals, more than 20% admitted to private, for-profit, institutions, and less than 1% admitted to state, municipal, and V.A. facilities (5, 6, 73). The differential use may reflect different facilities, but this explanation is inadequate when the population samples are examined closely. This is particularly true for the use of ECT among the elderly in state institutions. Because the risks of ECT are seen as materially greater among the elderly, many practitioners, particularly those who may not have secure medical positions in the medical hierarchy, may be reluctant to use ECT. The benefits of ECT are not universally accepted, and failing to use the procedure in suitable patients seldom subjects the physician to criticism. Some efforts must be made to make ECT more available to the elderly psychotic patients now resident in state and V.A. facilities, by education and by attention to the legal and insurance impediments to an optimal application of these treatments.

The benefits of ECT, particularly in patients with evidence of organic psychosis, are not so well defined as to be compelling in the selection of cases for ECT. For this reason, further study of the ECT process in the elderly is needed, focused on the predictors for a good behavioral response to ECT, particularly among patients with organic mental states. Studies are also needed to assess the relative merits of antidepressant drugs and ECT, the usefulness of unilateral and bilateral electrode placement, and the importance of brief stimuli for the induction current.

## MODE OF ACTION

Much has been written about the mode of action of convulsive therapy in depressive states. Some argue that the mechanism is unknown and that, in the absence of such knowledge, the treatments should not be given. Others emphasize psychological effects, and although these are surely contributory to the clinical state of the patient, it is clear that ECT is not effective because of amnesia, fear, or repression. Some argue that the biochemical effects in the brain are central, and each report emphasizes the biochemical system then under study. In the past decade, however, a number of reviews and conferences have assessed the present state of our knowledge, and some specific hypotheses have been formulated that are useful (74, 75). Among the current theories, the neuroendocrine hypothesis is of particular interest (5, 76).

This hypothesis suggests: *Hypothalamic dysfunction is central to endogenous depressive disease. Convulsive therapy increases the activity of hypothalamic-pituitary centers, releasing substances (probably peptides) that modify the mood, vegetative symptoms, and behavior associated with mood disturbances.* The hypothesis has much to support it, and the interested reader is referred to the original reviews for a detailed treatment of the theory and its evidence. For the present, it is sufficient to review some of the data that may be relevant to the management of depressed states in the elderly.

Neuroendocrine tests are often abnormal in patients with depressive disease, particularly those with prominent vegetative symptoms. Thyrotropin-releasing hormone (TRH) normally elevates pituitary thyroid-stimulating hormone (TSH) levels in plasma, but this response is obtunded or absent in patients with severe depression (77). The response returns in patients who improve with ECT (or tricyclic antidepressants) (78–81).

In patients with melancholia, particularly those with unipolar depression, the secretion of cortisol is elevated, its phasic rhythmicity is lost, and dexamethasone fails to suppress this secretion (82). With successful treatment, the basal levels fall, and both rhythmicity and the suppression after dexamethasone return. This is clearly demonstrated in case reports in which the response of cortisol to dexamethasone (dexamethasone suppression test, DST) paralleled the clinical course of depressed patients treated with ECT (83–86). Indeed, changes in cortisol levels and the response to the DST have been recommended as a guide to the end of a course of antidepressant drug therapy (85, 87, 88).

We, also, have found DST to be related to the outcome with ECT (86). We have examined the changes in DST in 14 patients with melancholia treated with ECT. Ten had an abnormal DST before treatment. Of these, DST was normalized in 6. In the 4 patients with a normal DST before ECT, it remained normal in 2 and became abnormal in 2. In a follow-up 1–9 months after the course of therapy, a favorable clinical state was reported in the 6 patients with a normalized DST, and an unfavorable state was reported in 8 patients—6 with abnormal DST and 2 with a normalized DST.

In the management of patients in ECT, particularly in those patients with complex medical conditions, and for research purposes, the DST and the TRH test may now be considered as useful adjuncts in the decision-making process.

## SUMMARY

Depressive disorders are common in the elderly, being both reactive to the stresses of aging and endogenous. The latter are particularly responsive to convulsive therapy, and should be considered in those patients with severe disability requiring hospitalization. ECT is a safe treatment, particularly when modern techniques of patient selection, anesthesia, hyperoxygenation, unilateral electrode placement, and monitoring of the seizure are used. The particular risks of combined ECT and other drugs are emphasized, and it is suggested that ECT be given without concomitant drug therapies unless required by the patient's medical illness. Recent determinations of abnormalities of neuroendocrine function in depressed patients lead to a neuroendocrine theory of the mode of action of ECT and to the suggestion that some tests of endocrine function may be useful in the management of ECT in complex cases.

## REFERENCES

    1. Ban, T. A. The treatment of depressed geriatric patients. *Amer. J. Psychother*. 32:93–104, 1978.

2. Goldfarb, A. I. Geriatric psychiatry. In: Freedman, A. M. and Kaplan, H. I. (eds.): *Comprehensive Textbook of Psychiatry*. Baltimore: Williams and Wilkins, 1564–1587, 1968.

3. Gaitz, C. M. Depression in the elderly. In: Fann, W., Karacan, I., Pokorny, A. D. and Williams, R. L. (eds.): *Phenomenology and Treatment of Depression*. New York: Spectrum, 153–166, 1977.

4. Pokorny, A. D. Suicide in depression. In: Fann, W., Karacan, I., Pokorny, A. D. and Williams, R. L. (eds.): *Phenomenology and Treatment of Depression* New York: Spectrum, 197–216, 1977.

5. Fink, M. *Convulsive Therapy: Theory and Practice*. New York: Raven Press, 1979.

6. A.P.A. *Electroconvulsive Therapy*. Task Force Report #14. Washington, D.C.: American Psychiatric Association, 1978.

7. Kalinowsky, L. and Hippius, H. *Pharmacological, Convulsive and Other Treatments in Psychiatry*. New York: Grune & Stratton, 1972.

8. Sargant, W. and Slater, E. *An Introduction to Physical Methods of Treatment in Psychiatry*. Baltimore: Williams & Wilkins, 1963.

9. Hordern, A., Holt, H. F., Burt, C. G. and Gordon, W. F. Amitriptyline in depressive cases. *Brit. J. Psychiat.* 109:815–825, 1963.

10. Glassman, A. H., Kantor, S. J. and Shostak, M. Depression, delusions and drug response. *Amer. J. Psychiat.* 132:716–719, 1975.

11. Davidson, J. R. T., McLeod, M., Kurland, A. A. and White, H. L. Antidepressant drug therapy in psychotic depression. *Brit. J. Psychiat.* 131:493–496, 1977.

12. Kantor, S. J. and Glassman, A. H. Delusional depressions: Natural history and response to treatment. *Brit. J. Psychiat.* 131:351–360, 1977.

13. Nelson, J. C. and Bowers, M. B. Delusional unipolar depression—Description and drug response. *Arch. Gen. Psychiat.* 35:1321–1328, 1978.

14. Minter, R. E. and Mandel, M. R. The treatment of psychotic major depressive disorder with drugs and electroconvulsive therapy. *J. Nerv. Ment. Dis.* 167:726–733, 1979a.

15. Minter, R. E. and Mandel, M. R. A prospective study of the treatment of psychotic depression. *Amer. J. Psychiat.* 136:1470–1472, 1979.

16. Kaskey, G. B., Nasr, S. and Meltzer, H. Y. Drug treatment in delusional depression. *Psychiat. Res.* 1:267–277, 1980.

17. Savitsky, N. and Karliner, W. Electroshock in the presence of organic disease of the nervous system. *J. Hillside Hosp.* 2:3–22, 1953.

18. Brown, G. L. Parkinsonism, depression, and ECT. *Amer. J. Psychiat.* 132:1084, 1975.

19. Lebensohn, Z. M. and Jenkins, R. B. Improvement of parkinsonism in depressed patients treated with ECT. *Amer. J. Psychiat.* 132:283–285, 1975.

20. Dysken, M., Evans, H. M., Chan, C. H., and Davis, J. M. Improvement of depression and parkinsonism during ECT: A case study. *Neuropsychobiology* 2:81–86, 1976.

21. Asnis, G. Parkinson's disease, depression, and ECT: A review and case study. *Amer. J. Psychiat.* 134:191–195, 1977.

22. Ananth, J., Samra, D. and Kolivakis, T. Amelioration of drug-induced parkinsonism by ECT. *Amer. J. Psychiat.* 136:1094, 1980.

23. Yudofsky, S. C. Parkinson's disease, depression and electroconvulsive therapy: A clinical and neurobiologic synthesis. *Comprehens. Psychiat.* 20:579–581, 1979.

24. Balldin, J., Eden, J., Granerus, A.-K, Modigh, K., Svanborg, A., Walinder, J. and Wallin, L. Electroconvulsive therapy in Parkinson's syndrome with "On-Off" phenomenon. *J. Neural Transmission* 47:11–21, 1980.

25. Roth, M. and Rosie, J. M. The use of electroplexy in mental disease with clouding of consciousness. *J. Ment. Sci.* 99:103–111, 1953.

26. Heilbrunn, G. and Feldman, P. Electro-shock treatment in general paresis. *Amer. J. Psychiat.* 120:78–79, 1963.

27. Tomlinson, P. J. Insulin and electric therapy in general paresis. *Psychiatr. Quart.* 18:413–421, 1943.

28. Solomon, H. C., Rose, A. S. and Arnot, R. E. Electric shock treatment in general paresis. *J. Nerv. Ment. Dis.* 107:377–381, 1948.

29. Dewhurst, K. Treatment of neurosyphilitic psychoses. *Acta Psychiat. Scand.* 45:63–74, 1969.

30. Mitchell, P. H. Electric convulsion therapy in treatment of prolonged stupor. *Brit. Med. J.* 1:535–538, 1952.

31. Roberts, A. H. The value of E.C.T. in delirium. *Brit. J. Psychiat.* 109:653–655, 1963.

32. Silverman, M. Organic stupor subsequent to severe head injury treated with ECT. *Brit. J. Psychiat.* 110:648–650, 1964.

33. Salzman, C. ECT and ethical psychiatry. *Amer. J. Psychiat.* 134:1006–1009, 1977.

34. Arneson, G. A. and Ourso, R. Bromide intoxication and electroshock therapy. *Amer. J. Psychiat.* 121:1115–1116, 1965.

35. Muller, J. D. ECT in LSD psychosis: A report of three cases. *Amer. J. Psychiat.* 128:351–352, 1971.

36. Dudley, W. H., Jr. and Williams, J. G. Electroconvulsive therapy in delirium tremens. *Compr. Psychiat.* 13:357–360, 1972.

37. Davis, R. A., Abrams, R. and Taylor, M. A. Failure of bromide psychosis to respond to ECT. *Brit. J. Psychiat.* 133:94, 1978.

38. Bodley, P. O. and Fenwich, P. B. C. The effects of electro-convulsive therapy on patients with essential hypertension. *Brit. J. Psychiat.* 112:1241–1249, 1966.

39. Youmans, C. R., Bourianoff, G., Allensworth, D. C., Martin, W. L. and Derrick, J. R. Electroshock therapy and cardiac pacemakers. *Amer. J. Surgery,* 118:931–936, 1969.

40. Abiuso, P., Dunkelman, R. and Proper, M. Electroconvulsive therapy in patients with pacemakers. *JAMA* 240:2459–2460, 1978.

41. Jauhar, P., Weller, M. and Hirsch, S. R. Electroconvulsive therapy for patients with cardiac pacemakers. *Brit. Med. J.* 1:90–91, 1979.

42. Yudofsky, S. C. and Rosenthal, N. E. ECT in a depressed patient with adult onset diabetes mellitus. *Amer. J. Psychiat.* 137:100–101, 1980.

43. Tsuang, M. T., Tidball, S. and Geller, D. ECT in a depressed patient with shunt in place for normal pressure hydrocephalus. *Amer. J. Psychiat.* 136:1205–1206, 1979.
44. Kalinowsky, L. Organic psychotic syndromes occurring during electric convulsive therapy. *Arch. Neurol. Psychiat.* 53:269–273, 1945.
45. Stainbrook, E. Shock Therapy: Psychologic theory and research. *Psychol. Bull.* 43:21–60, 1946.
46. Fink, M. and Kahn, R. L. Behavioral patterns in convulsive therapy. *Arch. Gen. Psychiat.* 5:30–36, 1961.
47. Harper, R. G. and Wiens, A. N. Electroconvulsive therapy and memory. *J. Nerv. Ment. Dis.* 161:245–254, 1975.
48. Squire, L. ECT and memory loss. *Amer. J. Psychiat.* 134:997–1001, 1977.
49. Summers, W. K., Robins, E. and Reich, T. The natural history of acute organic mental syndrome after bilateral electroconvulsive therapy. *Biol. Psychiat.* 14:905–912, 1979.
50. Holmberg, G. The factor of hypoxemia in electroshock therapy. *Amer. J. Psychiat.* 110:115–118, 1953.
51. Blachly, P. and Gowing, D. Multiple monitored electroconvulsive treatment. *Compr. Psychiat.* 7:100–109, 1966.
52. Cannicott, S. M. Unilateral electroconvulsive therapy. *Postgrad. Med. J.* 38:451–459, 1962.
53. Stromgren, L. S. Unilateral vs. bilateral electroconvulsive therapy. *Acta Psychiatr. Scand.* (Suppl.) 240:1–65, 1973.
54. d'Elia, G. and Raotma, H. Is unilateral ECT less effective than bilateral ECT? *Brit. J. Psychiat,* 126:83–89, 1975.
55. Fraser, R. M. and Glass, I. B. Recovery from ECT in elderly patients. *Brit. J. Psychiat.* 133:524–528, 1978.
56. Fraser, R. M. and Glass, I. B. Unilateral and bilateral ECT in elderly patients: A comparative study. *Acta Psychiat. Scand.* 62:13–31, 1980.
57. Pinel, J. P. J. and van Ooot, P. H. Generality of the kindling phenomenon: Some clinical implications. *Can. J. Neurol. Sci.* 2:467–475, 1975.
58. Weiner, R. D., Henschen, G. M., Dellasega, M. and Baker, J. S. Propranolol treatment of an ECT-related ventricular arrhythmia. *Amer. J. Psychiat.* 136:1594–1595, 1979.
59. Ciraulo, D., Lind, L., Salzman, C., Pilon, R., and Elkins, R. Sodium nitroprusside treatment of ECT-induced blood pressure elevations. *Amer. J. Psychiat.* 135:1105–1106, 1978.
60. Addersley, D. J. and Hamilton, M. Use of succinylcholine in ECT. *Brit. Med. J.* 1:195–197, 1953.
61. Seager, C. P. and Bird, R. L. Imipramine with electrical treatment in depression—A controlled trial. *J. Ment. Sci.* 108:704–707, 1962.
62. Wilson, I. C., Vernon, J. T., Guin, T. and Sandifer, M. G. A controlled study of treatments of depression. *J. Neuropsychiatry* 4:331–337, 1963.
63. Imlah, N. W., Ryan, E. and Harrington, J. A. The influence of antidepressant drugs on the response to electroconvulsive therapy and on subsequent relapse rates. *Neuropsychopharm.* 4:438–442, 1965.

64. Kay, D. W. K., Fahy, T. and Garside, R. F. A seven month double-blind trial of amitriptyline and diazepam in ECT-treated depressed patients. *Brit. J. Psychiat.* 117:667–671, 1970.

65. Arfwidsson, L., Arn, L., Beskow, J., d'Elia, G., Laurell, B., Ottosson, J.-O., Perris, C., Persson, G. and Wistedt, B. Chlorpromazine and the antidepressive efficacy of electroconvulsive therapy. *Acta Psychiat. Scand.* 49:580–587, 1973.

66. d'Elia, G., Lehmann, J. and Raotma, H. Evaluation of the combination of tryptophan and ECT in the treatment of depression. I. Clinical analysis. *Acta Psychiat. Scand.* 56:303–318, 1977.

67. Ray, I. Side effects from lithium. *CMA Jrl.* 112:417–418, 1975.

68. Hoenig, J. and Chaulk, R. Delirium associated with lithium therapy and electroconvulsive therapy. *CMA Jrl.* 116:837–838, 1977.

69. Remick, R. A. Acute brain syndrome associated with ECT and lithium. *Can. Psychiat. Ass. J.* 23:129–130, 1978.

70. Small, J. G., Kellams, J. J., Milstein, V. and Small, I. F. Complications with electroconvulsive treatment combined with lithium. *Biol. Psychiat.* 15:103–112, 1980.

71. Marco, L. A. and Randels, P. M. Succinylcholine drug interaction during electroconvulsive therapy. *Biol. Psychiat.* 14:433–445, 1979.

72. Reimherr, F. W., Hodges, M. R., Hill, G. E. and Wong, K. C. Prolongation of muscle relaxant effects of lithium carbonate. *Amer. J. Psychiat.* 134:205, 1977.

73. Asnis, G., Fink, M. and Saferstein, S. ECT in metropolitan New York Hospitals: A survey of practice, 1975–1976. *Amer. J. Psychiat.* 135:479–482, 1978.

74. Fink, M., Kety, S., McGaugh, J. and Williams, T. A. *Psychobiology of Convulsive Therapy.* Washington, D. C.: V. H. Winston & Sons, 1974.

75. Grahame-Smith, D. G., Green, A. R. and Costain, D. W. Mechanism of the antidepressant action of electroconvulsive therapy. *Lancet* 1:254–256, 1978.

76. Fink, M. and Ottosson, J.-O. A theory of convulsive therapy in endogenous depression: Significance of hypothalamic functions. *Psych. Res.* 2:49–61, 1980.

77. Loosen, P. T. and Prange, A. J., Jr. Thyrotropin releasing hormone (TRH) A useful tool for psychoendocrine investigation. *Psychoneuroendocrinol.* 5:63–80, 1980.

78. Kirkegaard, C. and Bjorum, N. TSH response to TRH in endogenous depression. *Lancet* 1:152 (letter), 1980.

79. Kirkegaard, C., Bjorum, N., Cohn, D., and Lauridsen, U. B. Thyrotropin-releasing hormone (TRH) stimulation tests in manic-depressive illness. *Arch. Gen. Psychiat.* 35:1017–1021, 1978.

80. Kirkegaard, C. and Smith, E. Continuation therapy in endogenous depression controlled by changes in the TRH stimulation test. *Psychol. Med.* 8:501–503, 1978.

81. Gold, M. S., Pottash, A. L. C., Ryan, N., Sweeney, D. R., Davies, R. K., and Martin, D. M. TRH-induced TSH response in unipolar, bipolar, and secondary depressions: Possible utility in clinical assessment and differential diagnosis. *Psychoneuroendocrinol.* 5:147–155, 1980.

82. Carroll, B. J., Greden, J. F., Feinberg, M., James, N. M., Haskett, R. F., Steiner, J., and Tarika, J. Neuroendocrine dysfunction in genetic subtypes of primary unipolar depression. *Psychiat. Res.* 2:251–258, 1980.

83. Dysken, M., Pandey, G. N., Chang, S. S., Hicks, R., and Davis, J. M. Serial postdexamethasone cortisol levels in a patient undergoing ECT. *Amer. J. Psychiat.* 136:1328–1329, 1979.

84. Albala, A. A. and Greden, J. F. Serial dexamethasone suppression tests in affective disorders. *Amer. J. Psychiat.* 137:383, 1980.

85. Greden, J. F., Albala, A. A., Haskett, R. F., James, N. M., Goodman, L., Steiner, M., and Carroll, B. J. Normalization of the dexamethasone suppression test: A laboratory index of recovery from endogenous depression. *Biol. Psychiat.* 15:449–458, 1980.

86. Papakostas, Y., Fink, M., Lee, J., Irwin, P., Johnson, L. Neuroendocrine measures in psychiatric patients: Course and outcome with ECT. *Psychiat. Res.* 4:55-64, 1981.

87. Brown, W. A., Johnston, R., and Mayfield, D. The 24-hour dexamethasone suppression test in a clinical setting: Relationship to diagnosis, symptoms, and response to treatment. *Amer. J. Psychiat.* 136:543–547, 1979.

88. Gold, M. S., Pottash, A. L. C., Extein, I. and Sweeney, D. R. Dexamethasone suppression tests in depression and response to treatment. *Lancet* 1:1190 (letter), 1980.

# CHAPTER 8

# Cardiac Effects of the Tricyclic Antidepressants: Clinical Implications for Treating the Elderly

Richard C. Veith, M.D.

Tricyclic antidepressant (TCA) treatment is believed to be potentially unsafe for the elderly or patients with preexisting heart disease. This perception, derived chiefly from the overdose setting where significant cardiotoxicity is well documented, presents a particular problem for clinicians treating elderly patients since the aged are at increased risk for both depression and cardiovascular disease. Although renewed interest in recent years has resulted in a more systematic investigation of the cardiovascular effects of TCAs, specific guidelines for the use of TCAs with high-risk patients have not yet been formulated. The purpose of this chapter is to review briefly recent findings in this area and to present preliminary results of our own ongoing studies. The implications of these findings for treating the depressed elderly patient are discussed.

## HISTORICAL PERSPECTIVE

Reports of electrocardiographic (ECG) abnormalities associated with TCA treatment emerged shortly after these agents achieved widespread clinical use. Early reports described reversible, usually benign, nonspecific ECG changes (1–4). With the increasing frequency of TCA overdose, it became apparent that these agents could be highly toxic at high doses, producing impairment of cardiac conduction and severe disturbances of cardiac rhythm (5–9).

Two surveys conducted by the Aberdeen General Hospitals Group (10–12) found an increased incidence of unexplained sudden death among cardiac patients receiving amitriptyline compared to a matched control group. Imipramine therapy was not associated with increased mortality. These findings have been criticized with regard to the adequacy of the matched control group (13) and were not confirmed by the Boston Collaborative Drug Surveillance Program (14). Nevertheless, the reports of the Aberdeen group are significant historically because they led to increased concern over the possible cardiotoxic risks of therapeutic doses of TCAs, and raised the possibility that clinically relevant differences may exist among TCAs with regard to cardiovascular toxicity.

Questions raised but unanswered by these early studies have been the subject of more systematic recent studies that have included the determination of TCA plasma levels. These studies have explored:

1. the relationship between TCA-induced ECG alterations and TCA plasma levels,
2. the possible differences in cardiotoxic effects among the TCAs,
3. the effects of TCAs on cardiac rhythm and myocardial performance,
4. the effects of TCAs on blood pressure, and
5. the relative risks of TCA cardiotoxicity for patients with cardiac disease.

## ELECTROCARDIOGRAPHIC EFFECTS OF TCAs: RELATIONSHIP TO PLASMA TCA LEVELS

Recent clinical studies, controlled for plasma TCA levels, have examined the electrocardiographic effects of TCAs following overdose and in the typical therapeutic setting. In a series of reports (15–17), Biggs and associates examined the effects of TCA overdose on cardiovascular function. They found that TCA levels greater than 1000 ng/ml were associated with an increased frequency of ventricular rate ($\geq$120 beats/minute), bundle branch block, cardiac arrhythmias, and cardiac arrest (17). Prolongation of the QRS interval ($\geq$100 milliseconds), present in all patients with plasma TCA levels >1000 ng/ml, was a useful clinical indicator of a serious TCA overdose. A significant correlation between QRS duration and total drug plasma level was found among their patients, but no correlation was noted between antidepressant plasma levels and maximum heart rate, PR interval or ST–T wave changes (15).

The ECG effects of TCAs for patients receiving typical clinical doses of those TCAs available in this country have been reported for nortripty-line (18–23), amitriptyline (24), imipramine (25–28), doxepin (18), and desipramine (DMI) (29, 30). Findings are generally in agreement and are best illustrated by a recent report describing the effects of DMI on gener-ally young, depressed patients free of known cardiovascular disease (29). In this study, patients were treated with progressively increasing doses of DMI to a maximum dose of 200 mg nightly. A 12-lead electrocardio-gram and plasma DMI levels were obtained at baseline and weekly throughout a 3-week trial. As noted in Table 8.1, compared to baseline, DMI produced a significant increase in heart rate and progressive prolon-gation of the P–R, QRS, and Q–T$_c$ intervals. In addition, progressive flattening of T wave amplitude was noted. Although these changes were highly significant statistically, most of the electrocardiographic effects of DMI would go unnoticed by routine ECG interpretation, and none was clinically significant.

The correlations between the weekly ECG variables and corre-sponding DMI levels during the trial are given in Table 8.2. Plasma DMI levels varied from 13.4 to 882.2 ng/ml. Although the correlation coeffi-cients between plasma DMI and the ECG variables were highly signifi-cant, DMI plasma levels accounted for a relatively small part of the variance. These findings are in agreement with other clinical trials of therapeutic doses of TCAs that have largely failed to demonstrate a sig-nificant relationship between TCA plasma levels and ECG variables.

Compared to human studies, the animal studies have demonstrated more impressive correlations between plasma TCA levels and electrocar-diographic alterations (31–33). This may reflect the larger doses and higher plasma levels utilized in the animal studies. A wide range of plasma TCA levels may be necessary to demonstrate significant quantita-tive relationships between plasma concentration and ECG variables. This possibility is supported by the fact that the only significant relationship, the correlation between QRS duration and plasma TCA (r=0.75; p<0.01) reported by Spiker, et al. (15), was noted in a series of TCA overdose patients whose plasma levels ranged from 90 to 2190 ng/ml. Individual differences in plasma protein-binding or differences in myocardial tis-sue–TCA binding affinity may also be relevant factors. In addition, TCA metabolites not measured in the clinical trials may account for some of the ECG changes noted during treatment. For example, 2-hydroxy-desipramine, although pharmacologically inactive, has been shown to be cardiotoxic, and may have played a role in producing the ECG changes noted above (34, 35).

In an interesting series of reports, Vohra and associates (18, 20, 21,

TABLE 8.1  ECG Alterations during Treatment with Desipramine ($\pm$ SEM, n = 26)

| Variable | Baseline | Week 1 | Week 2 | Week 3 |
|---|---|---|---|---|
| Heart rate (bpm) | 69.3±2.0 | 81.2±2.3[a] | 83.9±2.2[a] | 82.4±2.4[a] |
| PR interval (msec) | 150.0±2.0 | 154.0±3.0[b] | 158.0±3.0[c] | 159.0±2.0[a] |
| QRS interval (msec) | 73.0±2.0 | 77.0±2.0[b] | 79.0±2.0[a] | 82.0±2.0[a] |
| QT$_c$ interval | 408.0±6.0 | 419.0±5.0 | 429.0±5.0[a] | 432.0±8.0[a] |
| T wave amplitude V$_5$ (mm) | 3.8±0.3 | 3.0±0.2[a] | 2.5±0.2[a] | 2.7±0.3[a] |

[a]p=0.001, paired t test compared with baseline.
[b]p=0.05, paired t test compared with baseline.
[c]p=0.01, paired t test compared with baseline.

36) utilized histidine (His) bundle electrocardiography (HBE) to determine the site of the TCA-induced intracardiac conduction disturbance reflected in the prolongation of the PR and QRS intervals on the surface electrocardiogram. Compared to the routine 12-lead ECG, HBE more accurately defines intracardiac conduction. Briefly, intracardiac conduction normally originates in the sinoatrial (SA) node, which establishes the heart rate. The electrical impulse proceeds to the atrioventricular (AV) node, and is transmitted to the ventricular muscle tissue via the ventricular specialized conducting system (VSCS). The VSCS is composed of the bundle of His, the right and left bundle branches, and the peripheral Purkinje fibers. On the standard 12-lead ECG, the PR interval represents transmission from the SA node through the AV node and the VSCS. The QRS interval reflects activation of the ventricular muscle fibers and ventricular depolarization. HBE, performed during cardiac catheterization, can be used to further characterize this intracardiac conduction by

TABLE 8.2  Correlation (r) between ECG Variables and Plasma Desipramine Levels

| Variable | Week 1 (n=24)[a] | Week 2 (n=26) | Week 3 (n=26) | Weeks 0, 1, 2, 3 (n=102) |
|---|---|---|---|---|
| Heart rate | 0.202 | 0.468[b] | 0.342 | 0.405[c] |
| PR interval | 0.315 | −0.004 | 0.054 | 0.171 |
| QRS interval | 0.387 | 0.263 | 0.270 | 0.346[c] |
| QT$_c$ interval | 0.070 | 0.747[c] | 0.578[d] | 0.534[c] |
| T wave amplitude V$_5$ | −0.223 | −0.434[b] | −0.354 | −0.386[c] |

[a]Two samples lost during plasma analysis.
[b]p < 0.05.
[c]p < 0.001.
[d]p < 0.01.

defining transmission from the SA node through the AV node (A–H interval) and from the His bundle through the Purkinje fibers (H–V interval).

Vohra, et al. (36), found normal A–H conduction but reversible prolongation of the QRS interval and increased H–V conduction time in 3 of 4 patients following overdose with imipramine or nortriptyline. Of 12 patients receiving typical clinical doses of nortriptyline (≤150 mg/day), 5 patients, 4 of whom had plasma nortriptyline levels exceeding 200 ng/ml, had significant H–V interval prolongation (21). In 7 of 8 patients who overdosed with nortriptyline, amitriptyline, or imipramine, HBE also revealed H–V and QRS interval prolongation (21). Six other patients had normal H–V conduction time following doxepin overdose (21).

Pursuing the possibility that doxepin may be less cardiotoxic than nortriptyline, but recognizing that their findings may have simply reflected decreased potency of doxepin, these investigators performed a subsequent study attempting to control for plasma TCA levels (18). Seventeen depressed patients were treated in a crossover trial with doxepin and nortriptyline for a period of 3 weeks. Six of the patients on nortriptyline, compared to only 1 patient on doxepin, demonstrated significant prolongation of the QRS interval, but plasma levels of doxepin (52±6 ng/ml) were significantly lower than nortriptyline levels (196±29 ng/ml) during the trial. Thus, it appears that a TCA-induced impairment of intracardiac conduction in the distal ventricular specialized conducting system, the Purkinje fibers, accounts for many of the electrocardiographic changes observed in patients receiving the TCA. Whether doxepin is less toxic in this regard rather than simply less potent remains to be determined.

In general, the electrocardiographic and cardiovascular effects of TCAs described in human clinical studies are in agreement with studies in animals (31–35, 37–52). As recently reviewed by Spiker (52), TCAs appear to exert three major pharmacologic effects on the heart:

1. a sympathomimetic effect reflected in the potentiation of the pressor response to norepinephrine that can be reversed by β-adrenergic blocking drugs,
2. an anticholinergic effect that antagonizes the pressor response to acetylcholine and increases heart rate through antagonism of peripheral vagal tone, and
3. a "quinidine-like" effect characterized by prolongation of intracardiac conduction.

In low doses these drugs increase heart rate and produce a positive inotropic effect. At toxic concentrations, TCAs reduce heart rate, decrease cardiac output, and produce a progressive impairment of myocardial contractility and intracardiac conduction, ultimately leading to asystole, cardiovascular collapse, and death.

## EFFECT OF TCAs ON CARDIAC RHYTHM

It is commonly believed that TCAs can produce cardiac rhythm disturbances in toxic doses or in customary doses in patients with preexisting heart disease. However, as noted above, the ECG effects of TCAs suggest that these agents produce a "quinidine-like" action. Animal studies have demonstrated that in low doses TCAs increase ventricular automaticity (38), presumably through their adrenergic properties, and in toxic doses TCAs induce significant cardiac arrhythmias (33, 40, 45–47, 50–52). However, Wilkerson (39) and others (37, 44–46) have demonstrated that in doses comparable to and slightly above those used clinically, TCAs effectively *reduce* cardiac arrhythmias. The mechanism of this antiarrhythmic action remains unclear. Although a direct action on the myocardium may be involved (41), a recent report by Tobis and Aronow (43) suggests that the effects of TCAs on cardiac rhythm may be centrally mediated.

Postulating that the TCA might also exert a clinically useful "quinidine-like" antiarrhythmic property in therapeutic concentrations, Bigger, et al. (25), performed weekly 24-hour electrocardiographic Holter monitoring in 2 patients receiving up to 2.5 mg/kg of imipramine per day. They demonstrated a significant antiarrhythmic effect of imipramine on both atrial and ventricular arrhythmias. A subsequent study by this group extended their original findings in 44 patients, 16 of whom had preexisting heart disease (26). Eleven of the 44 patients had >10 premature ventricular contractions (PVCs)/hour in two 24-hour Holter recording control periods. Ten of these 11 patients had >90% reduction in ventricular arrhythmias during treatment with imipramine at plasma concentrations ranging between 100 and 302 ng/ml.

To further explore this area, at the Seattle V.A. Medical Center we are examining the safety and efficacy of TCAs among depressed cardiac patients. Study subjects are clinically depressed according to DSM-III criteria and have a history of either a previous myocardial infarction or coronary surgery. Study subjects receive a 4-week, double-blind, placebo-controlled trial of imipramine or doxepin beginning at 50 mg, increasing to a maximum daily dose of 150 mg. During a 2-week washout period prior to treatment and throughout the trial, patients are monitored weekly with a 24-hour Holter electrocardiographic recording and have plasma drawn for determination of TCA levels. In addition, a radio-nuclide exercise ventriculogram is performed prior to treatment and repeated during the fourth week of treatment.

The preliminary results of the Holter monitoring of the initial 12 subjects of this project are presented in Table 8.3. There was a trend toward a decrease in mean PVCs for the imipramine group and an increase for the doxepin group that reflected an apparent decrease and increase, respectively, for only 1 patient from each group. Compared to baseline levels, there was no change in the frequency of PVCs for the remaining 6 patients on active treatment. Similar results were obtained during an open trial of 8 imipramine-treated cardiac patients performed as a pilot project before initiating our current study. Although it would be premature to draw conclusions from such a limited sample, thus far, imipramine and doxepin appear to be well tolerated in this relatively high-risk group. Definitive statements regarding the efficacy of TCAs as antiarrhythmic agents and comparisons between the two drugs will require a larger sample size, an increased number of subjects with significant numbers of PVCs prior to treatment, and determination of plasma TCA levels.

## EFFECTS OF TCAs
## ON MYOCARDIAL PERFORMANCE

Although congestive heart failure occasionally follows TCA overdose, and occurs even less frequently in patients receiving customary doses of TCAs, the effects of TCAs on myocardial performance have not been systematically investigated in man (53–58). Animal studies have demonstrated a direct myocardial depressant effect of TCAs, but this appears to occur in doses that are clearly in the toxic range for humans (31, 35, 47–50, 52). Thorstrand performed right heart catheterization and measured

TABLE 8.3 Frequency of Premature Ventricular Contractions for 12 Depressed Cardiac Patients[a]

| | Baseline | | Treatment Week | | | |
|---|---|---|---|---|---|---|
| | 1 | 2 | 1 | 2 | 3 | 4 |
| Imipramine patients (n=4) | 30[b] | 25 | 8 | 9 | 8 | 10 |
| Doxepin patients (n=4) | 16 | 33 | 30 | 156 | 83 | 131 |
| Placebo patients (n=4) | 41 | 33 | 43 | 25 | 42 | 35 |

[a]Age range 42–73 years.
[b] $\bar{x}$ PVC/HR by 24° Holter recording.

cardiac output (dye dilution technique) in 10 patients following overdose with amitriptyline or nortriptyline, but found no evidence of impairment of myocardial performance. Cardiac output was greater, and hemodynamic findings suggested hyperkinetic circulation shortly after admission compared to repeat determinations performed on an average of 37 hours later. These alterations were thought to be the consequence of increased adrenergic stimulation.

Typical therapeutic doses of TCAS (particularly amitriptyline) and tetracyclic antidepressants have been reported to reduce myocardial contractility as determined by measurement of systolic time intervals (STI, simultaneous recording of the ECG, phonocardiogram, and carotid pulse wave) (54–57). Unfortunately, marked variability of study design makes comparison of these studies difficult. In addition, these investigations were performed using either healthy subjects or those for whom the presence and severity of cardiac disease is undefined.

We have measured the left ventricular ejection fraction (LVEF) as part of our investigation of depressed cardiac patients described above. The LVEF is a measure of left ventricular pump performance derived from a radionuclide ventriculogram, a noninvasive, sensitive, and reliable diagnostic technique (59). The LVEF obtained from this procedure correlates closely with the ejection fraction determined by x-ray contrast left ventricular cineangiography, and is a more reliable measure than the STI (59–61). The LVEF is measured at rest and during bicycle exercise, both at baseline and following 4 weeks of TCA treatment. Preliminary findings from our first 12 study subjects are presented in Table 8.4. Baseline resting LVEF determinations of our subjects ranged from 11% to 68% (normal>50%). To date, we have found no evidence that treatment with either imipramine or doxepin produces a significant negative inotropic effect compared to placebo. In addition, none of our subjects has developed clinical evidence of an exacerbation of left heart failure during treatment. These findings are particularly significant since several of our subjects had marked impairment of myocardial performance prior to treatment.

## EFFECTS OF TCAs ON BLOOD PRESSURE

Although TCAS occasionally cause a mild increase in blood pressure, more commonly they produce postural hypotension. More than 20% of patients receiving TCAS experience this adverse effect (19, 62–65). Although early studies emphasized that postural hypotension is a particular risk for the elderly and those with known heart disease, a recent

TABLE 8.4  Resting Left Ventricular Ejection
Fraction[a] for 12 Depressed Patients

| Patient | Baseline | Week 4 |
|---|---|---|
| **Imipramine** | | |
| 1 | 0.37 | 0.34 |
| 4 | 0.45 | 0.48 |
| 10 | 0.58 | 0.59 |
| 11 | 0.68 | 0.71 |
| $\bar{X}$ | 0.52±0.14 | 0.53±0.16 |
| **Doxepin** | | |
| 3 | 0.55 | 0.46 |
| 5 | 0.11 | 0.11 |
| 8 | 0.36 | 0.42 |
| 12 | 0.49 | 0.44 |
| $\bar{X}$ | 0.38±0.20 | 0.36±0.17 |
| **Placebo** | | |
| 2 | 0.34 | 0.29 |
| 6 | 0.67 | 0.71 |
| 7 | 0.28 | 0.25 |
| 9 | 0.19 | 0.16 |
| $\bar{X}$ | 0.37±0.21 | 0.36±0.24 |

[a]LVEF=end diastolic volume–end systolic volume/
end diastolic volume, normal value ≥ 0.50.

prospective study by Glassman and associates (64) revealed that imipramine-induced orthostatic hypotension was unrelated to age, dose, the presence of preexisting heart disease, or plasma imipramine level. In 44 patients, they noted a mean fall in systolic pressure of 26 mm Hg compared to 10.9 mm Hg before drug treatment and found that the best predictor of orthostatic hypotension during treatment was the degree of orthostatic hypotension prior to treatment.

Compared to the reports from the Glassman group (25, 26, 64, 65, 66), postural hypotension has proven to be a less significant problem than anticipated in our own series of TCA-treated cardiac patients. The mean arterial pressures for this group are presented in Table 8.5. There was a nonsignificant trend toward a reduction in both supine and standing blood pressure among the doxepin patients. None of our patients experienced clinically significant symptoms of postural hypotension during treatment. The absence of significant difficulties among our subjects compared to those of the Glassman group may reflect the lower total daily doses and more gradual increase in dose used in our study. Adequate comparisons between these two studies and between drug groups within our study will require larger patient samples and determination of the plasma TCA levels.

TABLE 8.5 Mean Arterial Blood Pressure[a] for 12 Depressed Cardiac Patients

| Position and Time | Imipramine | | Doxepin | | Placebo | |
|---|---|---|---|---|---|---|
| | Baseline | Week 4 | Baseline | Week 4 | Baseline | Week 4 |
| **Supine** | | | | | | |
| 30 minute | 90 | 93 | 94 | 89 | 92 | 93 |
| **Standing** | | | | | | |
| 2 Minute | 90 | 88 | 93 | 90 | 95 | 94 |
| 5 Minute | 91 | 90 | 94 | 87 | 95 | 94 |
| 10 Minute | 94 | 93 | 94 | 87 | 93 | 94 |

[a]mm/Hg.

# IMPLICATIONS FOR TREATING THE ELDERLY

In general, the more recent studies suggest that the risks of TCA-induced cardiotoxic adverse effects may have been overstated. Clinical assumptions based on anecdotal reports, uncontrolled trials, and extrapolations from the overdose setting are, to a large degree, inaccurate. The cardiovascular effects of the TCA appear to be relatively well tolerated by the elderly, even those with cardiac disease.

The adrenergic and anticholinergic effects of the TCA produce an increase in heart rate that may be poorly tolerated by patients with significant ischemic heart disease or uncontrolled angina, for whom an increase in heart rate may further compromise cardiac oxygenation. Although the adrenergic effects of TCAs may promote ventricular irritability, it increasingly appears that the predominate effect of these drugs on cardiac rhythm is a membrane-stabilizing, antiarrhythmic effect. Although this may justify less concern over producing arrhythmias in otherwise predisposed patients, the effects of TCAs on intracardiac conduction require that special care be exercised in treating patients with preexisting conduction disturbance or those receiving concomitant Class 1 antiarrhythmic agents—for example, quinidine. Should an arrhythmia or conduction disturbance develop during TCA treatment, the drug should generally be stopped if the disturbance is deemed clinically significant. Electroconvulsive therapy (ECT), which is safe and effective in cardiac patients, may be considered as alternative treatment. The emergence of clinically insignificant ECG alterations will frequently not preclude continued TCA therapy.

The hypotensive effects of TCAs are a particular risk for the elderly, for whom complications from trauma and falls may be catastrophic. This risk may be reduced through careful monitoring of pretreatment postural hypotension and cautious treatment, in other words, starting with low doses, progressing slowly, using divided doses, and avoiding high doses if possible.

We currently recommend against using the TCAs in the following clinical circumstances:

1. within 2 months after an acute myocardial infarction or significant change in cardiovascular function (major episode of congestive heart failure),
2. in patients with uncontrolled ventricular arrhythmias, uncontrolled angina, or poorly compensated congestive heart failure,
3. in patients with significant pretreatment, postural hypotension.

In addition, particular care must be taken in treating patients with preexisting intracardiac conduction disturbance.

We generally begin treatment with 25–50 mg of a selected agent, increasing in 25 mg increments at 3–5 day intervals, using divided doses when 100 mg h.s. is exceeded. Supine and standing blood pressure and a baseline electrocardiogram should be obtained prior to treatment and repeated as clinically indicated. Treatment can otherwise proceed as with patients at lower risk, increasing the dose until a beneficial effect or intolerable adverse effects occur. Although the relationship between plasma TCA levels and efficacy continues to be defined, plasma TCA levels may be useful for determining a rough gauge of absorption in patients at high risk prior to exceeding customary doses.

Definitive statements regarding the effects of TCAs on myocardial performance as well as possible clinically relevant differences among the TCAs must await completion of further studies, which, it is to be hoped, will be adequately controlled and systematically designed to allow for comparison among studies and extrapolation to the clinical arena. This knowledge and the availability of newer compounds that appear to be relatively free of cardiovascular effects, such as the tetracyclic antidepressant mianserin (67), may greatly reduce the risks of treating the aged depressed patient.

## REFERENCES

1. Muller, O. F., Goodman, N., Bellet, S.: The hypotensive effect of imipramine hydrochloride in patients with cardiovascular disease. Clin Pharmacol Ther 2:300–307, 1961.

2. Kristiansen, E. S.: Cardiac complications during treatment with imipramine (Tofranil). Acta Psychiat Neurol 36:427–442, 1961.
3. Schou, M.: Electrocardiographic changes during treatment with lithium and with drugs of the imipramine type. Acta Psychiat Scand 38:331–336, 1962.
4. Rasmussen, E. B., Kristjansen, P.: ECG changes during amitriptyline treatment. Am J Psychiat 119:781–782, 1963.
5. Rasmussen, J.: Amitriptyline and imipramine posioning. Lancet 2:850–851, 1965.
6. Gaultier, M., Boissier, J. R., Gorceix, A., et al.: The cardiotoxicity of imipramine in man and animals. Proc Eur Soc Drug Toxicity 6:171–178, 1965.
7. Barnes, R. J., Kong, S. M., Wu, R. W. Y.: Electrocardiographic changes in amitriptyline posioning. Br Med J 3:222–223, 1968.
8. Freeman, J. W., Mundy, G. R., Beattie, R. R., et al.: Cardiac abnormalities in poisoning with tricyclic antidepressants. Br Med J 2:610–611, 1969.
9. Noble, J., Matthew, H.: Acute poisoning by tricyclic antidepressants: clinical features and management of 100 patients. Clin Toxicol 2:403–421, 1969.
10. Coull, D. C., Crooks, J., Dingwall-Fordyce, I., et al.: Amitriptyline and cardiac disease: risk of sudden death identified by monitoring system. Lancet 2:590–591, 1970.
11. Moir, D. C., Dingwall-Fordyce, I., Weir, R. D.: Medicines evaluation and monitoring group: a follow-up study of cardiac patients receiving amitriptyline. Eur J Clin Pharmacol 6:98–101, 1973.
12. Moir, D. C., Crooks, J., Cornwell, W. B., et al.: Cardiotoxicity of amitriptyline. Lancet 2:561–564, 1972.
13. Wendkos, M. H.: Sudden Death and Psychiatric Illness. New York: Spectrum, 1979, p. 302–303.
14. Boston Collaborative Drug Surveillance Program: Adverse reactions to the tricyclic antidepressant drugs. Lancet 1:529–531, 1972.
15. Spiker, D. G., Weiss, A. N., Chang, S. S., et al.: Tricyclic antidepressant overdose: clinical presentation and plasma levels. Clin Pharmacol Ther 18:539–546, 1975.
16. Spiker, D. G., Biggs, J. T.: Tricyclic antidepressants: prolonged plasma levels after overdose. JAMA 236: 1711–1712, 1976.
17. Petit, J. M., Spiker, D. G., Ruwitch, J. F., et al.: Tricyclic antidepressant plasma levels and adverse effects after overdose. Clin Pharmacol Ther 21:47–51, 1977.
18. Burrows, G. D., Vohra, J., Dumovic, P., et al.: Tricyclic antidepressant drugs and cardiac conduction. Prog Neuro-Psychopharmac 1:329–334, 1977.
19. Freyschuss, U., Sjöqvist, F., Tuck, D., et al.: Circulatory effects in man of nortriptyline, a tricyclic antidepressant drug. Pharmacologia Clinica 2:68–71, 1970.
20. Vohra, J., Burrows, G. D., Sloman, G.: Assessment of cardiovascular side

effects of therapeutic doses of tricyclic antidepressant drugs. Aust NZJ Med 5:7–11, 1975.

21. Vohra, J., Burrows, G., Hunt, D., et al.: The effect of toxic and therapeutic doses of tricyclic antidepressant drugs on intracardiac conduction. Eur J Cardiol 3:219–227, 1975.

22. Ziegler, V. E., Co, B. T., Biggs, J. T.: Plasma nortriptyline levels and ECG findings. Am J Psychiat 134:441–443, 1977.

23. Reed, K., Smith, R. C., Schooler, J. C., et al.: Cardiovascular effects of nortriptyline in geriatric patients. Am J Psychiat 134:986–987, 1980.

24. Ziegler, V. E., Co, B. T., Biggs, J. T.: Electrocardiographic findings in patients undergoing amitriptyline treatment. Dis Nerv 38:697–699, 1977.

25. Bigger, J. T., Jr, Giardina, E. G. V., Perel, J. M., et al.: Cardiac antiarrhythmic effect of imipramine hydrochloride. N Engl J Med 296:206–208, 1977.

26. Giardina, E. V., Bigger, J. T., Jr. Glassman, A. H., et al.: The electrocardiographic and antiarrhythmic effects of imipramine hydrochloride at therapeutic concentrations. Circulation 60:1045–1052, 1979.

27. Kantor, S. J., Bigger, J. T. Jr., Glassman, A. H., et al.: Imipramine-induced heart block: a longitudinal case study. JAMA 231:1364–1366, 1975.

28. Winsberg, B. G., Goldstein, S., Yepes, L. E., et al.: Imipramine and electrocardiographic abnormalities in hyperactive children. Am J Psychiat 132:542–545, 1975.

29. Veith, R. C., Friedel, R. O., Bloom, V: Electrocardiogram changes and plasma desipramine levels during treatment of depression. Clin Pharmacol Ther 27:796–802, 1980.

30. Rudorfer, M. V., Young, R. C.: Desipramine: cardiovascular effects and plasma levels. Am J Psychiat 137:984–986, 1980.

31. Bianchetti, G., Bonaccorsi, A., Chiodaroli, A., et al.: Plasma concentrations and cardiotoxic effects of desipramine and protriptyline in the rat. Br J Pharmac 60:11–19, 1977.

32. Bonaccorsi, A., Dejana, E., Franko, R., et al.: Plasma levels and cardiotoxic effects of some antidepressant drugs in the rat, in Depressive Disorders. Ed. by Garattini S. Stuttgart: Schattauer, 1978.

33. Bonaccorsi, A., Franko, R., Garattini, S., et al.: Plasma nortriptyline and cardiac responses in young and old rats. Br J Pharmac 60:21–27. 1977.

34. Buckley, J. P., Steenberg, M. L., Jandhyala, B. S., et al.: Effects of imipramine, desmethylimipramine and their 2–OH metabolites on hemodynamics and myocardial contractility. Fed Proc 34:450, 1975.

35. Jandhyala, B. S., Steenberg, M. L., Perel, J. M., et al.: Effects of several tricyclic antidepressants on the hemodynamics and myocardial contractility of the anesthetized dog. Eur J Pharmacol 42:403–410, 1977.

36. Vohra, J., Hunt, D., Burrows, G., et al.: Intracardiac conduction defects following overdose of tricyclic antidepressant drugs. Eur J Cardiol 2:453–458, 1975.

37. Fekete, M., Borsy, J.: On the antiarrhythmic effect of some thymoleptics

(amitriptyline, imipramine, trimepropimine, and desmethylimipramine). Med Exp 10:93–102, 1964.

38. Baum, T., Peters, J. R., Butz, F., et al.: Tricyclic antidepressants and cardiac conduction: changes in ventricular automaticity. Eur J Pharmacol 39:323–329, 1976.

39. Wilkerson, R. D.: Antiarrhythmic effects of tricyclic antidepressant drugs in ouabian-induced arrhythmias in the dog. J Pharmacol Exp Ther 205:666–674, 1978.

40. Harvengt, C., Desager, J. P., Vanderbist, M., et al.: Sympathetic nervous system response in acute cardiovascular toxicity induced by amitriptyline in conscious rabbits. Toxical Appl Pharmacol 44:115–126, 1978.

41. Tamargo, J., Rodriguez, S., De Jalón, P. G.: Electrophysiological effects of desipramine on guinea pig papillary muscles. Eur J Pharmacol 55:171–179, 1979.

42. Cavero, I., Gomeni, R., Lefèvre-Borg, F., et al.: Comparison of mianserin with desipramine, maprotiline and phentolamine on cardiac presynaptic and vascular postsynaptic α-adrenoceptors and noradrenaline reuptake in pithed normotensive rats. Br J Pharmac 68:321–332, 1980.

43. Tobis, J. M., Aronow, W. S.: Effect of amitriptyline antidotes on repetitive extrasystole threshold. Clin Pharmacol Ther 27:602–606, 1980.

44. Baum, T., Eckfeld, D. K., Shropshire, A. T., et al.: Observations on models used for the evaluation of antiarrhythmic drugs. Arch Int Pharmacodyn 193:149–170, 1971.

45. Schmitt, H., Cheymol, G., Gilbert, J. A.: Effects anti-arythmisants et hémo-dynamiques de l'imipramine et de la chlorimipramine. Arch Int Pharmacodyn 184:158–174, 1970.

46. Baum, T., Shropshire, A. T., Rowles, G., et al.: Antidepressants and cardiac conduction: iprindole and imipramine. Eur J Pharmacol 13:287–291, 1971.

47. Kato, H., Noguchi, Y., Takagi, K.: Comparison of cardiovascular toxicities induced by dimetacrine, imipramine and amitriptyline in isolate guinea pig atria and anesthetized dogs. Japan J Pharmacol 24:885–891, 1974.

48. Sigg, E. B., Osborne, M., Koroc, B.: Cardiovascular effects of imipramine. J Pharm Exp Ther 141:237–243, 1963.

49. Langslet, A., Johnson, G., Ryg, M., et al.: Effects of dibenzepine and imipramine on the isolated rat heart. Eur J Pharmacol 14:333–339, 1971.

50. Laddu, A. R., Somani, P.: Desipramine toxicity and its treatment. Toxicol Appl Pharmacol 15:287–294, 1969.

51. Elonen, E., Mattila, M. J., Saarnivaara, L.: Cardiovascular effects of amitriptyline, nortriptyline, protripryline and doxepin in conscious rabbits. Eur J Pharmacol 28:178–188, 1974.

52. Spiker, D. G.: The cardiovascular toxicity of tricyclic antidepressants, in Animal Models in Psychiatry and Neurology. Ed. by Hanin I., Usdin E. New York, Pergamon, 1977.

53. Thorstrand, C.: Cardiovascular effects of poisoning with tricyclic antidepressants. Acta Med Scand 195:505–514, 1974.

54. Burgess, C. D., Turner, P., Wadsworth, J.: Cardiovascular responses to mianserin hydrochloride: a comparison with tricyclic antidepressant drugs. Br J Clin Pharmac 5:21S–28S, 1978.

55. Burckhardt, D., Raeder, E., Müller, V., et al.: Cardiovascular effects of tricyclic and tetracyclic antidepressants. JAMA 239:213–216, 1978.

56. Kopera, H., Fluch, N., Harpe, H., et al.: Cardiovascular effects of mianserin—a comparative study with amitriptyline and a placebo in healthy subjects. Int J Clin Pharmacol Ther Toxicol 18:104–109, 1980.

57. Raeder, E. A., Burckhardt, D., Neubauer, H., et al.: Long-term tri- and tetracyclic antidepressants, myocardial contractility, and cardiac rhythm. Br Med J 57:666–667, 1978.

58. Mielke, D. H., Koepke, R. P., Phillips, J. H.: A controlled evaluation of a tetracyclic (maprotiline) and a tricyclic (imipramine) antidepressant and their effects of the heart. Curr Ther Res 25:738–742, 1979.

59. Bodenheimer, M. M., Banka, V. S., Helfant, R. H.: Nuclear Cardiology. 1. Radionuclide angiographic assessment of left ventricular contraction: uses, limitations and future directions. Am J Cardiol 45:661–673, 1980.

60. Folland, E. D., Hamilton, G. W., Larsen, S. M., et al.: Radionuclide ejection fraction: a comparision of three radionuclide techniques with contrast angiography. J Nucl Med 18:1159–1166, 1977.

61. Sorensen, S. G., Ritchie, J. L., Caldwell, J. H., et al.: Serial exercise radionuclide angiography: validation of count-derived changes in cardiac output and quantitation of maximal exercise ventricular volume change after nitroglycerin and propranolol in normal men. Circulation 61:600–609, 1980.

62. Muller, O. F., Goodman, N., Bellet, S.: The hypotensive effect of imipramine hydrochloride in patients with cardiovascular disease. Clin Pharmacol Ther 2:300–307, 1961.

63. Jefferson, J. W.: Hypotension from drugs: incidence, peril, prevention. Dis Nerv Syst 35:66–71, 1974.

64. Hayes, J. R., Born, G. F., Rosenbaum, A. H.: Incidence of orthostatic hypotension in patients with primary affective disorders treated with tricyclic antidepressants. Mayo Clin Proc 52:509–512, 1977.

65. Glassman, A. H., Bigger, J. T., Jr., Giardina, E. V., et al.: Clinical characteristics of imipramine-induced orthostatic hypotension. Lancet 2:468–472, 1979.

66. Kantor, S. J., Glassman, A. H., Bigger, J. T., Jr., et al.: The cardiac effects of therapeutic plasma concentrations of imipramine. Am J Psychiat 135:534–538, 1978.

67. Brogden, R. N., Heel, R. C., Speight, T. M., et al.: Mianserin: a review of its pharmacological properties and therapeutic efficacy in depressive illness. Drugs 16:273–301, 1978.

# CHAPTER 9

# Dementias and Drugs Affecting Cerebral Blood Flow

Jerome A. Yesavage, M.D.

## RATIONALES FOR THE USE OF VASOACTIVE DRUGS IN THE ELDERLY

Controversy surrounds the rationales for the use of vasoactive medications in the elderly, and the rationales themselves change rapidly. Before we discuss the rationales for the various classes of medications, we should first review some general points about dementia and cerebral blood flow (CBF).

First of all, dementia is a term used to define a diffuse deterioration of cerebral function, primarily in thought and memory, and secondarily in affect and behavior (1). Although dementia may have a number of causes, this chapter concerns the common dementias of old age caused by atherosclerotic or degenerative disease. There is considerable debate concerning the prevalence of atherosclerotic vs. degenerative brain disease in the elderly. Degenerative brain disease in the elderly, or Alzheimer's type dementia, is marked by a slow, insidious onset and global intellectual decline. Atherosclerotic brain disease, on the other hand, may have a more abrupt onset, and it may be accompanied by focal neurological signs. Both processes may affect the same patient, but it is generally held that the degenerative type of dementia is probably twice as common as atherosclerotic dementia and that it especially affects women (2).

A second important point is that some of these "degenerative" dementias, at least in their early stages, have relatively well-preserved regulation of CBF with minimal loss of neurons (3–5). A considerable amount of work has related cerebral glucose metabolism, oxygen consumption, carbon dioxide production, regulation of CBF, and dementia (6). At mean blood pressures greater than 50 mm Hg, CBF is proportional to tissue metabolic activity: increased metabolic activity, for example during a seizure, requires more oxygen, produces more carbon dioxide, and leads to reflex vasodilatation and increased CBF. Investigators have correlated the decline of CBF with slowing of the electroencephalogram (EEG) and with degree of decline of intellectual function (7, 8). Thus, some argue that at least in certain dementias a primary disorder of neuronal metabolism may lead to both diffuse deterioration of cerebral function (including impairment of neurotransmitter synthesis), and decreased CBF.

Despite these arguments, there are investigators who stress the atherosclerotic component of dementias and feel that reduction of CBF is the primary cause of many senile dementias (9). The evidence for this argument is based on studies of CBF that demonstrate that many healthy elderly without evidence of atherosclerosis have rates of CBF and oxygen consumption unchanged from those of adults 50 years younger. Furthermore, some elderly with minimal asymptomatic atherosclerosis exhibited marked reduction of CBF, evidence of reduced oxygen tension in the brain, as well as some impairment on psychological testing, when compared with the healthy elderly without any evidence of atherosclerosis.

Clearly, the results are not yet such that a definitive answer can be given, and in any case it is probable that the majority of demented elderly have a combination of atherosclerotic and degenerative cerebral changes. Nonetheless, this pathological distinction can serve as a rational basis for at least separating in one's mind the two major classes of vasoactive medications used in the dementias.

## TYPES OF MEDICATIONS

This chapter does not discuss the ensemble of medications that have been claimed to have positive effects on mentation in the elderly. The reader is directed to reviews that concern neurotransmitter precursors, neuropeptides, and other agents that have rationales potentially as strong as vasoactive compounds for their use in dementias (10). It should also be mentioned that careful differential diagnosis and the judicious use of neuroleptics and antidepressants are essential to the proper pharmacological treatment of dementias (11). Nonetheless, what are the types of vasoactive compounds that have been proposed as treatments for dementias? (See Table 9.1.)

TABLE 9.1. Cerebrally Vasoactive Drugs by Class

| |
| --- |
| PRIMARY VASODILATORS (Primary action on vasculature) |
|     Cyclandelate |
|     Papaverine |
|     Nylidrin |
|     Isoxsuprine |
|     Cinnarizine |
|     Bencyclane |
|     Betahistine Hydrochloride |
| SECONDARY VASODILATORS (Primary action on metabolism) |
|     Dihydroergotoxine Mesylate       Vinca Alkaloids |
|     Naftidrofuryl |
|     Pyritinol |
|     Piracetam |

It is useful to distinguish between drugs that appear to have an effect primarily on vasculature (i.e., smooth muscle dilators, to be called primary or pure vasodilators) and drugs that primarily appear to have an effect on cerebral metabolism and that secondarily induce an increase in CBF (secondary vasodilators, or drugs with mixed effects). Although there are medications that may overlap this classification, this distinction is useful: in a review of 102 studies of both types of agents, the drugs with mixed effects, as a class, had significantly more positive double-blind clinical trials in dementias than did the drugs with purely vasoactive effects (12). Let us now discuss specific agents in each class.

## PRIMARY VASODILATORS

Such medications have been studied at least since the turn of the century, when the transient effects of niacin (nicotinic acid) were tried in elderly subjects. Currently, a wide variety of these medications is in use; what follows is a discussion of each.

### Cyclandelate

Cyclandelate is probably the most widely used medication in the class, and is available in the United States. There have been at least 7 double-blind studies of cyclandelate (13–19) in demented elderly subjects. Six of these (13–18) found some positive effects. However, there was considerable question about the practical use of the medication (19). Some have suggested that the medication may have a prophylactic effect, but this claim needs more study for documentation (14). Future studies with this medication will center upon identifying a susceptible patient population. Studies to date have not been able to correlate this medication's positive results with clinical measures of atherosclerosis.

## Papaverine

It was recently reported by the Food and Drug Administration's Peripheral and Central Nervous System Drugs Advisory Committee that " . . . there is no body of evidence that will support the effectiveness of papaverine and ethaverine for any of their claimed indications" (20). This report cited questions of bioavailability as well as a lack of positive double-blind reports. There have been 5 direct comparisons of papaverine with dihydroergotoxine mesylate; the latter was superior in all 5 studies (21–25).

## Nylidrin and Isoxsuprine

These structurally similar sympathomimetic amines have been used primarily in peripheral vascular disease. Cerebrovascular disease studies with isoxsuprine have been less encouraging than those with nylidrin. A recent double-blind, placebo-controlled trial of nylidrin in senile dementias found positive results in all 11 centers of a multicenter trial involving over 500 subjects (26). This study appears to be the best documentation presently available for clinical efficacy of any primary vasodilator. The medication's structure leads one to speculate whether it has central nervous system stimulant effects in addition to its peripheral beta receptor activity.

## Cinnarazine

This piperazine derivative and its analogue flunarizine are potent primary vasodilators (12). The medication's use in dementia is difficult to evaluate since many of its studies have been in patients with transient ischemic attacks or Meniere's disease. It is presently under investigation in the United States for its use in multi-infarct dementias.

## Other Primary Vasodilators

Two other primary vasodilators have had too few studies to assess them properly. Bencyclane has had 4 clinical trials with mixed results. Betahistine hydrochloride has had 1 positive trial in patients with vertebrobasilar artery insufficiency (12).

A recent review has listed a host of other compounds that are potential cerebral vasodilators. These include: xanthinol niacinate, vasolantin, proxazole and vitamin E. This review also discusses the use of anticoagulants to increase CBF (27).

## SECONDARY VASODILATORS

Several types of medications available in other countries are claimed to be stimulants of cerebral metabolism and secondary cerebral vasodilators. Such medications have been under investigation since the first serious studies of ergotoxine in 1906 (28).

### Dihydroergotoxine Mesylate

Dihydroergotoxine mesylate (DEM) is the world's most widely prescribed medication for the indication of dementia. It is not widely used in the United States, where clinicians remain skeptical of its clinical effects. Nonetheless, at least 22 double-blind, placebo-controlled studies have shown it to be superior to placebo in this indication (12). Skeptics argue that the medication may improve some psychological tests inconsistently across studies but that the perceived improvements remain quite small. Optimists argue that any change in demented subjects should be seen as miraculous. Present research is examining the use of higher doses of the medication, and the combination of the medication with psychotherapy (29, 30), in an effort to augment response. At present, it is the only such agent available for clinical use in the United States.

### Naftidrofuryl

This synthetic molecule does not have the long history of ergot alkaloids; however, in its country of origin, France, it outsells DEM for use in dementias. The medication is at present under investigation in the United States, where 1 positive double-blind study has been added to the 8 positive well-controlled studies the medication has had in Europe (12). The use of this medication is open to the same criticisms of the clinical importance of its effect already noted for DEM. Also, as in the case of DEM, the optimal dosage for this medication remains unclear. Its usual dose in Europe is 300 mg per day, but ongoing testing in the United States is using higher dosages. At these higher dosages, biochemical effects (reduction of the lactate:pyruvate ratio) consistent with a stimulant effect on cerebral metabolism has been noted in spinal fluid samples in humans (31).

## Vinca Alkaloids

These compounds are used widely in Europe for the same indications as the ergot alkaloids. Although their clinical and biochemical effects seem well documented, they have been studied less than the ergot alkaloids (32). At present, the medication is not slated for testing in the United States.

## Piracetam

This European synthetic compound has been shown to have biochemical effects consistent with stimulation of cerebral glucose metabolism. A recent review of the literature of this medication has documented its clinical usefulness to a degree similar to DEM or naftidrofuryl (33); however, in a particularly elegant primate model of aged impairment of memory function, piracetam was shown to be superior to other stimulants of cerebral metabolism, the ergot and vinca alkaloids (34). The medication is currently under investigation in the United States.

## Pyritinol

This medication, available only in Europe, is claimed to have metabolic effects similiar to those of DEM or naftidrofuryl. However, the medication has less-well-documented results. Its usual formulation is in combination with pyridylcarbinol, a precursor of nicotinic acid (12).

## CONCLUSION AND CLINICAL POINTS

This chapter has briefly reviewed the pathophysiology of dementias and examined in more depth the two types of medications most widely used to treat dementias. Clearly, there are limitations in our understanding of both the pathophysiology and the treatment of dementia. Nonetheless, it is remarkable to note there are substantial numbers of positive studies both for drugs with primary vasodilating action and for those with mixed metabolic and vasoactive effects.

It should be noted that, despite some promising recent studies with primary vasodilators (especially nylidrin), the studies taken as a whole are more frequently positive for drugs with mixed effects than for primary vasodilators. This may be because the metabolic causes of dementia are more frequent than the purely vascular. Furthermore, it is still difficult to conceive how a purely vasoactive compound might increase CBF in atherosclerotic vessels or areas where there is already ischemia and substantial autoregulated vasodilation. In addition, there is the potential of reducing CBF by increasing peripheral pooling with such agents, though this has not been experimentally demonstrated with the commonly used primary vasodilators. Perhaps there is a small subgroup of dementias that have reversible vasospasm as a component, or perhaps some "purely" vasoactive medications have unrecognized CNS stimulant effects. In any case, no studies of either primary or secondary vasodilators have yet identified the optimal target population on any basis, let alone the patient's hypothesized cerebral pathology.

In the clinical realm, one is therefore left with the evidence that drugs with mixed metabolic and vasoactive properties have a better overall record than purely vasoactive drugs. But which one of the mixed drugs should one choose for a particular patient? In the United States, the choice is quite simple since there is only one such medication, DEM, available on the market. In Europe, there are several such agents available; but since there have been no direct comparisons between these drugs in humans, relative efficacy cannot be assessed.

The clinician should be aware that there are several points that may help in the effective use of agents such as DEM. First, he or she should make a proper differential diagnosis of the elderly with impaired cognitive function. This has been discussed at length elsewhere and has been facilitated by the use of mnemonic devices (35). Depression can be confused with dementia. This differential diagnosis has also been discussed at length (36).

Second, it is important to recognize that the optimal dosages for compounds such as DEM have not been fixed. Neuroleptics and antidepressants have wide ranges of serum levels, and the serum levels are better correlated with therapeutic effects and side effects than are oral doses. At present, there are no studies of serum levels of medications like DEM, naftidrofuryl, or piracetam and wide ranges of oral dosages are prescribed. The standard dose for DEM in the United States is 3 mg per day orally, but the common dosage used in Europe is 4.5 mg per day, and ongoing trials are using 6 mg per day. The clinician should be aware of this dosage problem and attentive to future research in this area that may change approved dosages or make serum-level monitoring more practical.

A third point about the use of such medications is the necessity for careful monitoring of results. Most of the metabolically active medications take at least 12 weeks for an effect to be seen, and the effects are usually modest. Hence, careful documentation of baseline functioning and changes seen over the trial period are necessary, otherwise one simply will not recognize the changes. The clinical course can be monitored using a simple rating scale such as the Sandoz Clinical Assessment Geriatric, commonly called the SCAG. This form, Which has been tested for validity and reliability (37), may be quickly completed after a clinical interview.

A final point is that although the best population for such medications has not been perfectly identified, there is some evidence that subjects who have relatively mild symptoms respond better than those with advanced disease (12). This is consistent with the concept that for any psychotropic medication to work, one must have at least some neurons and receptors. This may not be the case in advanced cases of Alzheimer's type dementias, where there is severe cerebral atrophy. Thus, one might be more likely to see an effect in subjects with dysfunctional, rather than absent, neurons.

# REFERENCES

1. Wells, C.: Dementia. Philadelphia: F. A. Davis, 1971.
2. Wells, C. E.: Geriatric organic psychoses. Psychiatr Ann 8:57–73, 1979.
3. Simard, D., Oleson, J., Paulson, O. B., et al.: Regional cerebral blood flow and its regulation in dementia. Brain 94:273–288, 1971.
4. Treff, W. M.: Das involutionsmuster des nucleus dentatus cerebelli. Altern Entwickl. pp 37–54, 1974.
5. Maker, H. S., Lehrer, G. M., Weiss, C.: DNA content of mouse cerebellar layers. Brain Res 50:226–229, 1973.
6. Meier-Ruge, W., Enz, A., Gygax, P., et al.: Experimental pathology in basic research of the aging brain, in Aging Vol. 2. Ed. by Gershon S., Raskin A. New York, Raven Press, 1975, pp. 55–126.
7. Kety, S. S.: Human cerebral blood flow and oxygen consumption as related to aging. Res Publ Assoc Res Nerv Ment Dis 35:31–45, 1956.
8. Obrist, W. D., Chiviane, E., Crouquist, S., et al.: Regional cerebral blood flow in senile and presenile dementia. Neurology 20:315–322, 1970.

9. Sokoloff, L.: Cerebral circulation and metabolism in the aged, in Aging Vol. 2. Ed. by Gerson S., Raskin A. New York: Raven Press, 1975, pp 45–54.
10. Yesavage, J.: Pharmacotherapy of the aged central nervous system. Clinical Neuropharmacology IV. New York: Raven Press, 1979, pp 199–220.
11. Hollister, L. E.: Drugs for mental disorders of old age. JAMA 234:195–198, 1975.
12. Yesavage, J., Tinklenberg, J., Berger, P., et al.: Vasodilators in senile dementias: A review of the literature. Arch Gen Psychiat 36:220–223, 1979.
13. Fine, E. W.: The use of cyclandelate in chronic brain syndrome with arteriosclerosis. Curr Ther Res 13:568–574, 1971.
14. Hall, P.: Cyclandelate in the treatment of cerebral arteriosclerosis. J Am Geriatr Soc 24:41–45, 1976.
15. Eichorn, O.: The effect of cyclandelate on cerebral circulation—a double-blind trial with clinical and radiographic investigations. Vasc Dis 2:305–315, 1965.
16. Alderman, M., Giardina, W. J., Loreniowski, S.: Effect of cyclandelate on perception, memory and cognition in a group of geriatric subjects. J Am Geriatr Soc 20:268–271, 1972.
17. Ball, J. A. C., Taylor, A. R.: Effect of cyclandelate on mental function and cerebral blood flow in elderly patients. Br Med J 3:525–528, 1967.
18. Young, J., Hall, P., Blakemore, C. B.: Treatment of the cerebral manifestations of arteriosclerosis with cyclandelate. Br J Psychiatry 124:177–180, 1974.
19. Westreich, G., Alter, M., Lundgren, S.: Effects of cyclandelate on dementia. Stroke 6:535–538, 1975.
20. F.D.A. Drug Bulletin. Nov 1979.
21. Baso, A. J.: An ergot preparation (Hydergine) versus papaverine in treating common complaints of the aged: Double-blind study. J Am Geriatr Soc 21:63–71, 1973.
22. Einspruch, B. C.: The elderly patient and the nursing home: Therapeutic compatibility. Scientific Exhibit, Am Geriatr Soc, Toronto, Canada, April 17–18, 1974.
23. Nelson, J. J.: Relieving select symptoms of the elderly. Geriatrics 30:133, 1975.
24. Rosen, H. J.: Mental decline in the elderly: Pharmacotherapy (ergot alkaloids versus papaverine). J Amer Geriatr Soc 23:169, 1975.
25. Winslow, I. E.: The hospitalized geriatric patient, guidelines for effective therapy. Scientific Exhibit, Am Med Assoc Portland, Ore, Nov 30, 1974.
26. Gaitz, C. M., Garetz, F. K., Goldstein, S. E., et al.: Scientific Exhibit Am Gerontological Soc, Washington DC, Nov 1979.
27. Sathananthan, G. L., Gershon, S.: Cerebral vasodilators: A review, in Aging Vol. 2. Ed. by Gershon S., Raskin A. New York: Raven Press, 1975.
28. Dale, H. H.: On some physiologic actions of ergot. J Physiol 34:163–206, 1906.
29. Yesavage, J., Burian, E., Hollister, L.: Hydergine in senile dementias, 6

mg versus 3 mg dosage: A preliminary report. J Am Ger Soc 27:80–84, 1979.

30. Yesavage, J., Westphal, J., Rush, L.: Combined pharmacological and psychological treatment for dementias. Accepted for publication, J Am Ger Soc, 1980.

31. Yesavage, J., Tinklenberg, J., Berger, P., et al.: CINP Congress, Goteborg, Sweden, June 1980.

32. Theil, P.: La Perivincamine Dans le Mond La Medicine Practicienne. No. 571, Jan 1975.

33. Reisberg, B., Ferris, S., Gershon, S.: Psychopharmacologic aspects of cognitive research in elderly: Some current perspectives. Interdisc Topics Geront 15:132–152, 1979.

34. Bartus, R.: Four stimulants of the central nervous system: Effects on short-term memory in young versus aged monkeys. J Am Ger Soc 27:289–297, 1979.

35. Yesavage, J.: Drugs to alter cognitive function in the elderly. Geriatrics, Sept 1979.

36. Wells, C. E.: Pseudodementia. Am J Psychiat 136:895–900, 1979.

37. Shader, R. I., Harmatz, J., Salzman, C.: A new scale for clinical assessment in geriatric populations: Sandoz Clinical Assessment–Geriatric (SCAG). J Am Geriatr Soc 22:107–113, 1974.

# CHAPTER 10

# Lithium Treatment of the Aged

David L. Dunner, M.D.

Lithium carbonate has been proven to be effective in treating acute manic states of bipolar manic depressive illness. Furthermore, the frequency and severity of recurrent episodes of both mania and depression are reduced when lithium is given on a maintenance basis to bipolar manic depressive patients (1). Since bipolar illness affects people of all ages, lithium treatment is increasingly used among aged patients, both for treatment of acute episodes and for maintenance therapy. In addition, recent studies have suggested that lithium may be of some use in the control of behavioral consequences of organic mental syndromes among the aged (2). In spite of the increasing clinical use of lithium in the aged, however, there is a paucity of data concerning precautions regarding lithium use among the elderly as well as pharmacokinetic aspects of lithium therapy. This chapter discusses the pharmacokinetics and metabolism of lithium carbonate, indications for lithium use in the elderly, side effects, and special precautions regarding the use of lithium carbonate in elderly patients.

## PHARMACOKINETICS AND METABOLISM OF LITHIUM

Lithium is rapidly absorbed from the gastrointestinal tract. Plasma lithium peaks 1–3 hours after an oral dose. The usual biological "half-life" of lithium is 24 hours. Lithium is primarily excreted into the urine, with very small percentages being excreted in the feces and sweat. During steady state conditions, there is lithium balance; that is, the amount of lithium ingested equals or nearly equals the amount of lithium excreted in the urine on a daily basis. The renal excretion of lithium is dependent upon an adequate sodium and fluid intake.

During steady state conditions, the plasma lithium concentration (8–24 hours after a dose) will be relatively constant from day to day. Similarly, the cellular lithium concentration, as reflected by the erythrocyte:lithium concentration, will be relatively constant. Although lithium is commonly measured in plasma, it should be noted that the clinical effects (and toxic effects) of lithium are probably related to intracellular, rather than extracellular, lithium concentrations.

Recent studies have suggested that intracellular lithium concentration (using the erythrocyte model) is regulated by an energy-dependent process that has been termed the "lithium pump" (3, 4). A constant ($\kappa 0$) rate for lithium efflux from the erythrocyte can be determined in erythrocytes from persons who have not been treated with lithium. $\kappa 0$ is decreased during lithium treatment and further decreased during lithium toxic states (5). A proposed model relates $\kappa 0$ to calcium ATPase activity, although further work is clearly necessary to establish the mechanism of lithium efflux (6).

Alterations of lithium steady state will result in changes in intracellular lithium concentration. The important clinical points for alteration of lithium steady state are intake of lithium, alterations in renal (glomerular) function, and alterations in reabsorption.

A decrease in intake will result in efflux of lithium from cells. An increase in intake will result in greater lithium urinary excretion and increased intracellular lithium. Lithium administration results in a temporary natriuresis, kaliuresis, and diuresis (7). Lithium toxicity can result from continued increased intake because of at least 2 mechanisms. The buildup of intracellular lithium will increase $\kappa 0$ inhibition, and the natriuresis will result in increased lithium reabsorption by the renal tubule. Both mechanisms increase cellular lithium.

Decreases in glomerular filtration (due to dehydration or acute renal disease) can result in lithium toxicity if the lithium dose is maintained. The cellular concentration will increase in response to an increase in plasma concentration.

Alterations in reabsorption can be due to renal disease, ureteral block, or changes in sodium intake. Diuretics will result in an increase in lithium in cells since more lithium is reabsorbed when conditions of reduced sodium reabsorption exist. A sudden decrease in sodium intake can result in a similar increase in lithium reabsorption. In addition, sodium loss (sweating) can also result in lithium toxicity through these mechanisms.

The lithium toxic patient has high cellular lithium with impaired ability for cellular excretion of lithium. The toxic patient may be dehydrated (secondary to polyuria) and may have a lowered total body potassium (reflecting kaliuresis and the fact that potassium is largely an intracellular ion).

During steady state conditions, lithium plasma concentrations are 0.8–1.2 mEq/L, and erythrocyte lithium concentrations are about 50% of the plasma concentrations. During lithium toxicity the erythrocyte: plasma lithium ratio is increased, but the cellular lithium concentration is rarely above 2 mEq/L. In contrast, intracellular potassium is about 70 mEq/L, and even during lithium toxic states, lithium accounts for considerably less than 5% of intracellular cation concentration. Thus, the neurotoxic signs and symptoms of lithium toxicity are probably related to indirect (rather than direct) effects of increased intracellular lithium, possibly through an alteration of intracellular calcium metabolism.

Although the mechanisms discussed above have largely been established in studies of younger patients, the principles apply to the elderly. Furthermore, it should be clear that the elderly are at greater risk of lithium toxicity than younger patients because of several factors, including greater prevalance of renal disease and impaired sodium and fluid intakes. The margin of safety for lithium is considerably less in older than in younger patients.

## CLINICAL INDICATIONS FOR LITHIUM IN THE ELDERLY

Lithium is clearly indicated for the treatment of acute mania and for maintenance treatment in bipolar manic depressive patients. Lithium is frequently used for the prevention of recurrent unipolar depression, but although this indication is supported by research data, it was not approved by the FDA as of 1981. The use of lithium in other psychiatric conditions is essentially not approved, although lithium may be of benefit in the treatment of behavioral disturbances associated with some organic mental syndromes (2).

Manic depressive illness is characterized by periods of mania and depression. Manic episodes are characterized by change in mood and by symptoms such as increased activity, decreased need for sleep, grandiosity, rapid thinking, rapid speech, and impulsive behavior. Depressive episodes are characterized by low mood, loss of interest, hopelessness, helplessness, trouble concentrating, feeling suicidal, suicide attempts, loss of energy, and sleep disturbance. Data support the notion that patients who exhibit a manic syndrome complicated by Schneiderian first rank symptoms should be diagnosed as having manic depressive illness (8, 9). What is not clear is how to classify patients who have an acute psychosis not characterized by symptoms of mania or depression. Research suggests that such patients do not have schizophrenia. However, the absence of inclusion criteria for bipolar affective disorder makes the diagnosis of manic depressive illness in such patients problematic. This is one of the groups whose manic depressive illness may be overdiagnosed and to whom lithium treatment may be given, perhaps, on an appropriate basis. It should be noted that the number of patients who become toxic with any given treatment increases in proportion to the number of patients who receive that treatment. Thus, the increase in use of lithium will undoubtedly result in a greater number of patients becoming toxic or suffering adverse side effects during lithium treatment.

Knowledge of the clinical course of manic depressive illness may be important in determining which patient should receive lithium treatment. For example, approximately 40% of patients with 1 manic depressive cycle will not have a recurrence of this cycle over a long period of time (10). Although episode frequency may be quite variable in a given patient, on the average, the episodes tend to increase in frequency with age. The average frequency of episodes is 3–4 per 10 years, and patients with a late age of onset seem to have the same episode frequency as patients with an early age of onset (11). Thus, lithium maintenance treatment in the aged may not be warranted unless there is a history of cyclical behavior of sufficient episode frequency to justify the treatment.

## USE OF LITHIUM IN ACUTE DEPRESSION

Once patients are begun on lithium maintenance, treatment should be continued indefinitely (12). Thus, there will be an increasing number of elderly patients whose lithium maintenance was begun earlier in life. If the use of lithium is approved for conditions other than bipolar illness, the numbers of lithium-treated elderly patients may be extraordinary.

Recently, lithium has been used and been reported to be effective in the control of behavioral manifestations of organic mental syndromes, particularly in elderly patients (2). The literature has been composed primarily of individual case reports. Our experience with lithium use for this purpose has mixed results. For example, we admitted a patient this past year who was maintained on lithium for control of agitated behavior. He was found to be lithium responsive by treating him with lithium and then withholding lithium and noting subsequent behavioral change. However, during a year of maintenance therapy, he developed lithium toxicity.

## SIDE EFFECTS OF LITHIUM
## AND LITHIUM TOXICITY

Lithium is generally well tolerated, even by the elderly. The usual side effects of lithium include nausea, vomiting, diarrhea, tremor, slight polyuria, and thirst. Most patients tolerate these side effects extremely well. Lithium toxicity, on the other hand, can be fatal. It is characterized by an increase in polyuria with excretion of body fluids, resulting in dehydration and salt depletion, particularly of sodium and potassium. There are behavioral disturbances, notably confusion, and neurotoxicity is also evidenced by hyperactive reflexes, delirium, coma, and at times seizures.

Other medical consequences of lithium treatment include hypothyroidism. Lithium has an antithyroid effect that can become clinically significant in a small percent of patients (13). Cardiac sinus node dysfunction may also result from lithium treatment. It was noted in a previous study that cardiac sinus node dysfunction seemed limited to elderly patients and that the mechanism for this was probably to bring about an earlier clinical manifestation of cardiac dysfunction in patients who were probably predisposed to it (14). Interestingly enough, the cardiac sinus node is a calcium-dependent group of cells, and the fact that lithium inhibits these cells gives some support to the notion of lithium efflux being related to a calcium-dependent process. At any rate, we have recommended that patients undergoing lithium treatment receive a thorough medical evaluation, including an ECG. Baseline kidney function is also important. There has been recent concern that maintenance lithium treatment may result in chronic renal disease, although the clinical significance of the renal abnormalities associated with lithium maintenance is in dispute (15, 16).

## COMPLICATIONS OF TREATMENT

Complications of treatment can be separated into complications of initiating treatment, complications due to development of medical problems, and complications relating to maintenance treatment (17, 18). In considering the complications of initiating treatment, it should be noted that older patients are more likely to have medical problems, including cardiac and renal disease, than are younger patients. In addition, hypertension is a fairly frequent problem among older patients, and this is often treated with diuretics. Since diuretics change sodium metabolism, we have suggested that patients be switched to nondiuretic antihypertensives because the change in sodium metabolism resulting from concomitant use of lithium and diuretics effectively reduces the safety margin for lithium. Furthermore, there are many older patients who are on sodium restrictive diets, and this should be noted by the treating physician. In beginning older patients on lithium, it may be advisable to hospitalize the patient to initiate treatment. The baseline medical workup can be done best in the hospital, and the dose:blood-level relationships of lithium can be determined better in the hospital in older patients. It is important to keep in mind that the doses given to older patients should be quite low, and blood levels should be taken frequently in order to determine safety parameters. It should be noted that manic patients often take in a greater amount of fluids and salts when manic than when depressed, and it may be necessary to give older acutely manic patients higher doses of lithium and to be careful to decrease the dose after they become depressed. Another complicating factor is that patients, as they become depressed, may restrict their caloric and fluid intake, and may develop toxicity just because of reduction in salt intake.

## COMPLICATIONS CAUSED BY DEVELOPMENT OF MEDICAL PROBLEMS

Most patients who are on lithium develop stable blood levels in relation to their dose, and this is certainly true of older patients as well as younger ones. Older patients are maintained at lower plasma lithium concentrations than younger patients. However, since older patients are more prone to medical problems than younger patients, any change in the medical condition of patients may result in a change in lithium metabolism. For example, the development of medical illness that may entail a change in food (sodium, fluid) intake could result in the older patient developing lithium toxicity. Furthermore, the patient should be advised to decrease or stop lithium intake prior to any surgical procedure involving general anesthesia.

We have found that many internists and family doctors are not familiar with the relationship of lithium balance and sodium balance, and may advise the patient to decrease the sodium intake or may advise the patient to begin treatment with a diuretic. It should be emphasized that any change in sodium intake or excretion may result in a change in lithium balance, usually toward the development of lithium toxicity.

## COMPLICATIONS OF MAINTENANCE TREATMENT

Complications of maintenance treatment include development of sinus node dysfunction, lithium toxicity itself, and the problem of lack of a supporting social environment in which to take lithium. Sinus node dysfunction occurs largely among elderly patients. Furthermore, in assessing electrocardiograms of patients over the age of 60 in the lithium clinic in New York, we found that a number of these patients had an increase in the PR interval. Our impression is that sinus node dysfunction is a medical condition that occurs with a certain frequency and that by chance occurs in a lithium-treated population, perhaps accentuated by lithium treatment.

Lithium toxicity is an important consideration since this condition can be fatal. Surviving patients may have long-term renal side effects. Over half of the cases of lithium toxicity we observed in New York were patients over 60. Also, it is important to note that these patients had toxic side effects at much lower plasma concentrations than younger patients. A third complication relates to the fact that many elderly patients live alone and may have difficulty in taking a medication regularly or maintaining a normal diet, both of which are quite important regarding lithium treatment.

There is a good deal of concern about chronic renal effects of lithium. Although this area is still being investigated, it seems likely that patients who develop renal disease of any clinical severity with lithium are patients who would have been prone to develop renal disease without lithium. However, it should be noted that many patients develop a mild polyuria during lithium treatment.

In summary, lithium can be a very safe and useful drug in the treatment of bipolar manic depressive illness in older patients. Perhaps lithium is also of use in the treatment of confusional states. However, the clinician should carefully consider the use of lithium in an older patient, taking into account the patient's medical history and social circumstances before prescribing this drug. Blood checks should be made at least at monthly intervals. Furthermore, the patient may need to be hospitalized to begin treatment. Lithium toxicity often begins rather abruptly in older patients, and the patient's family should be advised

144

fully of the symptoms of lithium toxicity before lithium treatment is initiated. Other medical problems, such as sinus node dysfunction, may be more frequent among the elderly, who may require medical monitoring on a routine basis. In spite of these precautions, lithium may be of particular benefit to older patients because of the increasing frequency of episodes of manic depressive illness with advancing age.

## REFERENCES

1. Dunner, D. L., Fieve, R. R.: "The effect of lithium in depressive subtypes" in *Neuropsychopharmacology* Deniker, P., Radouco-Thomas, C., Villeneure, A., eds., 1978, Pergamon Press, New York pp 1109–1115.
2. Rosenbaum A. H., Barry M. J., Jr.: Positive therapeutic response to lithium in hypomania secondary to organic brain syndrome. *Amer. J. Psychiat.* 132:1072–1073, 1975.
3. Meltzer, H. L., Rosoff, C., Kassir, S., et al.: Active efflux of lithium from erythrocytes of manic-depressive subjects. *Life Sci. 9:* 371–380, 1976.
4. Dunner, D. L., Meltzer, H. L., Fieve, R. R.: Clinical correlates of the lithium pump. *Amer. J. Psychiat.* 135:1062–1064, 1978.
5. Meltzer, H. L., Kassir, S., Dunner, D. L., et al.: Repression of a lithium pump as a consequence of lithium ingestion by manic-depressive subjects. *Psychopharmacology* 54:113–118, 1977.
6. Meltzer, H. L.: Personal communication.
7. Baer, L., Platman, S. R., Kassir, S., et al.: Mechanisms of renal lithium handling and their relationship to mineralocorticoids: A dissociation between sodium and lithium ions. *J. Psychiat. Res.* 8:91–105, 1971.
8. Dunner, D. L., Rosenthal, N. E.: Schizoaffective states. *Psychiat. Clin. North Amer.* 2:441–448, 1978.
9. Rosenthal, N. E., Rosenthal, L. N., Stallone, F., et al.: Toward the validation of RDC schizoaffective disorder. *Arch. Gen. Psychiat.* 37:804–810, 1980.
10. Pollock, H. M.: Recurrence of attacks in manic-depressive psychoses. *Amer. J. Psychiat* 11:562–573, 1931.
11. Dunner, D. L., Murphy, D, Stallone, F, et al.: Episode frequency prior to lithium treatment in bipolar manic-depressive patients. *Compr. Psychait.* 20:511–515, 1979.
12. Fleiss, J. L., Prien, R., Dunner, D. L., et al.: Actuarial studies of the course of manic-depressive illness. *Compr. Psychiat.* 19:335–362, 1978.
13. Cho, J. T., Bone, S., Dunner, D. L., et al.: The effect of lithium treatment on thyroid function in patients with primary affective disorder. *Amer. J. Psychiat.* 136:115–116, 1979.
14. Roose, S. P., Nurnberger, J. I., Dunner, D. L., et al.: Cardiac sinus node dysfunction during lithium treatment. *Amer. J. Psychiat.* 136:804–807, 1979.

15. Jenner, F. A.: "Lithium and the kidney" in *Lithium/Controversies and Unresolved Issues*, Cooper T. B., Gershon S., Kline N. S., et al., eds, Excerpta Medica, Amsterdam, 1979, pp. 567–577.
16. Colt, E. W. D., Igel, G., Fieve, R. R., et al.: Lithium associated neuropathy. *Amer. J. Psychiatr. 136:*1098–1099, 1979.
17. Roose, S. P., Bone, S., Haidorfer, C., et al.: Lithium treatment in older patients. *Amer. J. Psychiat. 136:*843–844, 1979.
18. Dunner, D. L., Roose, S. P., Bone, S.: "Complications of lithium treatment in older patients" in *Lithium/Controversies and Unresolved Issues*, Cooper T. B., Gershon S., Kline N. S., et al. eds, Excerpta Medica, Amsterdam, 1979, pp. 427–431.

# CHAPTER 11

# Psychotropic Drug Side Effects in the Elderly

Carl Salzman, M.D.

As people age, they are increasingly likely to experience side effects of drugs of all kinds, including psychotropic drugs (1–3). Clinical experience suggests that these older psychotropic drug recipients are also more likely to experience adverse effects (4–6). The most common psychotropic drug side effects in the elderly are neurological (sedation, confusion, extrapyramidal) and cardiovascular (hypotension, arrythmias) (see Table 11.1).

The elderly are predisposed to adverse drug reactions because of three age-related changes (see Table 11.2). First, the body's ability to metabolize and excrete drugs decreases with age. This leads to higher circulating levels of the unmetabolized drug and a prolonged sojourn of this drug in the body (altered pharmacokinetics). Second, there is a tendency for increased central nervous sensitivity to psychotropic drugs so that older people often become toxic on doses that are routinely prescribed to younger adults (increased receptor site sensitivity). Third, older people are more likely to be taking a variety of drugs for treatment of age-related medical illness (polypharmacy). The interaction between medical, over-the-counter, and psychotropic drugs often results in severe drug toxicity.

Since adverse drug effects in the elderly are common to different classes of psychotropic drugs, this chapter is organized according to the category of side effect. An attempt is made to compare different drugs within each category of side effect, and within the context of clinical medical and psychiatric practice.

TABLE 11.1 Common Side Effects of Psychotropic Drugs in the Elderly

| Drug Effect | Symptoms |
| --- | --- |
| Decreased central nervous system arousal level | Sedation, apathy, withdrawal, depressed mood, disinhibition, confusion |
| Peripheral anticholinergic blockade | Dry mouth, constipation, atonic bladder, aggravation of narrow-angle glaucoma, and prostatic hypertrophy |
| Central anticholinergic blockade | Confusion, disorientation, agitation, assaultiveness, visual hallucinosis |
| Alpha-adrenergic blockade and central pressor blockade | Orthostatic hypotension |
| Quinidine effect, anticholinergic effect, decreased myocardial contractility | Tachycardia, cardiac arrhythmia, heart block, increased P–R interval and widening of QRS complex, decreased ionotropic effect, heart failure |
| Dopaminergic blockade | Extrapyramidal symptoms, (?) tardive dyskinesia |

TABLE 11.2 Etiology of Psychotropic Drug Side Effects in the Elderly

| Change | Result | Clinical Consequence | References |
| --- | --- | --- | --- |
| Altered pharmaco-kinetics | Decreased protein binding, excretion, and metabolism; increased distribution | Prolonged action of toxic levels of psychotropic drug | (34–38) |
| Decreased dopamine and choline acetyl-transferase in CNS | Increased sensitivity to receptor blockade; Increased clinical sensitivity | Increased extrapyramidal symptoms; increased anticholinergic toxicity; need lower doses | (2, 11, 31, 39, 40) |
| Polypharmacy and drug-drug interactions | May alter kinetics and/or receptor sensitivity | Increased toxic consequences of common drug interactions | (1, 2, 12, 13, 14, 34, 41) |

# SEDATION

A variety of psychotropic drugs may cause daytime drowsiness and sedation in the elderly patient (see Table 11.3). These include benzodiazepines (7–11), sedating neuroleptics such as chlorpromazine and chlorprothixene (see Table 11.6), and sedating tricyclic antidepressants such as amitriptyline and doxepin (see Table 11.7) (2, 3). In older patients, sedation may be misinterpreted by the physician as depression. Day-

TABLE 11.3 Psychotropic Drugs Commonly Associated with Sedation in the Elderly

| Neuroleptics | All benzodiazepines |
|---|---|
| Chlorpromazine | |
| Thioridazine | |
| Chlorprothixene | |
| | |
| Tricyclic antidepressants | All hypnotics |
| Amitriptyline | |
| Doxepin | |

time sedation may cause nighttime insomnia, or may contribute to a decline in the older patient's contact with his or her environment. This, in turn, may lead to a sense of isolation, helplessness, and depression and to a decline in cognitive performance (see "Confusion," below).

In older medical or surgical patients, psychotropic drugs may augment the sedation produced by medical drugs. It is not uncommon to encounter an elderly patient who is receiving a narcotic and/or analgesic for pain, in combination with one or more sedating psychotropic drugs. In one survey, for example, at least 1 narcotic (often more than 1) was prescribed to three-quarters of elderly patients who were receiving a hypnotic drug or tricyclic (usually amitriptyline). Narcotics were also prescribed to 9 out of 10 diazepam recipients and to half of those older patients who received a neuroleptic (12, 13).

## CONFUSION

Confusion in the older person taking psychotropic drugs may result from three causes:

1. decreased central nervous system arousal levels (sedation)
2. anticholinergic toxicity
3. lithium toxicity (see Table 11.4)

Confusion that results from a decrease in central nervous system arousal levels (i.e., sedation) resembles Sundowner's syndrome. In mild forms, the older person may be restless and have trouble concentrating or recalling recent information. In more severe cases, there may be agitation, misidentification of familiar people, wandering, and assaultiveness. This syndrome is worse when there is a lack of familiar orienting stimuli.

TABLE 11.4 Psychotropic Drug Causes of Confusion in the Elderly

| Type | Drug | Reference |
|---|---|---|
| Decreased CNS arousal levels | Any sedating psychotropic drug; reported with benzodiazepines | (8–10) |
| Anticholinergic activity | Tricyclic antidepressants, especially amitriptyline; neuroleptics, especially thioridazine; anticholinergic drugs | (2, 42) (43) (43) |
| Lithium | Confusion even at relatively low blood levels | (44) |

Older patients who have been recently hospitalized, or have moved, or have entered a nursing home are particularly susceptible. The syndrome is seen in its most severe form in the hospital intensive care unit. Here the older patient frequently tries to climb out of bed; tries to pull out tubes, catheters, and sutures; and becomes frightened, paranoid, and assaultive. Although sedation is often necessary for such a patient, care must be taken not to further aggravate confusion with additional drug toxicity.

Confusion caused by lithium is common in the elderly (14). It is similar to Sundowner's syndrome, but may also include other signs and symptoms of lithium toxicity such as tremor, increased fluid intake, and increased urine output.

Confusion caused by anticholinergic toxicity is more common and more severe in older people (2). In mild forms, it also resembles Sundowner's syndrome. In more severe cases, it includes repetitive stereotyped behavior, delerium, and assaultiveness. In very severe cases of toxicity, these symptoms may be life-threatening. For example, an older person may not be able to eat or conduct self-care activities, and may become self-mutilating. In the hospital, he or she may interfere with medical and nursing care, and become almost unmanageable. In the nursing home, the patient may attack other residents, staff, and family members.

Among the antidepressants, amitriptyline is the most anticholinergic, followed by imipramine, doxepin, and nortriptyline. Desipramine is the least anticholinergic tricylic (see Table 11.7). Maprotiline is a tetracyclic antidepressant reputed to have low anticholinergic properties. However, this drug has not been studied in older patients. Among the neuroleptic drugs, thioridazine and chlorpromazine have the strongest anticholinergic effects (see Table 11.6).

In older medical or surgical patients, severe anticholinergic toxicity may result from the interaction of these psychotropic drugs with medical drugs that also have anticholinergic properties (14). Meperidine (Demerol), for example, or atropine or atropine-like drugs are commonly used in association with surgery. Over-the-counter sleeping and antihistamine preparations also have anticholinergic properties. Antiparkinson drugs such as trihexyphenidyl (Artane) or benztropine (Cogentin) are used to treat endogenous parkinsonian symptoms as well as the extrapyramidal effects of neuroleptics (see below). It is not uncommon for the older patient to be taking at least one of these drugs in association with an anticholinergic tricyclic or neuroleptic medication. Since there is an increased sensitivity in the aging central nervous system to cholinergic blockade, the result of this poylpharmacy is often severe toxicity.

## ORTHOSTATIC HYPOTENSION

Orthostatic hypotension probably results from blockade of cerebral vasomotor centers, peripheral alpha-adrenergic blockade, as well as decrease in myocardial contractility (4, 15).

In the elderly patient, orthostatic hypotension is a frequent drug side effect that may precipitate falls with fractures, strokes, or even heart attacks. The drugs most responsible for producing hypotension are neuroleptics and tricyclics. Forty percent of geriatric patients in one survey complained of dizziness and falling. Seventeen percent of these patients were taking a phenothiazine, 11% a tricyclic alone and 23% a tricyclic with another drug. Patients who suffered from cervical osteoarthritis of low cardiac output were especially vulnerable (16). Orthostatic hypotensive episodes commonly occur at night, when the older person awakens to urinate. Older patients who take a psychotropic drug that produces hypotension should be advised, therefore, to arise slowly from the recumbent position (17). Supportive stockings may be used, but drugs that elevate blood pressure, such as amphetamines, may aggravate psychosis and should be avoided. Epinephrine will further lower blood pressure due to beta receptor activity, and should also be avoided (4).

If milligram equivalent doses of neuroleptic drugs are compared in elderly patients, chlorpromazine and thioridazine are more likely to produce orthostatic hypotension than other neuroleptic drugs (2, 3, 5). Drugs of the piperazine type of phenothiazines (acetophenazine, perphenazine, trifluoperazine, and fluphenazine) or butyrophenone (haloperidol) are less likely to cause a decrease in blood pressure (18). Since neuroleptic drugs that produce orthostatic hypotension also are sedating, the selection of a sedating neuroleptic for clinical purposes may entail a concomitant risk of a drop in blood pressure (see Table 11.6).

Potential drop in blood pressure with tricyclic antidepressants is not age related, but its consequences may be more severe in the elderly. Orthostatic hypotension is probably the most common cardiovascular side effect of imipramine (19), and is particularly dangerous in older patients with preexisting cardiovascular disease (20). Eleven percent of elderly patients receiving tricyclics alone were reported to experience orthostatic hypotension; this rose to 23% when taken with other drugs, particularly thiazide diuretics (16). (In general, volume-depleting diuretics will exacerbate tricyclic-induced orthostatic hypotension [21].)

Orthostatic hypotension has also been observed in patients receiving amitriptyline, desipramine, and doxepin (see Table 11.6) (22). Recent evidence suggests that nortriptyline may be relatively free of this side effect, and suggests an advantage for this tricyclic in elderly patients with preexisting cardiac disease (2, 22). Monoamine oxidase inhibitors have also been associated with orthostatic hypotension (16, 23), although a recent study of phenelzine and tranylcypromine in the elderly did not mention hypotension as a side effect (24).

At therapeutic levels, lithium does not seem to have an effect on blood pressure in humans, although there have been no specific studies of lithium effects on blood pressure in the aged (25).

## CARDIAC SIDE EFFECTS

Cardiac side effects of psychotropic drugs consist of alterations of rate, rhythm, and the force of myocardial contraction. There are only a few published case reports of these effects in the elderly. It is not clear, therefore, whether or not cardiac toxicity is correlated with increasing age, as it is with increasing dose (21). It seems certain, however, that these side effects are more hazardous in the patient with preexisting cardiac pathology (26). Since older people tend to be more likely to have cardiac disease than younger people, they may be more susceptible to serious cardiac toxicity of psychotropic drugs.

Most cardiac effects of psychotropic drugs are seen with neuroleptics, tricyclic antidepressants, and lithium. Benzodiazepines do not affect cardiac function, and there are no data implicating monoamine oxidase inhibitors in producing any effects other than blood pressure changes.

Neuroleptics and tricyclics cause tachycardia probably as a consequence of anticholinergic effects and direct effect on intraventricular conduction (15). Ventricular tachycardias may be due to the occurrence of a premature ventricular contraction during cardiac repolarization (27).

Neuroleptic and tricyclic alterations in conduction have been associated with atrial and ventricular arrhythmias and varying degrees of heart block (15, 21, 23, 27).

These alterations in rate and rhythm are reflected in characteristic ECG changes. In general, neuroleptics and tricyclics prolong the P–R and Q–T interval, widen the QRS complex, depress the S–T segment, and depress and notch the T wave (15, 28). There have not been specific studies of these changes in elderly patients, but examples of clinical reports of ECG changes in the elderly are shown in Table 11.5. Tricyclic antidepressants probably should be avoided in an elderly patient with prolonged Q–T$_c$ intervals or bundle branch block, unless cautiously treated in collaboration with a cardiologist.

Tricyclics and neuroleptics may have a direct effect on myocardial function as suggested by several studies (15, 21, 29). In the clinical setting, tricyclics have been associated with complete heart failure (25)

TABLE 11.5 Examples of ECG Changes in Elderly Patients Associated with Therapeutic Doses of Psychotropic Drugs

| Drug and Patient(s) | Effect | Reference |
|---|---|---|
| **Amitriptyline** | | |
| 65 patients, average age 65 | ST depressed; extra systoles | (45) |
| 73-year-old woman | Complete heart block | (46) |
| **Nortriptyline** | | |
| 65-year-old man | 1st degree heart block | (47) |
| 73-year-old woman | Complete heart block | (46) |
| **All tricyclics** | | |
| Elderly patients | Increased heart rate | (15) |
| **Imipramine** | | |
| 74-year-old man with right bundle branch block | 2:1 A-V block | (48) |
| **Lithium** | | |
| 65-year-old woman | A-V dissociation, PVC's | (49) |
| **Thioridazine** **Mesoridazine** | | |
| 64-year-old woman | Complete A-V block; bigeminy and ventricular fibrillation | (28) |
| **Chlorpromazine** | | |
| 73-year-old woman | Left bundle branch block | (28) |

and with the aggravation of preexisting congestive heart failure (30). As a general principle, therefore, tricyclics should not be given to elderly patients in congestive heart failure.

## EXTRAPYRAMIDAL SYMPTOMS

The extrapyramidal symptoms that result from neuroleptic medication tend to be more frequent and more severe in the elderly (4). This may be caused by altered pharmacokinetics of the neuroleptics, leading to higher blood levels and prolonged effect, as well as to decreased levels of dopamine in the aging nigrostriatal tract of the central nervous system. As many as 50% of all patients between 60 and 80 years old who receive neuroleptics develop extrapyramidal symptoms (31). The extrapyramidal symptoms that are commonly seen in the elderly are akathisia, parkinsonism, akinesia, and the Pisa syndrome.

Akathisia resembles agitation. The elderly patient with akathisia cannot sit still, sits and stands frequently, and paces. The patient may have "restless legs," and describes his muscles as tense or jittery. There also may be choreiform movements of the hands and trunk. Akathisia symptoms in the elderly may be misinterpreted as agitation. More neuroleptic is then given, which only worsens the symptoms. Parkinsonian symptoms resemble those of the clinical illness—shuffling gait, pill-rolling tremor, cog-wheel rigidity. Drug-induced parkinsonian side effects aggravate preexisting parkinsonism, and may disable a functioning older person. The peak incidence of drug-induced parkinsonism is in the eighth decade (32). Akinesia is an extrapyramidal side effect seen more

TABLE 11.6 Relative Side Effects of Representative Neuroleptic Drugs for the Elderly Patient

| Generic and Trade Names | Relative Incidence of Side Effects | | | |
|---|---|---|---|---|
| | Sedative | Hypotensive | Extrapyramidal | Anticholinergic |
| Chlorpromazine (Thorazine, Chlor-P2) | marked | marked | moderate | strong |
| Thioridazine (Mellaril) | marked | marked | mild–moderate | very strong |
| Acetophenazine (Tindal) | mild | mild | moderate | moderate |
| Trifluoperazine, thiothixene (Stelazine, Navane) | mild | mild | marked | mild |
| Haloperidol (Haldol) | minimal | minimal | very marked | mild |

TABLE 11.7 Relative Side Effects of Tricyclic Antidepressants for the Elderly Patient

| Tertiary Amine | Secondary Amine | Trade Name | Sedation | Hypotension | Anticholinergic | Arrhythmias |
|---|---|---|---|---|---|---|
| **Imipramine** | | Tofranil Immavate Antipress Janimine Presamine sk-Pramine | mild | moderate | moderate | moderate |
| | Desmethylimipramine | Norpramin Pertofrane | mild | mild | mild | mild |
| **Doxepin** | | Sinequan Adapin | moderate | moderate | moderate | mild |
| | Desmethyldoxepin | — | — | — | — | — |
| **Amitriptyline** | | Elavil Amitril Endep | strong | moderate | very strong | strong |
| | Nortriptyline | Aventyl Pamelor | mild | mild | moderate | mild |
| | Protriptyline | Vivactil | mild | mild | strong | mild |

TABLE 11.8  Symptoms of Tardive Dyskinesia

---

Vermicular (wavy) movements of tongue when at rest or protruded; "fly-catching"

Tongue pouching in cheek; (bon-bon sign)

Snorting, blowing, chewing (rhythmical)

Blinking

Choreiform movements of trunk, arms, big toe

Gait disturbances

---

commonly in older people that consists of decreased energy, decreased speech, and depressed or mask-like facies. The older patient may appear apathetic, withdrawn, and depressed; akinesia is often misdiagnosed as depression. The Pisa syndrome refers to a drug-induced dystonic reaction in geriatric patients in which the trunk is flexed to one side (33).

Although extrapyramidal symptoms can be treated with anticholinergic drugs such as trihexyphenidyl (Artane) or benztropine (Cogentin), these symptoms are best treated by lowering the dose of the neuroleptic or by switching to a drug that produces a lower incidence of extrapyramidal symptoms (see Table 11.6).

Tardive dyskinesia is a syndrome that may appear after a patient has received neuroleptics for more than a year. Although its appearance is not strictly correlated with advanced age, it is seen in older, chronically ill patients because they are likely to have been taking neuroleptics for a long time.

The syndrome consists of involuntary movements of the tongue, mouth, and face, with peripheral choreoathetoid components. In the older patient, the mouth movements are sometimes confused with the "gumming" movements of the edentulous person. The movements are made worse when the patient is distracted (see Table 11.8). There is no treatment for tardive dyskinesia, but neuroleptics should be stopped, if possible, to see whether the symptoms diminish.

# REFERENCES

1. Lamy, P. P.: Prescribing for the elderly. Littleton, Mass.: PSG Publishing, 1980.
2. Salzman, C.: A primer on geriatric psychopharmacology. Submitted for publication.
3. Salzman, C.: Geriatric psychopharmacology. In *Textbook of Geriatric Medicine*. ed. by J. R. Rowe and R. Besdine. Boston: Little, Brown, in press.
4. Salzman, C., Shader, R. I., Pearlman, M.: Psychopharmacology and the

elderly. In *Psychotropic Drug Side Effects*. ed. by R. I. Shader and A. DiMascio. Baltimore: Williams and Wilkins, 1980, pp 261–279.
5. Salzman C., Shader, R. I., van der Kolk, B. A.: Clinical psychopharmacology and the elderly patient. NY State J of Med 76:71–77, 1976.
6. Salzman, C.: Update on geriatric psychopharmacology. Geriatrics 34:87–90, 1979.
7. Boston Collaborative Drug Surveillance Program: Clinical depression of the central nervous system due to diazepam and chlordiazepoxide in relation to cigarette smoking and age. N. E. J. Med. 288:277–280, 1973.
8. Glascow, J F T. A neurological disorder associated with chlordiazepoxide therapy. Clin Toxicol 2:456–462, 1969.
9. Evans, J. G., Jarvis, E. H.: Nitrazepam in the elderly. Brit Med J 4:487–489, 1972.
10. Greenblatt, D. J., Allen, M. D., Shader, R. I.: Toxicity of high-dose flurazepam in the elderly. Clin Pharmac and Therap 21:355–361, 1977.
11. Castleden, C. M., George, C. F., Marcer, D., et al.: Increased sensitivity to nitrazepam in old age. Br Med J 1:10–12, 1977.
12. Salzman, C., van der Kolk, B. A.: Psychotropic drug prescriptions to elderly patients in a general hospital. J Am Geriat Soc 28:18–22, 1980.
13. Salzman, C., van der Kolk, B. A.: Psychotropic drugs and polypharmacy in elderly patients in a general hospital. J Geriat Psychiatry 12:167–176, 1979.
14. Salzman, C.: Polypharmacy and drug-drug interactions in the elderly. In *Geriatric Psychopharmacology*. ed. by K. Nandy. New York: Elsevier-North Holland, 1979, pp. 117–126.
15. Stimmel, B.: *Cardiovascular Effects of Mood-altering Drugs*. New York, Raven Press, 1979, pp 133–166.
16. Blumenthal, M. D., Davie, J. W.: Dizziness and falling in elderly psychiatric outpatients. Am J Psychiatry 137:203–206, 1980.
17. Salzman, C., van der Kolk, B. A., Shader, R. I.: Psychopharmacology and the geriatric patient. In *Manual of Psychiatric Therapeutics*. ed. by R. I. Shader. Boston: Little, Brown, 1975, pp 171–184.
18. Ban, T. A.: *Psychopharmacology for the Aged*. Basel, Karger, 1980.
19. Kantor, S. J., Glassman, A. H., Bigger, J. T., et al.: The cardiac effects of therapeutic concentrations of imipramine. Am J Psychiatry 135:534–538, 1978.
20. Mueller, O. E., Goodman, N., Bellett, S.: The hypotensive effect of imipramine hydrochloride in patients with cardiovascular disease. Clin Pharmacol Ther 2:300–307, 1961.
21. Kantor, S. J., Glassman, A. H.: The use of tricyclic antidepressant drugs in geriatric patients. In *Psychopharmacology of Aging*. ed. by C. Eisdorfer and W. E. Fann. New York: Spectrum, 1980, pp 99–117.
22. Roose, S., Glassman, A. H., Siris, S., et al.: Tricyclic antidepressant-induced postural hypotension: Comparative studies. Presented at the Annual Meeting, American Psychiatric Association, San Francisco, May 8, 1980.

23. Ebert, M. H., Shader, R. I.: Cardiovascular effects. In *Psychotropic Drug Side Effects*. ed. by R. I. Shader and A. DiMascio. Baltimore: Williams and Wilkins, 1970, pp 149–163.
24. Ashford, J. W., Ford, C. V.: Use of MAO inhibitors in elderly patients. Am J Psychiatry 136:1466–1467, 1979.
25. Jefferson, J. H., Greist, J. H.: The cardiovascular effects and toxicity of lithium. In *Psychopharmacology Update*. ed. by JM Davis and D. Greenblatt. New York: Grune and Stratton, 1979, pp 65–79.
26. Swett, C. P. Jr., Shader, R. I.: Cardiac side effects and sudden death in hospitalized psychiatric patients. Dis Nerv Syst 38:66–72, 1977.
27. Hollister, L. E.: Clinical pharmacology of psychotherapeutic drugs. New York: Churchill Livingstone, 1978, p 111.
28. Fowler, N. O., McCall, D., Chou, T. C. et al.: Electrocardiographic changes and cardiac arrythmias in patients receiving psychotropic drugs. Am J Cardiology 37:223–230, 1976.
29. Bigger, J. T., Kantor, S. J., Glassman, A. H., et al.: Cardiovascular effects of tricyclic antidepressant drugs. In *Psychopharmacology: A Generation of Progress*. ed. by M. A. Lipton, A. DiMascio, and K. F. Killam. New York: Raven Press, 1978, pp 1033–1046.
30. Edelstein, E. L.: Antidepressant drugs. In *Meyler's Side Effects of Drugs* ed. by M. N. G. Dukes. Amsterdam, Excerpta Medica, 1980, pp 21–42.
31. Hamilton L. D.: Aged brain and the phenothiazines. Geriatrics 21:131–138, 1966.
32. Ayd, F. J. Jr: Tranquilizers and the ambulatory geriatric patient. J Am Geriat Soc 8:909–914, 1960.
33. Sovner, R., DiMascio, A.: Extrapyramidal syndromes and other neurological side effects of psychotropic drugs. In *Psychopharmacology: A Generation of Progress*. ed. by M. A. Lipton, A. DiMascio, and K. F. Killam. New York: Raven Press, 1978, pp 1021–1032.
34. Salzman, C.: Key concepts in geriatric psychopharmacology: Altered pharmacokinetics and polypharmacy. *Psychiat. Clin. North Amer*. ed. by L. Jarvik. Philadelphia, W. B. Saunders, in press.
35. Hicks, R., Davis, J. M.: Pharmacokinetics in geriatric psychopharmacology. In *Psychopharmacology of Aging*. ed. by C. Eisdorfer and W. E. Fann. New York: Spectrum, 1980, pp 169–212.
36. Israili, Z. H.: Age-related change in pharmacokinetics of some psychotropic drugs and its clinical implications. In *Geriatric Psychopharmacology*. ed. by K. Nandy. New York: Elsevier-North Holland, 1979, pp 31–62.
37. Triggs, E. J., Nation, R. L.: Pharmacokinetics in the aged: A review. J. Pharmaco Biopharm 3:387–418, 1975.
38. Friedel, R. O.: Pharmacokinetics in the geropsychiatric patient. In *Psychopharmacology: A Generation of Progress*. ed. by M. A. Lipton, A. DiMascio, and K. F. Killam. New York: Spectrum, 1980, pp 1409–1505.
39. Samorajski, T.: Neurochemical changes in the aging human and nonhuman primate brain. In *Psychopharmacology of Aging*. ed. by C. Eisdorfer and W. E. Fann. New York: Spectrum, 1980, pp 145–168.

40. Siede, H., Mueller, H. F.: Choreiform movements as side effects of pheno-
    thiazine medication in geriatric patients. J Am Geriat Soc 15:517–522,
    1967.
41. Blashke, T. F., Cohen, S. N., Tatro, D. S. et al.: Drug-drug interactions
    and aging. In *Clinical Pharmacology and the Aged Patient.* ed. by L. F.
    Jarvik. New York: Raven Press, 1981, pp 11–26.
42. Davies, R. K., Tucker, G. J., Hanaco, M. et al.: Confusional episodes and
    antidepressant medication. Am J Psychiatry 131:127–131, 1971.
43. Snyder, S. H., Yamamura, H. I.: Antidepressants and the muscarinic ace-
    tylcholine receptor. Arch Gen Psychiatry 34:236–239, 1977.
44. Davis, J. M., Fann, W. E., El-Yousef, M. K. et al.: Clinical problems in
    treating the aged with psychotropic drugs. In *Psychopharmacology and
    Aging.* ed. by C. Eisdorfer and W. E. Fann. New York: Plenum Press,
    1973, pp 111–128.
45. Rasmussen, E. B., Kristjansen, P.: EKG changes during amitriptyline treat-
    ment. Am J Psychiatry 119:781–782, 1963.
46. Smith, R. R., Rusbatch, B. J.: Amitriptyline and heart block. Brit Med J
    3:311, 1967.
47. Ziegler, V. E., Co, B. T., Biggs, J. T.: Plasma nortriptyline levels and EKG
    findings. Am J Psychiatry 134:441–443, 1977.
48. Kantor, S. J., Bigger, T., Glassman, A. G. et al.: Imipramine-induced heart
    block. JAMA 231:1364, 1975.
49. Tseng, H. L.: Interstitial myocarditis probably related to lithium carbonate
    intoxication. Arch Pathology 92:444–446, 1971.

CHAPTER 12

# Drug Treatment in Elderly Psychiatric Patients

Monica D. Blumenthal, M.D., PH.D.

## INTRODUCTION

All of us are very much aware of the importance of the physician-patient relationship in good medical care. The last 40 years have brought enormous increases in our ability to combat disease, reduce disability, and promote health, but medicine remains as much an art as a science. It is to the art of prescribing medication to elderly patients that I wish to address myself here. Although we acknowledge the importance of viewing the patient as a person, the value of the physician-patient relationship, and the idiosyncracies of the individual case, we are all inclined to view drugs mainly in relationship to disease, pathophysiology, and pharmacology, kinetic and dynamic. In spite of the firm scientific underpinnings that anchor our pharmacotherapies, the personal characteristics of the patient and the physician-patient relationship remain indispensable ingredients in the success or failure of drug treatment. In dispensing drugs, the older patient teaches us over and over again the importance of dealing with the person whom the disease inhabits.

## PHYSICAL BARRIERS TO COMPLIANCE

When we prescribe drugs, the first thing we need to know is whether the patient is able to take the drugs as we prescribe them. In the younger patient, such considerations rarely require a second thought. In the older patient, numerous barriers may preclude the patient's ability

159

to comply, even though he desires to do so. The first barrier to compliance is simple and mechanical. Bubble packs may be extremely difficult for the elderly patient (1, 2). Many older patients cannot open the child-proof caps that are standard packaging for most medication. In fact, the caps that are meant to foil small and nimble fingers are probably a far greater barrier to the elderly individual with arthritic joints, poor proprioception, limited eyesight, and enfeebled muscles. Not all pharmacists honor requests for nonpediatric caps, although printed requests on your prescription pad can be helpful. Inspection of the patient's medication bottles and a call to the pharmacist can be more persuasive than a printed message, and are sometimes necessary.

The second possible barrier to the patient's taking medication lies in the patient's ability to recognize the medication and see the instruction. Many older patients suffer from poor vision. Proper labeling of bottles and large lettering is essential (3). White on a black background is most visible, although we rarely have the option of such elegant choices. For those whose vision is particularly poor, color coding may improve recognition of medications and, hence, compliance with the regimen (4). In all cases, it is essential that medication bottles be adequately labeled. Each medication should contain the name of the drug, the use for which it is prescribed, and explicit directions as to how the drug should be taken. For example, in prescribing the antidepressant amitriptyline, the bottle should read "amitriptyline 10 mg, for depression, one tablet, three times a day." It must always be kept in mind that the elderly patient is likely to be taking several medications for several illnesses; it is of utmost importance to assist him in differentiating between these medications in every way possible. No prescription should ever read "Use as directed," and "p.r.n." prescriptions are to be avoided whenever possible.

## MENTAL BARRIERS TO COMPLIANCE

A third factor that may interfere with the patient's ability to comply with the physician's regimen is the patient's mental status. It cannot be taken for granted that the older patient's mental functioning is sufficiently intact to allow him or her to follow instructions even if he or she is capable of reading them. It is estimated that among patients who are 80 years of age or older, 20% suffer from severe chronic organic brain syndromes. Such patients are not always easily recognized. In one British study, it was estimated that general practitioners failed to recognize dementia in 80% of their patients who were so affected (5).

A useful adjunct to any kind of medical treatment in the elderly is a brief mental status examination, which allows the practitioner to evaluate the patient's memory function, his ability to manipulate time, and his ability to make simple calculations. The mini mental status examination (6) is one example of an easily used screening test. In addition, it is essential for the practitioner to know whether or not the patient is able to exert sufficient initiative to manage his own medications. Many patients with minimal organic brain syndromes are disabled by the inability to initiate appropriate actions. This lack of initiative may be completely out of proportion to other cognitive disabilities, and cannot be measured on the usual mental status test. Ancillary history from a relative is very helpful in assessing this characteristic. Indeed, for many geriatric patients, the presence of a relative to corroborate and amplify the history is essential.

Most of us are inclined to think of the taking of medication as a relatively uncomplicated behavior. We write prescriptions, and the patient takes them. Unfortunately, medication-taking behaviors are not nearly as simple as one might think. The strikingly low compliance rates that have been discovered in a number of studies are ample testimony to the lack of simplicity of drug-taking behaviors (7). Let us consider for a moment the cognitive skills that are necessary to correct medication taking. First, it is necessary for the patient to be able to recognize the pills. This involves the use of vision, the ability to read, the ability to integrate visual materials, and the ability to follow written instructions. Of course, some people rely on their memory for instructions, but this often leads to unwanted complications.

The art of taking medication also requires that the patient have a reasonably intact memory and a good sense of the passage of time. Neither of these characteristics are easily come by. In order to take medication on a regular basis, it is necessary to remember how often you are to take it and when you last took it. This problem becomes considerably more complex when one is taking 3 or 4 medications, as many older people are; more so if one is taking 8 or 9, as do a considerable number of the elderly; let alone the 25–54 medication regimens that one occasionally encounters in the older individual. No one ought to be taking 25 or 50 medications, but some patients are nevertheless maintained on such regimens and are unable to remember the multitude of instructions and schedules. Each pill generates the problem of remembering whether or not one took it this morning at breakfast, or whether it was breakfast yesterday. The longer the medication has been prescribed, and the more medications there are, the more difficult it becomes to remember (8).

There are a variety of devices to assist the patient with these problems. There are 7-day pill containers into which the appropriate pills for
the day can be counted. One can give the patient a check sheet to mark
off when his pills have been taken, or the patient can be given a tear-off
calendar (9). These devices are useful, but they require a fairly compulsive individual to utilize them, and not every patient can be persuaded
to take such elaborate measures. Prepackaged labeled bubble containers
are often difficult for elderly patients to open, and hence are not as
useful as they might be in spite of the fact that some come labeled with
day and time of day when the pill is to be taken. A pill identification
card that has the medication pasted on the card next to the instruction
for how it is used can be very helpful. When a patient can neither
remember nor record having taken a pill, the problem of errors in
self-medication becomes serious. Fortunately, most patients are not as
vested in taking their pills as their physicians would like them to be, so
they are more likely to forget to take them than to take too many.
Nevertheless, we have seen serious overdoses occur precipitated by
repetitive drug-taking behaviors in patients who could not remember
taking their last pill. One rather hypochondriacal lady, with poor recent
memory and back pain, took sufficient aspirin-containing medication to
give herself a gastrointestinal bleed, all the while explaining vigorously
that she never took any medication because her caretakers wouldn't let
her have it. Eventually, this lady's medication had to be stored in a
locked cabinet.


## PATIENT EDUCATION AND DRUG-TAKING

In addition to good recent memory, another cognitive factor important
in medication-taking behavior is that the patient must be able to understand the nature of the pill he is taking and the medical indications for
it. I have always believed in patient education, and I have always spent
a considerable amount of time talking to my patients about the drugs
they are taking, what we expect from them, and what their side effects
are. I have been amazed and dismayed over and over again to find out
how little our patients understood about their medications and how
poorly equipped they were to participate in the collaborative relationship that is implicit in the care of chronic illness. In my experience,
patients have particular difficulty in understanding the relation between
drug effects and side effects; between necessary dietary compliance and
insulin or monoamine oxidase inhibitors, and with the necessity of re-
porting serious side effects such as falling. Nevertheless, a basic

knowledge of the medication and the pathophysiology is essential for the patient to collaborate. This is especially true for drug regimens in which the drug must be taken in spite of the fact that the patient feels relatively well, as is true in the treatment of hypertension and the maintenance treatment of affective disorders. Medication errors by the elderly are more common than not, and at least one study shows that 30–40% do not understand their medications (10, 11). Lack of understanding of the medication and its mechanism of action has caused several patients of mine to take antidepressants on a p.r.n. basis when they felt particularly badly, rather than as I prescribed them. As you might expect, such regimens tend to end in "treatment failure." Lack of understanding of medication also causes patients to terminate antidepressants when they start to feel well, often leading to relapse. Careful monitoring by the physician of how the patient is taking the prescribed medication is essential to effective treatment.

## SIMPLIFICATION OF DRUG REGIMENS

Simplification of the patient's drug regimen is undoubtedly the first step in trying to establish an optimal routine for the patient with long-term or psychiatric illness. We find many patients taking multiple medications often prescribed by a variety of physicians. The first approach to these patients is to discontinue as many drugs as possible since medication errors are related to the number of drugs prescribed (12). It is absolutely amazing what people can do without. Often, the indications for a particular drug in a particular patient are not clear. In such cases, the drug is best discontinued. If the patient truly requires the medication in question, the patient's subsequent course will amply demonstrate that fact, and the drug can be started again. Of course, it is essential to monitor a patient after a drug has been removed so that resurgence of disease or symptoms will be promptly dealt with.

Often, physicians will add drugs if one is not working properly. So it is not unusual to find patients on several pain medications, tranquilizers, or hypnotics, which taken together may have a cumulative effect. Obviously, a better route is to find a single drug that works. Many patients are on drugs of dubious merit such as papaverine. Other patients have complicated regimens for constipation. We see a small but very definite number of patients who are anticoagulated for long periods of time for unclear indications. Clearly, the best procedure in such cases is to review the indications for the medication with the internist and reduce the medication whenever possible. We see a large number of patients on second-order antihypertensives whose hypertension appears to respond very adequately to diuretics alone or even to no medication at all. The first question that the physician must ask himself when dealing with medication regimens, then, is whether or not drug therapy is required at all. Often, the answer will be no (13).

When a physician is adding a drug to control the side effect of another drug, as is frequently the case when psychotropics are prescribed, the question should always be considered whether the patient could do with a smaller dose of the primary drug or perhaps could do without the primary drug altogether. When the question arises of whether or not a patient requires an antidepressant, the question must always be asked whether or not the patient would do as well if a suitable schedule of activities were arranged. Would a friendly visitor, transportation to the senior citizens' center, or involvement by the patient's church make the patient less lonely and hence less depressed? Although many older patients require psychotropics, manipulation of the environment is often a crucial prerequisite to successful drug treatment, and may obviate the necessity for drug treatment in some patients.

When the physician asks whether or not drug therapy is required, he should always ask himself whether or not a nondrug regimen could serve the same purpose. If a patient is not sleeping well, could the insomnia be controlled by a regular prescribed exercise such as a daily walk, a glass of warm milk at bedtime, and an empty bladder and bowel on retiring? Does the patient have a comfortable bed? Has the patient avoided caffeinated beverages after lunch? Does the patient take long naps in the afternoon? Often, regulation of the patient's daily routine will produce sleep more satisfactorily than the use of any hypnotic. Attention to general principles of hygiene is a vital part of prescribing drugs to the old.

When the physician decides that a patient may do without a drug, or several drugs, he must then develop a plan for how to remove the medication. It is best to manipulate one drug at a time, and it is usually wise to taper the drug rather than discontinue it abruptly. Drugs should be tapered not only for physiological reasons, such as the avoidance of withdrawal effects, but also because many patients are psychologically dependent on their drugs and fearful of doing without them. This is particularly true of potent drugs such as digoxin or antihypertensives, for which the patient may have been given stern warnings about compliance by other physicians. If the drug is reduced in several steps, the patient can see that no harm results and develops confidence in the medication reduction plan.

After the physician has decided that the patient does actually re-

quire the drug, he must decide how the drug is to be divided throughout the day. Many drugs have longer half-lives in older people than they
do in the young. Drugs that must be given to young people in divided
doses can conveniently be given once daily to patients who are older
(14). Librium is a good example of such a drug. Other drugs such as
tricyclics, which we commonly give in single daily doses to young
people, are better given in divided doses to older people to minimize
acute side effects which are poorly tolerated. Nevertheless, the physician should aim for the fewest possible daily doses. Once a day is best,
followed by twice a day, and so on. If the patient is taking several drugs,
it is ideal if the patient is on the same drug regimen for all of them. If
the physician has a choice about whether to give a drug in two or more
doses, it is helpful to the patient if the schedules for the varying drugs
are all the same. Schedules that include a mixture of drugs given q.d.,
b.i.d., t.i.d., and q.i.d. are difficult—if not impossible—for the patient
to manage.

The physician who is asked to deal with an elderly patient with
psychiatric symptoms often finds himself in the position of having to
simplify and manage the patient's overall drug regimen. By far, the most
common problems seen in a geriatric psychiatry clinic are organic behavioral syndromes, depression, and paranoias. All three of these conditions can be caused by commonly used drugs (15–17), and the first step
in the treatment of these conditions is always to remove the patient from
drugs that might be a source of the behavioral syndrome. This invariably
means that the physician must assume an active and detailed interest in
all of the patient's medications and all of the patient's illnesses.

The physician who is trying to simplify the drug regimen of an
elderly patient soon will be confronted by the intricacies of the American medical care system—or noncare system, as some have called it.
The elderly patient, as we all know, is likely to suffer from several
chronic illnesses. He or she is also likely to have these illnesses treated
by several physicians. The American patient is accustomed to looking for
the care of a specialist. By the time the patient is 70 years old, he or she
may very well have several specialists. The patient who arrives complete
with surgeon, cardiologist, dermatologist, general family physician, and
gynecologist is not at all infrequent. The difficulty here is that while you
are trying to consolidate and reduce the patient's medications, some
other physician, unaware of your efforts, may be increasing them. Patients don't necessarily tell us about these things spontaneously, and
sometimes don't tell us even when we ask them. It is helpful, however,
to review the patient's medications with him or her, and to ask on each
visit if anything new has been added. It is also helpful to ask the patient

to bring in all medication bottles periodically for a detailed review. When a patient has several physicians, contact among them is important to the successful work of each.

## GENERIC VS. BRAND NAMES

We are becoming aware that all drugs are not alike and that in some cases—for example, Lanoxin and digoxin, amitriptyline and Elavil (18)—bioavailability may not be the same. So there may be pharmacologic reasons for not prescribing generic drugs. There are, however, an increasing number of laws that allow the pharmacist to make generic substitutions, and the generic drugs often have the advantage of being cheaper than the brand-name drugs. There are, however, several problems with the generic drugs in addition to the question of bioavailability. Generic drugs are likely to come in different shapes, sizes, and colors, from the brand-name drugs and from other generics of the same formula. This can be extremely confusing to the patient who identifies a medication as the little blue pill or the little red pill. It obviates the use of a pill card as an aid in compliance. For patients who are not as mentally alert as they might be, the variability in size and shape of generic drugs may present a major difficulty, and for this group prescribing by the brand name may be best. Patients also have the disconcerting habit of using pill boxes or, worse, placing all their medications in one bottle. The bottle may be an old one that happens to have a screw top, and no medication in the bottle may match the label. Under these circumstances (and it is extremely difficult to talk patients out of doing this), the additional variety produced by generic prescribing is most unwelcome. In addition, the patient may not understand that the brand name and the generic name are the same drug and, of course, the brand and generic drug will not look alike. Consequently, the patient may believe the pills represent entirely different drugs. Recently, I had an elderly patient with a very serious depression for which she was eventually hospitalized. She was discharged from the hospital on 75 mg of Tofranil daily. I followed her as an outpatient, and prescribed for her 75 mg of imipramine daily. The patient, unbeknownst to me, continued to have her Tofranil prescription filled while she also complied with my imipramine regimen. She developed a series of falls that she did not report, and eventually fractured her wrist, undoubtedly a complication of tricyclic overdosage caused by confusion of brand and generic name. The problem of patient confusion caused by different professionals using different names for the same drug has been noted by others (19). The physician should be aware that the pharmacist may sometimes substitute a brand for a generic name on the bottle, compounding the confusion that may exist between physician and patient.

## MEDICATION MANAGEMENT FOR THE CONFUSED PATIENT

So far we have been talking about general aspects of drug taking in the patient who is motivated to take medication and is cognitively able to comply. That brings us to further problems: first, the patient who cannot manage his medication and, second, the patient who is not motivated to comply. The first case is relatively simple. When the patient is not able to take his own medication, some arrangement must be made for the patient's medication to be supervised. The supervision may be provided by a spouse, a child, or other relative, or by a professional such as a visiting nurse or a caseworker. When the medication is supervised by a relative who is also elderly, the same assessment of cognitive skill of the relative must be undertaken as must be made of the older patient. It is not unusual to find that the relative of a mentally impaired older patient is also somewhat mentally disabled and is not able to supervise a complicated medical regimen. When the patient lives alone, the problem is more complex. Unless a willing relative will help, there may be serious difficulties, since few American agencies will provide daily care.

## THE NONCOMPLIANT PATIENT

Equally difficult is the case of patients who are not motivated to comply with the physician's regimen. Older people often have very strong feelings about their drugs. Some of them are dependent on their medication and extremely fearful if medication is removed: others are extremely reluctant to take medication. Somehow, they feel, they ought to be able to manage by themselves without having to rely on crutches such as pills. Pill-taking becomes the symbol of ill health, and the patient may feel better about himself if he is not taking any medication, even though he may not actually be doing as well on a physiological level. Such patients are likely to abandon medication regimens prematurely, to fail to comply with drug increases, and to take medication on a p.r.n. basis rather than continually, as prescribed. The physician can keep informed of whether or not the patient is in compliance by writing prescriptions that are not refillable, keeping track of the number of pills that have been prescribed, and calculating whether the patient has run out at the appropriate time or not. Engaging in an occasional pill count can also be useful. We have found regular pill counts more difficult than they sound in theory because patients often forget to bring their bottles to the clinic. In addition, patients miss appointments, and friendly pharmacists refill prescriptions even when there is no order to do so. I am aware of no way to make the noncompliant patient comply 100% of the time. I do know that in order to manage the noncompliant patient, it is essential for the physician to recognize that the patient is not taking the medication properly. The physician must then convey to the patient that the drug is essential to the treatment and that the physician expects the patient to comply. An important ingredient in obtaining the patient's compliance is the patient's understanding of the nature of the drug and its expected action. Unfortunately, patients with organic behavioral syndromes and serious depressions in old age are often not able to understand the nature of the information that the physician is trying to impart; patients with organic behavioral syndrome suffer cognitive limitations; patients with depressive disorders are intensely preoccupied with their own troubles and worries and, in some cases are cognitively impaired as well. The paranoid patient may very well misinterpret the meaning of the drug because of the nature of his illness. Repeated explanations may be necessary, and a continuing dialogue about the drug and its nature may be an essential part of the treatment process. In the long run, patient compliance is based on trust, and any effort that the physician makes to increase the level of trust between himself and the patient will increase the likelihood of good patient compliance. In the final analysis, many patients do the things we tell them not because they understand or because they profoundly believe that it is the best course of action but because they trust us and wish to please us. This is the most powerful tool we have.

## PSYCHOTROPIC DRUGS IN THE ELDERLY

This discussion has concentrated on the clinical aspects of drug taking in general rather than the specifics of managing psychotherapeutic drugs in the geriatric psychiatry patient. This is because I very firmly believe that geriatric psychiatry cannot be practiced unless the patient is viewed as a whole. When we concern ourselves with drugs in the geriatric psychiatric patient, we must concern ourselves with all aspects of that problem. I do wish, however, to make some specific comments about the use of psychotropic drugs in the elderly patient. The first maxim is, of course, to "start low, go slow." The second is that patients with organic brain syndromes, irrespective of etiology, are particularly sensitive to psychotropic drugs of all kinds. Whether this is due to a relative decrease in the number of receptors in the brain or to imbalance in neurotransmitters or to some other reason, I have not the slightest notion. Nevertheless, I believe it to be true clinically, and I believe that one must show particular caution when one is dealing with such patients.

The fundamental principal in administering psychotropic medications to elderly patients is to remember that there is enormous variation in dose and that each patient must be titrated to his optimal drug level individually. Titration of the patient involves obtaining an optimal beneficial effect with a minimal amount of side effect. The first rule is to do no harm. In considering side effects, it must be kept in mind that some are trivial and others are extremely damaging. The array of what is trivial or damaging is not the same for the old as it is for the young, nor for one person as for another: I tend to use very little of the benzodiazepines and no propanediols or barbiturates. It has been my experience that most of the effect that one could expect from a properly used benzodiazepine can be obtained just as well by regular supportive therapy and telephone consultation. We have, however, seen a considerable number of older patients who had developed psychological and even physiological dependence on these drugs. Many of the problems that precipitate anxiety reactions in the elderly are rather long-term problems that are not easily solved; to use minor tranquilizers under such circumstances is likely to produce little result other than drug dependence. In addition to the problem of drug dependence, we have seen a number of older people who developed apparent cognitive impairment while taking these drugs, and a number in whom such drugs appeared to be a contributing factor in the development of depression. The unwanted side effects seem to outweigh the benefit for too many patients.

In the case of the tricyclics, the problem is somewhat different. These drugs are major treatment modalities for many older patients. My group has developed a tendency to use amitriptyline less than the other tricyclics because early in the development of our program we encountered a number of patients who had developed anticholinergic psychosis on amitriptyline. I am sure that other tricyclic antidepressants are capable of causing this situation, but in our experience, amitriptyline is far more likely to do so than any of the other tricyclic antidepressants, and it is true that amitriptyline is the most anticholinergic of the tricyclics available on the American market (20). An anticholinergic confusional state is probably the most undesirable side effect of the antidepressants, and is to be avoided at all costs. It is not common, but in my clinical experience it has been more common than urinary obstruction, the precipitation of glaucoma, ileus, or other major anticholinergic side effects of these drugs. The second major side effect that must be taken into account in titrating a person to an adequate drug dose of antidepressant is the problem of orthostatic hypotension, dizziness, and falling. Most elderly patients on tricyclic medication develop orthostatic hypotension. We generally increase drug dose until the patient has developed a drop of 20 ml Hg systolic with symptoms of dizziness or 40 ml Hg if the patient does not complain of dizziness on standing, unless, of course, the patient gets better before these levels of orthostatic hypotension are reached. Usually, these drug doses are well below doses that are normally used in young people. The problem of dizziness and falling is a major one for older people (21, 22). If they become symptomatic in this way, they are very likely to reduce their activities and decrease their ability to manage the tasks of daily living. Falls are often disastrous in this age group, and may be lethal. The minor side effects of the tricyclics such as a dry mouth, blurred vision, and sweating are uncomfortable, but most patients manage to tolerate them quite well.

A great deal has been written about the relationship between tricyclic antidepressants and the heart. There are very few absolute contraindications for the tricyclics in the patient with heart disease, although we do not give tricyclics to patients who are in active congestive heart failure or are less than 6 months postmyocardial infarction. We tend to avoid giving tricyclics to patients who have left bundle branch block, although we have done so in the hospital with repeated ECG monitoring. Depressions can be devastating illnesses in older people; perhaps the most serious cases occur in this age group. Situations arise in which the patient cannot be managed by ECT because of a tendency to relapse rapidly after treatment and in which the MAOIs are not effective. In such cases, tricyclics may be tried in the hospital with frequent ECG monitoring and the assistance of an internist. In the case of one elderly lady with a left bundle branch block who suffered from repeated severe suicidal depressions and who had extremely rapid relapses after ECT (she was unable to tolerate tricyclics because she developed complete heart block on small doses), we eventually had a pacemaker implanted so that the patient could be maintained on tricyclic antidepressants. The key to success in titrating antidepressant medication in the older person is careful monitoring.

Similar comments can be made about the use of the neuroleptics. Here the problems are somewhat different, but again, the object is to produce a good result without damaging the patient through intolerable side effects. In the case of the neuroleptics, the most common serious side effects are confusional states (these are most likely to appear when the patient has also been placed on an anticholinergic to control basal ganglion symptoms), parkinsonian symptoms, and orthostatic hypotension. Not all neuroleptics are equally likely to cause these side effects. Haloperidol has been implicated in the development of reversible dementias, and we have seen such cases in our own experience. Thioridazine and chlorpromazine are most likely to cause orthostatic hypotension, and least likely to produce parkinsonian syndromes.

We have become so accustomed to dealing with massive basal ganglion symptoms secondary to neuroleptics in young people that we think very little of it. In older people, however, parkinsonian symptoms can be quite damaging. They often include retropulsion, propulsion, and falling, symptoms more typical of idiopathic Parkinson's disease than the rigidity and oculogyric crisis that one so commonly sees in younger patients on neuroleptics. I have the impression that neuroleptic drugs in old people sometimes unmask idiopathic Parkinson's disease, which is quite difficult to treat and persists long after the neuroleptic drugs have been discontinued. For this reason, we are careful to avoid symptoms of parkinsonism as much as possible. Because of the danger of developing anticholinergic psychoses in these patients, we are more likely to control the development of parkinsonism by the reduction of drugs, or a change in drug type, for example, from haloperidol to thioridazine, than to control them with the anticholinergic agents.

Sedation is another limiting side effect of the neuroleptic agents. In older people, sedation may appear with almost any of the neuroleptics. Although nighttime sedation may be a desirable side effect, particularly in the confused, organically impaired patient who suffers from day/night confusion, daytime sedation is undesirable and should be avoided. Often, daytime sedation will result in a decline rather than an improvement in the level of functioning of the patient.

In the case of all the psychotropic medications, different patients will develop different limiting side effects. The side effect must always be weighed against the benefit of the drug. When a side effect begins to impair fuction, it should be considered limiting, and drug dosage should generally be reduced. One is always tempted to treat side effects with more drugs; for example, the dry mouth of which patients often complain when taking tricyclic antidepressants can be managed very nicely with bethanechol chloride. There are, however, real problems associated with maintaining elderly patients on multiple medications, and this practice is best avoided. Usually, a single drug can be found that will do the trick, and it is worth the trouble of finding it. Less is more in the geriatric population, and more is less. Maximal function with minimal pharmacological intervention is not only possible, but practical as well.

## REFERENCES

1. Davidson, J. R.: Presentation and packaging of drugs for the elderly. Journal of Hospital Pharmacy 31:180–184, 1973.
2. Atkinson, L., Gibson, I. I. J. M., and Andrews, J.: The difficulties of old people taking drugs. Age & Ageing 6:144–150, 1977.
3. Leader: Keep on taking tablets. British Medical Journal 1:793, 1977.
4. Davie, J. W.: Personal communication, 1980.
5. Arie, T.: Issues in the psychiatric care of the elderly. In: Exton-Smith A. N. and Evans, J. G. (eds.): Care of the Elderly: Meeting the Challenge of Dependency. London, England: Academic Press, 1977.
6. Folstein, M. F., Folstein, S. E. and McHugh, P. R.: "Mini-Mental State." A practical method for grading the cognitive state of patients for the clinician. J Psychiatr Res 12:189–198, 1975.
7. Stewart, R. B. and Cluff, L. E.: A review of medication errors and compliance in ambulant patients. Clin Pharmacol Ter 13:463–468, 1972.
8. Haynes, R. B.: A critical review of patient compliance with therapeutic regimens. In: Sackett, D. L. and Haynes, R. B. (eds.): Compliance with Therapeutic Regimens. Baltimore: John Hopkins University Press, 1976.
9. Wandless, I. and Davie, J. W.: Can drug compliance in the elderly be improved? Br Med J 1:359–361, 1977.
10. Schwartz, D., Wang, M., Zeitz, L., et al.: Medication errors made by elderly, chronically ill patients. Am J Public Health 54:2018–2029, 1962.
11. Neely, E. and Patrick, M. L.: Problems of aged persons taking medications at home. Nurs Res 17:52–55, 1968.
12. Parkin, D. M., Henney, C. R., Quirk, J., et al.: Deviation from prescribed drug treatment after discharge from hospital. Br Med J 2:686–688, 1976.
13. Judge, T. G. and Caird, F. I.: Drug Treatment of the Elderly Patient. Kent, England: Pitman Medical, 1978.
14. Vestal, R. E. Drug use in the elderly: a review of problems and special considerations. Drugs 16:358–382, 1978.
15. Cummings, J., Benson, D. F., LoVerme, S.: Reversible dementia. JAMA 243:2434–2439, 1980.
16. Blumenthal, M. D.: Depressive illness in old age: getting behind the mask. Geriatrics 35:34–43, 1980.
17. Bridge, T. P. and Wyatt, R. J.: Paraphrenia: paranoid states of late life. I. European research. II. American Research. J Am Geriatr Soc 28:193–205, 1980.
18. Biological therapies in psychiatry. Massachusetts General Hospital Newsletter 3:5–6, 1980.

19. Ewy, G. A., Marcus, F. I., Fillmore, S. J., et al.: Digitalis intoxication—diagnosis, management and prevention. Cardiovasc Clin 6:153–174, 1974.
20. Snyder, S. H. and Yamamura, H. I.: Antidepressants and the muscarinic acetylcholine receptor. Arch Gen Psychiatry 34:236–239, 1977.
21. Blumenthal, M. D. and Davie, J. W.: Dizziness and falling in elderly psychiatric outpatients. Am J Psychiatry 137(2):203–206, 1980.
22. Davie, J. W., Blumenthal, M. D., and Robinson-Hawkins, S: A model of risk for psychogeriatric patients. Arch Gen Psychiatry, 38:463–467, 1981.

# CHAPTER 13

# Treatment of Alzheimer's Disease: A Cholinergic Strategy

Kenneth L. Davis, M.D.
Richard C. Mohs, PH.D.
Gordon S. Rosenberg, B.A.
Bonnie M. Davis, M.D.
Thomas B. Horvath, M.D.
Yvonne De Nigris, M.A.
Alison Ross, B.A.
Thomas Cummings, B.A.
Michael Levy, M.D.

## INTRODUCTION

Neurochemical and pharmacological investigations of human memory and aging provide evidence to suggest an approach to the treatment of the Alzheimer's type of dementia. Neurochemical studies indicate that Alzheimer's disease is a primary degenerative nerve cell disorder that specifically impairs the functioning of neocortical cholinergic neurons (1–7). The cholinergic defect is manifested by a significant reduction in the level of choline acetyltransferase (CAT) activity, as well as acetylcholinesterase (AChE) activity (1, 2, 4, 5, 8, 9). The CAT deficiency has been positively correlated with the degree of intellectual impairment, formation of senile plaques, and in vitro reduction of acetylcholine syn-

Supported in part by the Veterans Administration Research Funds, a grant from the National Institute on Aging, grant No. 79–141 PS/VA, and NIH grant RR–71, Division of Research Resources, General Clinical Research Centers Branch.

thesis from cortical biopsy samples (10, 11). The extent to which muscarinic receptor binding is altered in cases of Alzheimer's disease has not been definitively determined (5), although several studies suggest that it remains unchanged (3, 4, 10, 12).

A wide range of pharmacological investigations has further implicated cholinergic neurotransmission in human memory. Drug-induced alterations in cholinergic transmission have been shown to underlie disordered or impaired memory functioning. The anticholinergic drug scopolamine, when administered to young normal subjects, produces a memory deficit that is strikingly similar to the cognitive profile of drug-free Alzheimer's patients (13). That this effect is induced specifically by the anticholinergic properties of scopolamine is supported by the finding that amphetamine is unable to reverse this memory impairment (14). Two cholinergic agonists, physostigmine and arecoline, when given in moderate doses, have enhanced memory performance. Interestingly, the aspect of memory that was improved by physostigmine and arecoline was similar to that aspect of memory impaired by scopolamine (15, 16). This finding is most critical, for it suggests that cholinomimetics might be able to enhance those memory functions which are at a greatest deficit in patients with Alzheimer's disease.

The possibility that cholinomimetic agents might be of benefit to patients with Alzheimer's has led many investigators to treat this condition with choline or lecithin (17–23). Occasionally, a few subjects demonstrated a mild improvement in memory, but such improvement was not of a degree to be clinically meaningful in patients with Alzheimer's disease.

To further test the efficacy of choline as a cholinomimetic agent affecting memory, a study was designed to assess choline's potential for reversing a scopolamine-induced memory deficit in young normal subjects (24). Second, since physostigmine had previously been shown to enhance memory in young normal subjects, a trial was designed to test the effect of physostigmine on memory in subjects with Alzheimer's type dementia (25, 26). This chapter reports the findings of these 2 studies.

## Study I

Twenty normal, healthy, male subjects participated in this 3-day drug study. On each of 3 nonconsecutive days, subjects received 1 of the following drug combinations in a double-blind, randomized fashion:

1. Placebo (quinine sulfate) 8 gms P.O. Placebo (saline) 0.43 mg S.C.
2. Placebo (quinine sulfate) 8 gms P.O. Scopolamine 0.43 mg S.C.
3. Choline 8 gms P.O. Scopolamine 0.43 mg S.C.

Choline or quinine sulfate was administered orally to subjects 45 minutes before receiving an injection of scopolamine or placebo. Thirty minutes after the injection of scopolamine or placebo, a psychologist who was blind to the drug regimen administered a series of cognitive tasks to the subject, including a digit-span task and word-recall test. These cognitive tasks required that the subjects learn a different list of 24 nouns in each drug condition. Lists were composed of 12 high-imagery words (e.g., house, clock) and 12 low-imagery words (e.g., faith, trauma). The ability to recall 24 words was assessed over 6 consecutive trials. After each trial, the subjects were reminded of the words that they did not recall, and were informed of those responses not contained in the original list of words.

## Study II

Nine patients with Alzheimer's disease between the ages of 50 and 68 years participated in this study. The diagnosis of Alzheimer's disease was made with the aid of CAT scan, brain scan, skull films, CSF analysis, serum analysis, a careful history, and a physical exam. Particular care was given to ruling out cases of multi-infarct dementia. All patients had a Memory and Information Test (MIT) score greater than 10 and/or Dementia Rating Scale (DRS) score less than 4. These criteria have been shown to select patients with a high probability of Alzheimer's disease as verified by histopathological examination upon autopsy (28).

Drug administration was divided into two phases. In the first—or dose-response—phase, subjects received under double-blind conditions either 0 mg, 0.125 mg, 0.25 mg, or 0.50 mg of physostigmine in a random order. The drug was dissolved in 100 cc of saline and administered at a constant rate for 30 minutes. In the second—or replication—phase of the study, the dose of physostigmine associated with the best performance on cognitive tests involving long-term memory (LTM) storage was readministered (29, 30), as was the placebo 0.0 mg infusion. The order of these two infusions was also randomized, and the conditions of administration double-blind. Subjects' memory functioning was addressed by cognitive tasks administered in the following order:

1. famous-faces test (31),
2. digit-span task, and
3. modified Buschke test (32, 33) consisting of a 24-word or 24-picture recognition task (34).

Testing was begun 5 minutes after the infusion began, and was concluded 10 minutes after the infusion had ended. The more-demented subjects were assessed using the picture recognition task, and the less-demented subjects were assessed using the word-recognition task. Three trials were completed.

The purpose in these modifications of the Buschke paradigm was to produce a task with the following characteristics:

1. It measured the ability of the subject to encode information into LTM.
2. It would be sensitive to an improvement or worsening in performance.
3. It was comprehensible to the subject, and could be completed in the time period of physostigmine's biological activity.
4. Roughly equivalent or multiple forms of the test could be readily constructed.

## RESULTS

### Study I

Scopolamine administration significantly impaired the subjects' ability to recall 24 words over 6 trials when compared to the control day ($p < 0.01$). Choline administration did not produce a significant reversal of this effect. However, as Table 13.1 illustrates, an analysis of subjects' ability to recall only high-imagery words shows that choline did have a significant effect in partially reversing the scopolamine-induced deficit ($p < 0.05$). In contrast, choline did not reverse the effects of scopolamine on recall of low-imagery words.

### Study II

Of the 9 patients with Alzheimer's disease, 3 required concomitant neuroleptic medication in the form of daily oral haloperidol administration in an attempt to control their psychosis, agitation, and uncooperative-

Table 13.1  Ability of Choline to Reverse
Scopolamine-Induced Amnesia in Recall of High-Imagery
Words

| Treatment | Average Number of Words Recalled Over 6 Trials |
|---|---|
| 1. Placebo 8 gm P.O., and Placebo 0.43 mg S.C. | 8.11 SEM± 0.41 |
| 2. Placebo 8 gm P.O., and Scopolamine 0.43 mg S.C. | 5.96 SEM± 0.46 |
| 3. Choline 8 gm P.O., and Scopolamine 0.43 mg S.C. | 6.59 SEM± 0.34 |

[a]Analysis of varients (ANOVA) ($p<0.05$) for Group 2 vs. Group 3.

ness. As a result of inconsistencies in those patients' cooperation, their data has been presented separately from that of the 6 neuroleptic-free subjects.

Table 13.2 describes the effects of physostigmine upon the ability of subjects to store information into LTM As determined during the dose-response phase of the study, all neuroleptic-free subjects had their best performance in ability to encode information into LTM. on some dose of physostigmine rather than the placebo saline infusion. Two of the 3 neuroleptic-treated subjects similarly responded best to a dose of physo-stigmine. In all of these patients, the best dose of physostigmine varied among 0.125 mg, 0.25 mg, and 0.50 mg. During the replication phase of the study, all 6 of the neuroleptic-free subjects again demonstrated a physostigmine-related improvement in LTM encoding ($p<0.01$). Again, the results of these tests in neuroleptic-treated subjects was less consistent. These effects are presented in Table 13.3.

It should be noted that whenever the improvement in performance was approximately 10% or greater, both the subject and the experimenter were aware of a marked, clinically meaningful difference in the subject's qualitative performance. The administration of physostigmine did not produce a consistent effect upon either the digit-span task or the famous-faces test. It appears that the enhancement in memory performance was limited specifically to the encoding process of long-term memory.

Table 13.2  Dose Response Characteristics of Physostigmine in Alzheimer's Patients

| Patient | % Correct Placebo | % Correct Physostigmine | % Correct Increment over Placebo |
|---|---|---|---|
| **Neuroleptic-Free Patients** | | | |
| WD | 45.83 | 69.46 | 23.63 |
| UG | 75.00 | 90.29 | 15.29 |
| RC | 73.67 | 79.17 | 5.50 |
| MM | 65.29 | 66.67 | 1.38 |
| VB | 75.00 | 87.50 | 12.50 |
| LF | 59.71 | 81.96 | 22.25 |
| X̄ | 65.73 | 79.18 | 13.43 |
| **Neuroleptic-Treated Patients** | | | |
| JB | 76.38 | 76.38 | 0.00 |
| SB | 56.96 | 65.29 | 8.33 |
| TH | 75.00 | 84.71 | 9.71 |
| X̄ | 69.45 | 75.46 | 6.01 |

## DISCUSSION

The effect of low doses of physostigmine to improve transiently the ability of Alzheimer's patients to encode information into long-term memory is consistent with similar effects of physostigmine and arecoline in young normal subjects (15, 16). Subjects who are demented, however, show a greater variability in the dose of physostigmine that enhances memory. A similar variability has been shown in the response of elderly primates to physostigmine (35). The ability of physostigmine to enhance LTM appears to be quite specific. Since only those cognitive tasks involving encoding processes were affected by physostigmine, it is not likely that the improvement seen in this study reflects a more general change in attention or performance. Furthermore, it has been demonstrated that attentional changes that can be detected in the Sternberg paradigm (36) remain unchanged by physostigmine (15). These results provide more convincing evidence to support the hypothesis that cholinergic neurons are critically involved in the encoding of information into LTM (14).

Though previous studies utilizing cholinergic precursors were not suggestive of a beneficial treatment in Alzheimer's disease, the present results suggest that the cholinergic deficiency can in fact be partially corrected by physostigmine, an acetylcholinesterase inhibitor. Most of our patients who did not require neuroleptics and whose duration of

TABLE 13.3 Replication: Physostigmine vs. Saline in Alzheimer's Patients

| Patient | % Correct Placebo | % Correct Physostigmine | % Correct Increment over Placebo |
|---|---|---|---|
| **Neuroleptic-Free Patients[a]** | | | |
| WD | 58.33 | 68.04 | 9.71 |
| UG | 83.33 | 97.21 | 13.88 |
| RC | 55.54 | 73.62 | 18.08 |
| MM | 55.54 | 63.88 | 8.34 |
| VB | 76.38 | 79.17 | 2.79 |
| LF | 65.29 | 75.00 | 9.71 |
| X̄ | 65.74 | 76.15 | 10.42 |
| **Neuroleptic-Treated Patients** | | | |
| JB | 72.21 | 72.21 | 0.00 |
| SB | 59.71 | 62.50 | 2.79 |
| TH | 62.50 | 59.71 | −2.79 |
| X̄ | 64.81 | 64.81 | 0.00 |

[a]Two-tailed paired T-test, t=4.9, p<0.01.

dementia was less than 2 years (four patients) demonstrated a clinically significant improvement in their memory functioning while receiving an infusion of physostigmine. The fact that duration of dementia might predict treatment responsiveness could indicate that as continued degeneration of cholinergic neurons occurs, anticholinesterase administration becomes a less viable strategy to increase cholinergic neurotransmission. In contrast, 1 patient with a duration of dementia longer than 6 years demonstrated a marked response to physostigmine. Should muscarinic receptors remain unaltered in Alzheimer's disease, administration of a muscarinic cholinergic agonist may provide an improvement in memory performance in patients with a prolonged period of illness.

The oral administration of choline to young normals partially reversed the amnesia caused by scopolamine. These results suggest that increases in dietary choline can increase cholinergic activity under conditions of cholinergic blockade. Neurochemical studies have demonstrated that the availability of exogenous choline does play a role in the pharmacological responsiveness of cholinergic neurons to the anticholinergic agent atropine. Specifically, the acetylcholine-depleting action of atropine is reduced when exogenous choline supplies are administered in rats (37). Though the results in the present study were not dramatic, the ability of choline to reverse partially the amnesia caused by scopolamine may reflect a blockade of the ability of scopolamine to deplete fully the availability of acetylcholine for neurotransmission. If Alzheimer's disease reflects a degeneration of the presynaptic receptor or a defect in the rate-limiting step of acetylcholine synthesis (probably the high-affinity uptake system for choline [38]), then it should not be surprising that precursor loading with choline and lecithin would be ineffective in treating this disease.

When physostigmine is administered intravenously its duration of action is very short. Thus, an effective therapeutic intervention for Alzheimer's disease that augments central cholinergic transmission must await the development of an oral long-acting cholinomimetic agent. However, the present results do suggest that investigators can be encouraged by the fact that a rational course of treatment for Alzheimer's disease, based on reversing the cholinergic deficit, can be followed.

# REFERENCES

1. Bowen, D. M., Smith, C. B., White, P., and Davison, A. N., Neurotransmitter-related enzymes and indices of hypoxia in senile dementia and other abiotrophies, Brain 99:459, 1976.
2. Davies, P., and Maloney, A. J. F., Selective loss of central cholinergic neurons in Alzheimer's disease (letter), Lancet 2:1403, 1976.
3. Perry, E. K., Perry, R. H., Blessed, G., and Tomlinson, B. E., Necropsy evidence of central cholinergic deficits in senile dementia, Lancet 1:189, 1977.
4. White, P., Hiley, C. R., Goodhardt, M. J., Carrasco, L. H., Keet, J. P., Williams, I. E. I., and Bowen, D. M., Neocortical neurons in elderly people, Lancet 1:668, 1977.
5. Reisine, T. D., Yamamura, H. E., Bird, E. D., Spokes, E., Enna, S. J., Pre and postsynaptic neurochemical alterations in Alzheimer's disease, Brain Res 159:477, 1978.
6. Bowen, D. M., Spillane, J. A., Gurzon, G., Meier-Ruge, W., White, P., Goodhardt, M. J., Iwangoff, P., and Davison, A. N., Accelerated ageing or selective neuronal loss as a important cause of dementia, Lancet 1:11 1979.
7. Richter, J. A., Perry, E. K., Tomlinson, B. E. Acetylcholine and choline levels in postmortem human brain tissue: Preliminary observations in Alzheimer's disease, Life Sci 26:1683–1689,1980.
8. Perry, E. K., Gibson, P. N., Blessed, G., Perry, R. H., Tomlinson, B. E., Neurotransmitter enzyme abnormalities in senile dementia, J Neurol Sci 34:247, 1977.
9. Davies, P., Neurotransmitter-related enzymes in senile dementia of the Alzheimer type, Brain Res 171:319, 1979.
10. Perry, E. K., Tomlinson, B. E., Blessed, G., Bergman, K., Gibson, P. H., and Perry, R. H., Correlation of cholinergic abnormalities with senile plaques and mental test scores in senile dementia, Brit Med J 2:1457, 1978.

11. Sims, N. R., Smith, C. C. T., Davison, A. N., Bowen, D. M., Flack, R. H. A., Snowden, J. S. and Neary, D., Glucose metabolism and acetylcholine synthesis in relation to neuronal activity in Alzheimer's disease, *Lancet* 1:333, 1980.

12. Davies, P., Regional distribution of muscarinic acetylcholine receptors in normal and Alzheimer's type dementia brain, *Brain Res* 138:385, 1978.

13. Drachman, D. A., and Leavitt, J., Human memory and the cholinergic system, *Arch Neurol* 30:113, 1974.

14. Drachman, D. A., Memory and cognitive function in man: does the cholinergic system have a specific role? *Neurology* 27:783, 1977.

15. Davis, K. L., Mohs, R. C., Tinklenberg, J. R., Pfefferbaum, A., Hollister, L. E., and Kopell, B. S., Physostigmine: Improvement of long-term memory processes in normal humans, *Science* 201:272, 1978.

16. Sitaram, N., Weingartner, H. and Gillian, J. C., Human serial learning: Enhancement with arecoline and choline impairment with scopolamine, *Science* 261:274, 1978.

17. Boyd, W. D., Graham-White, J., Blackwood, G., Glen, I., and McQueen, J., Clinical effects of choline in Alzheimer senile dementia, *Lancet* 2:711, 1977.

18. Spillane, J. A., Goodhart, M. H., White, P., Bowen, D. M. and Davison, A. N., Choline in Alzheimer's disease, *Lancet* 2:711, 1977.

19. Signoret, J. L., Whitely, A., Lhermitee, F., Influence of choline on amnesia in early Alzheimer's disease, *Lancet* 2:837, 1978.

20. Ferris, S. H., Sathananthan, G., Reisberg, B., Gershon, S. Long-term choline treatment in memory impaired elderly patients. *Science* 205:1039–40 1979.

21. Christie, J. E., Blackburn, E. M., Glen, A. I. M., Zeisel, S., Shering, A. and Yates, C. M., Effects of choline and lecithin on CSF choline levels and on cognitive function in patients with presenile dementia of the Alzheimer's type *in* "Nutrition and the Brain" (A. Barbeau, J. H. Growdon, and R. J. Wurtman, eds). Vol. 5, Raven Press, New York 1979.

22. Peters, B. H., and Levin, H. S., Effects of physostigmine and lecithin on memory in Alzheimer's disease, *Ann Neurol* 16:219, 1979.

23. Caine, E. D.: Cholinomimetic treatment fails to improve memory disorders. *N. Engl J Med* 303:585, 1980.

24. Davis, K. L., Mohs, R. C., Tinklenberg, R., Hollister, L. E., Pfefferbaum, A., and Koppell, B. S., Cholinomimetics and memory: The effect of choline chloride, *Arch Neurol* 37:49, 1980.

25. Mohs, R. C., Davis, K. L., Tinklenberg, J. R., Hollister, L. E., Yesavage, J. A., and Koppell, B. S., Choline Chloride treatment of memory deficits in the elderly, *Am J Psychiatry* 136:10, 1979.

26. Mohs, R. C., and Davis, K. L., Choline chloride effects on memory: Correlation with the effects of physostigmine, *Psychiatry Res* 2:149, 1980.

27. Mohs, R. C., Davis, K. L., Tinklenberg, M. R. and Hollister, L. E.,

Choline chloride effects on memory in the elderly, *Neurobiology of Aging* 1:21–25, 1980.

28. Kay, D. W. K., The Epidemiology and identification of brain deficit in the elderly, *in* "Cognitive and Emotional Disturbance in the Elderly" (C. Eisdorfer and R. O. Friedel, eds), pp. 11–26, Year Book Medical Publishers, Chicago, 1977.

29. Atkinson, R. C., and Shiffrin, R. M., Human memory: a proposed system and its control processes, *in* "The Psychology of Learning and Motivation: Advances in Research and Theory" (K. W. Spence, and J. T. Spence, eds), pp. 89–195, Academic Press, New York, 1968.

30. Atkinson, R. C., and Shiffrin, R. M., The control of short term memory, *Sci Am* 224:82, 1971.

31. Marslen-Wilson, W. D., and Teuber, H. L., Memory for remote events in anterograde amnesia: Recognition of public figures from news photographs, *Neuropsychologia* 13:353, 1975.

32. Buschke, H., Selective reminding for analysis of memory and learning, *J Verb Learn Verb Behav* 12:543, 1973.

33. Buschke, H., and Fuld, P. A., Evaluating storage, retention, and retrieval in disordered memory and learning, *Neurology* 24:1019, 1974.

34. Shepard, R. N., Recognition memory for words, sentences and pictures, *J Verb Learn Verb Behavior*, 6:156, 1967.

35. Bartus, R. T., Aging in the rhesus monkey: Specific behavioral impairments and effects of pharmacological intervention, *Excerpta Medica*, Tokyo, XI International Congress of Geronotology, 1978, 1979.

36. Sternberg, S., Memory scanning: mental processes revealed by reaction-time experiments, *Am Sci*, 57:421, 1969.

37. Wecker, L. and Schmidt, D. E.: Neuropharmacological consequences of choline administration. *Brain Res* 184:231–238, 1980.

38. Yamamura, H. and Snyder, S., High affinity transport of choline into synaptosomes of rat brain *J Neurochem* 21:1355, 1977.

# CHAPTER 14

# Paranoid Syndromes in the Elderly

Murray Raskind, M.D.

Paranoid symptoms are prominent features of several important psychopathologic syndromes in the elderly. Paranoid patients suffer from excessive suspiciousness, and usually believe they are being attacked, harassed, cheated, persecuted, conspired against, or unfairly treated. Although paranoid symptomatology is commonly present in older patients whose psychiatric disease began in early life (such as those with chronic schizophrenia), the focus of this chapter is the diseases in which paranoid symptomatology is the dominant feature or a prominent complication of psychiatric illnesses that begin in later life. The most important of these geropsychiatric disorders are paraphrenia, dementia, and delirium. In paraphrenia, paranoid symptoms are the core manifestations of the illness; in dementia and delirium, paranoid symptoms are common complicating problems that require careful management.

## PARAPHRENIA

Paraphrenia has been well described in the British literature (1–3), but has only recently received attention in this country (4–6). It is a dramatic psychosis of later life, the onset of which is rare before the age of 60. Women are far more commonly affected than men. When one combines Kay and Roth's series from England and Sweden (1), there were 87 women and only 12 men. In our smaller series from Seattle, Washington, there were 23 women and 3 men (6). The striking preponderance of women sustaining this disorder is unusual in psychiatry, and is matched only by the sex distribution in somatization disorder (hysteria or Briquet's syndrome) (7). Although premorbid traits such as eccentric-

ity, sensitivity, obstinacy, and a higher than expected incidence of un-
married status in early life have been noted by several authors, the
consensus (3) is that these premorbid personality "difficulties" are less
remarkable than the often-satisfactory life adjustment many paraphrenic
patients were able to achieve prior to the onset of their illness. In fact,
these patients frequently retain their social graces and function quite
well in areas uncontaminated by persecutory ideation.

The core manifestations of paraphrenia are persecutory delusions.
Hallucinations are usually, but not invariably, present. These delusions
and hallucinations clearly cannot be interpreted in terms of depression
or elation. These symptoms are usually bizarre, and frequently include
primary delusions, delusions of influence and passivity, and hallucinations of voices communicating about the patient in the third person.
Patients complain that persons in their environment are plotting to hurt,
kill, or sexually abuse them. They may be convinced that they are being
spied upon, that persons repeatedly enter their living quarters by mys-
terious means at night, that lethal gases are pumped into their homes,
or that food and water are poisoned. Telepathic experiences are common, as are feelings of being controlled by demonic instruments or
machines. Patients complain of being stabbed, cut, irradiated, or otherwise bodily manipulated by persons in distant settings. The variety of
delusions and hallucinations is endless, but frequent themes are plots
involving sexual molestation, poisoning, and other bodily harm.

Many of the above symptoms have been considered pathognomonic
of schizophrenia by some authorities (8). In striking contrast to schizophrenia, however, paraphrenia is not accompanied by deterioration of
personality, loosening of associations, affective incongruity and blunting,
or the loss of volition. Thus, the phenomenology of paraphrenia both
resembles and differs from schizophrenia, and a considerable controversy
has existed in the European literature as to the proper classification of this
disorder. The controversy has not been resolved by the third edition of
the *Diagnostic and Statistical Manual of Mental Disorders* (DSM-III),
which lists the term "paraphrenia" in the index (7), and refers the reader
to a discussion of paranoid disorder. DSM-III then describes paranoid
disorder (7) as an illness of onset in middle or later life manifested by
persistent persecutory delusions or delusional jealousy. Unfortunately,
exclusion criteria for paranoid disorder (i.e., bizarre delusions and prominent hallucinations) are the very core manifestations of paraphrenia. Paraphrenia is also poorly accommodated by the DSM-III category of schizophrenia, which is described as an illness with an onset before age 45 (7).
Rather than dwelling upon apparently unresolvable nosologic issues, it
appears reasonable to accept the suggestion of Ridge and Wyatt (5) that

the separate diagnostic category of paraphrenia is a useful one that should receive greater attention from American psychiatrists.

Several other features of the paraphrenic syndrome deserve comment. The first is the relationship of sensory deficits, particularly deafness, to the etiology of the disorder. Although deficient vision was found in 15% of Kay and Roth's paraphrenic patients (1), this was not more frequent than in the control groups of comparable age. On the other hand, some impairment of hearing was found in 40% of their paraphrenic patients, and was of marked degree in 15% of the paraphrenics. This incidence of hearing impairment was larger than that in a roughly comparable group of elderly patients with affective disorder, but sensory testing was not done in a rigorous manner. Furthermore, control patients were somewhat younger than the paraphrenics. Cooper (9) has studied this issue in a more systematic manner, and again finds a modestly increased incidence of socially important hearing impairment in paraphrenic patients compared to either affective controls or elderly normals. On the other hand, these differences were not striking, and it is clear that the majority of paraphrenic patients have relatively well-preserved vision and hearing.

The relationship of paraphrenia to organic mental disorders, particularly dementia, has also received attention. Paraphrenic patients rarely manifest disorders of memory or other cognitive/intellectual functions, nor do they have an increased incidence of focal cerebrovascular disease. Roth (10) has carefully followed the course of hospitalized paraphrenic patients in terms of life expectancy. Despite the chronicity of these patients' illness, their life expectancy was normal for their age. This longevity was in striking contrast to that of demented patients, whose life expectancy was approximately 20% that of normal people of the same age. When paraphrenic patients do develop dementia, they do so at no higher frequency than do normal elderly persons. Although it may be tempting to assume that any behavioral disorder in later life is secondary to degenerative brain disease, this does not appear to be the case for paraphrenia.

Prognosis and treatment will be discussed together because recent psychopharmacologic advances have affected the prognosis of this disorder. It should be stated at the outset that our knowledge of the prognosis and natural course of paraphrenia is obtained from patients who were hospitalized because the severity of their symptoms made further existence in the general community impossible, at least in the context of Great Britain in the period before 1970. This sample may be atypical as to severity, and it is quite plausible that patients with mild paraphrenia could function reasonably well in a tolerant community setting and never come to the attention of physicians. In this hospitalized population, however, prognosis for recovery was poor. Although Post states that patients rarely suffered personality deterioration with volitional changes or affective incongruity, those who finally required psychiatric hospital admission were rarely discharged (3). In Kay and Roth's series of hospitalized paraphrenics, only one was known to have made a lasting recovery (1). In others, spontaneous remissions and those induced by electroconvulsive therapy were almost always followed by recurrence.

With the advent of the antipsychotic medications, an effective symptomatic treatment for paraphrenia is now available. Post (3) has studied a series of hospitalized paraphrenic patients treated with trifluoperazine (Stelazine) or placebo. In a group of patients followed for 3 years, 25 of 28 patients treated with adequate doses of antipsychotic medication showed improvement, and 14 of the 25 patients recovered completely so long as the medication regimen was maintained. In contrast, only 4 of 23 inadequately or placebo-treated patients had lasting remissions. It is also clear that antipsychotic medications do not change the underlying course of the disorder. Only 6 patients in Post's series continued in remission when antipsychotic medications were discontinued. Most relapsed as soon as the dosage was allowed to drop below an individually determined maintenance level or was discontinued completely.

Recent changes in public policy concerning involuntary psychiatric hospitalization have created new problems in the management of the acutely psychotic paraphrenic patient, at least in many states in this country. Prior to the early 1970s, these suspicious, frightened, and usually uncooperative patients, who lacked insight concerning the nature of their illness, were involuntarily hospitalized. Recent changes in public policy, legal statutes, and treatment philosophy have created a situation in which these patients rarely meet stringent legal criteria for involuntary hospitalization, despite being involved in crisis situations caused by their florid paranoid symptoms. In these situations, treatment must be delivered by primary care physicians with whom the patient has had long-standing relationships or by outreach psychiatric teams. In either case, outpatient treatment is often associated with poor medication compliance and subsequent poor response to the prescribed regimen. Raskind et al. (6) found that fluphenazine enanthate, a depot parenteral antipsychotic preparation, was effective in such crisis intervention treatment of outpatient paraphrenics who were involved in traumatic and chaotic situations but who did not meet stringent criteria for involuntary hospitalization. Fluphenazine enanthate in an average dose of 5 mg every 2 weeks was significantly superior to haloperidol prescribed as a regimen of 2 mg orally 3 times daily. Eleven of 13 patients in the

188 — Treatment of Psychopathology in the Aging

fluphenazine group improved, compared to only 3 of 13 patients in the oral antipsychotic drug group. It is extremely likely that the poor results in the oral antipsychotic drug group were attributable to poor patient compliance.

Although the paraphrenic patient appears not to respond well to traditional insight-oriented psychotherapy, this does not obviate the need for an interpersonal and environmental approach to management of these patients. Antipsychotic drugs will work only if the patient will ingest them. A trusting relationship with the health care provider is therefore an essential ingredient of successful management. The physician who treats the paraphrenic patient must also be skillful at dealing with significant others in the patient's environment. Neighbors, apartment house managers, and other persons involved with the patient need reassurance that despite the patient's bizarre and often frightening behavior, he or she is rarely dangerous and will respond to an effective treatment program.

## PARANOID SYMPTOMS IN DEMENTIA

Dementia (chronic organic brain syndrome) is the most devastating behavioral disorder of later life. Primary neuronal degeneration of the Alzheimer's type and cerebrovascular disease (multiple infarctions) account for the majority of cases. Whatever the etiology, the essential feature of the dementia syndrome is loss of intellectual abilities of sufficient severity to interfere with social or occupational functioning. Although memory loss is the central behavioral symptom, impairment of judgment, impairment of abstract thinking, and personality disintegration usually occur.

Paranoid symptoms can complicate dementia, causing distress to the patient and difficult management problems for the physician and the persons with whom the patient resides. The most common problem is delusions of theft. The dynamics of these delusions appear reasonably clear. The mildly demented patient misplaces an article and assumes that some other person must have taken it from its customary place. As memory for recent events grows worse, a long-since-discarded article of clothing or piece of household furniture exists in an old memory trace as a current possession. When this long-discarded article cannot be located, it is not unreasonable for the patient to assume that it has been stolen. The objects of the patient's accusations are usually persons in the immediate environment. Neighbors, apartment house custodians, teenagers, and nursing aides in long-term care facilities are frequently objects of suspicion. Although the demented patient can sometimes be persuaded that a theft has not actually occurred, it is common for these beliefs to assume an unshakable delusional intensity. Of course, it must be borne in mind that the object or possession in question may actually have been stolen. The forgetful elderly patient can be a tempting target for an unscrupulous person. At any rate, accusations of theft must be given at least a respectful and careful hearing by the treating health professional before an assumption is made that the accusation is a paranoid symptom. It is only the minority of demented patients who develop delusions of theft. It appears that patients with premorbid personality traits of compulsivity, suspiciousness, and litigiousness in earlier life will probably develop delusions of theft as dementia develops.

The treatment of delusions of theft may be difficult. Data concerning the efficacy of antipsychotic drugs in the treatment of simple theft delusions is not available. They have not proved very helpful in my clinical experience, unless the delusions assume broader, more schizophreniform proportions. More effective are interpersonal and environmental strategies. First, the persons who are objects of the patient's accusations as well as others in the environment must be given attention. If they fail to understand the dynamics of the patient's paranoid beliefs, they may react with anger and resentment, which will further stress the patient and intensify his or her fearfulness. The persons in the environment must be taught to assume a nonjudgmental attitude toward the patient and be made aware of the etiologic role of memory loss in the patient's paranoid beliefs. Rather than confronting the patient's delusions, the persons involved with the patient must seek ways to decrease the patient's anxiety and confusion and to create as secure an atmosphere for the patient as possible. Delusions of theft wax and wane with the patient's anxiety level. As a more predictable and secure environment is created, the emotional urgency of paranoid ideation and even false beliefs themselves can fade away.

Another paranoid syndrome may occur in demented patients as their disease progresses. The patient fails to recognize the persons with whom he or she has been living for many years (usually a spouse, but occasionally children or acquaintances), becomes terrified that "strangers" are living with him or her, and believes that the strange persons are trying to do mischief or harm. In the most pathetic of these cases, an elderly spouse of a severely demented patient is rejected as an interloping stranger. Such spouses are often devastated, particularly after having devoted so much time and energy to the care of their demented spouse in the early stages of the disease. In such situations, a tremendous amount of supportive psychotherapy must be directed towards the healthy spouse. Such periods of nonrecognition of the spouse complicated by paranoid delusional beliefs concerning the "stranger" tend to be self-limited.

## PARANOID SYMPTOMS IN DELIRIUM

Delirium (acute organic brain syndrome) is manifested by a clouded state of consciousness with reduced clarity of awareness of the environment. A disorder of attention is the central feature. The patient suffers from sensory misperceptions and disordered thought processes. Sleep-wakefulness disturbances and abnormalities of psychomotor activity are common. The onset is usually rapid with a fluctuating course, and although the patient can remain delirious for significant periods of time, the duration of the disorder is typically brief. Vivid threatening hallucinations and poorly systematized persecutory delusions are common. Fear secondary to these phenomena can present a significant management problem. Delirium can coexist with dementia, and this brief discussion of paranoid symptoms in delirium can apply to both the demented and nondemented patient.

The presence of delirium implies an acute change in brain physiology. Such changes may include acute physical insults to the brain (stroke or head trauma), general medical illnesses, drug intoxication (or drug withdrawal in the addicted patient), postoperative states, and less-well-understood phenomena such as sensory deprivation and diurnal rhythm phenomena. A careful search for and treatment of a reversible etiology of delirium is therefore the primary management objective (11).

Not uncommonly, especially in the demented patient with frequent episodes of delirium, a specific etiology will not be found. In these cases, and even in those in whom the etiology of delirium is clear, symptomatic management of paranoid delusions and threatening hallucinations is necessary. Reassurance and structuring the environment so as to provide constancy of moderate stimulation are helpful. High-potency antipsychotic medication with low anticholinergic and low antiadrenergic activity (thiothixene, haloperidol, or perphenazine) are preferable if antipsychotics are necessary. Dosage should be kept low, and must be carefully individualized.

## CONCLUSIONS

Although the paranoid syndromes cause significant morbidity in later life, they are also among the most treatable geropsychiatric disorders. A successful clinical intervention can dramatically improve the quality of life for the paranoid patient and those in his or her environment. These disorders also pose exciting research questions. Is paraphrenia a valid diagnostic entity? What premorbid personality variables will predict paranoid symptoms complicating the dementia syndrome? Are antipsychotic medications effective in the treatment of delusions of theft? Hypotheses concerning these issues have been presented in this chapter, but much work will be needed before the answers are acceptably clear.

## REFERENCES

1. Kay, D. W. K., Roth, M.: Environmental and hereditary factors in the schizophrenias of old age (late paraphrenia) and their bearing on the general problem of causation in schizophrenia. J Ment Sci 107:649–686, 1961.
2. Post, F.: Persistent Persecutory States of the Elderly. Oxford: Pergamon Press, 1966.
3. Post, F.: The Clinical Psychiatry of Late Life. Oxford: Pergamon Press, 1965.
4. Bridge, T. P., Wyatt, R. J.: Paraphrenia: paranoid states of late life. I. European research. J Am Geriatrics Soc 28:193–200, 1980.
5. Bridge, T. P., Wyatt R. J.: Paraphrenia: paranoid states of later life. II. American research. J Am Geriatrics Soc 28:201–205, 1980.
6. Raskind, M. A., Alvarez, C., Herlin, S.: Fluphenazine enanthate in the outpatient treatment of late paraphrenia. J Am Geriatrics Soc 27:459–463, 1979.
7. Task Force on Nomenclature and Statistics, American Psychiatric Association: Diagnostic and Statistical Manual of Mental Disorders (Third Edition). Washington, D. C., American Psychiatric Association, 1980.
8. Schneider, K.: Clinical Psychopathology. Translated by Hamilton MW, New York: Grune & Stratton, 1959.
9. Cooper, A. F., Curry, A. R., Kay, D. W. K., et al.: Hearing loss in paranoid and affective psychoses of the elderly. Lancet 2:851–854, 1974.
10. Roth, M.: The natural history of mental disorder in old age. J Ment Sci 101:281–301, 1955.
11. Raskind, M. A.: The organic mental disorders, in Handbook of Geriatric Psychiatry. Ed. by Busse, E. W., Blazer D. G. New York: Van Nostrand Reinhold, 1980.

# CHAPTER 15

# Issues in Psychological Diagnosis and Management of the Cognitively Impaired Aged

Donna Cohen, PH.D.

This chapter examines several important issues in the treatment and management of older persons with dementing disorders during the various stages of the illness and the phases in the family reaction, the range of available therapeutic options in the psychological management of the cognitively impaired adult and his or her family, and areas for future research. Although a great deal can be done to treat, manage, and rehabilitate individuals with irreversible dementia, the implementation of new research programs and innovative clinical services will have profound implications for the future well-being of the elderly.

## DIMENSIONS OF THE PROBLEM

Dementing disorders have become a significant problem not only because of their catastrophic effect on health and quality of family life but because of their prevalence and resultant social and economic impact on our society at large (1–4). Through improved sanitation, antibiotics, and immunizations, infectious diseases are no longer the major killers in our society. Cardiovascular diseases and cancers are the major causes of death in the United States today, and both groups of diseases are being subjected to intensive investigation. However, the brain diseases of middle and later life—Alzheimer's disease, multi-infarct dementia, and related disorders—are as yet little understood.

The result of major advances in our understanding, treatment, and prevention of cardiovascular disease and cancer, as well as our success in keeping more people alive longer, may have the serious consequence of increasing the prevalence of brain disorders in later life. The risk for dementing disorders increases with advancing age after age 65; at age 85, the risk is 40–50%. Dementing disorders may well be the fourth major killer of people over age 65 (5).

## Normal Aging vs. Dementia

Profound intellectual or cognitive losses are not the inevitable consequence of growing old. They are the result of progressive degenerative neuronal pathology in the nervous system. Unfortunately, the popular use of the term "senility" has implied that dementia is the same as being old, and that inevitable mental changes occur with advancing age. Not only is there the belief that "senility" is inevitable, but the term also carries with it the implication that diagnosis and treatment of these victimized older adults is a waste of time. Thus, these myths about aging have had a significant negative impact on older patients, their families, and caregivers.

Changes in personality and intellect occur in many older people, but aging does not cause these losses. When signs of cognitive or emotional disturbances are apparent, it is important first to diagnose whether there are reversible and treatable causes of the decline. One-third of all persons presenting with intellectual disturbances have an underlying cause that may be treatable and reversible, if diagnosed properly (6–8). Infections, metabolic disorders, poor nutritional habits, circulatory and pulmonary diseases, drug effects, social isolation, depression, and alcohol and drug abuse are all possible causes of intellectual change. Many other factors besides health have a significant impact on behavior, including motivation to perform, feelings of self-worth and competence, the ability to work or use time effectively, finances, independence and mobility, and experience. These are often difficult to evaluate without a careful interview with the individuals, their families, and significant other persons in their lives.

## Forms of Dementia

Not all intellectual changes are reversible (9). There are a group of brain diseases or dementing illnesses in which intellectual functioning, personality, and the ability for self-care deteriorate progressively in middle-aged and older adults. Dementias are characterized by deterioration in a number of cognitive abilities that inevitably interfere with social and occupational performance. Many conditions may cause intellectual dysfunction, and these include metabolic and vascular disorders, hypoxia and anoxia, nutritional deficiency, alcohol and drug abuse, toxic substances such as metals (lead, mercury) or carbon monoxide, brain tumors, trauma (head injuries, heat strokes), infections, and a variety of diseases such as multiple sclerosis. There are also several diseases of the central nervous system whose primary symptoms are dementia or cognitive dysfunction. These include Alzheimer's disease, Pick's disease, Huntington's chorea, Creutzfeldt-Jakob disease, and some forms of Parkinson's disease.

Alzheimer's disease is the most common form of dementing illness, affecting more than 50–60% of the total number of people with dementia. The second most important nonreversible disorder is vascular dementia, which is actually caused by multiple small strokes, and which accounts for another 20%. Vascular dementias are also called multi-infarct dementias, referring to the many small infarcts in the brain tissue. Another 10–15% of individuals with dementia show a mixture of Alzheimer's disease and multi-infarct dementia. The remaining individuals are affected by a variety of other conditions related to alcoholism, multiple sclerosis, Huntington's chorea, viruses, metabolic disease, head trauma, and so on.

## How Does Dementia Affect Behavior?

The individual with dementia develops deficits in areas of memory, learning, attention, communication, and a range of cognitive skills. In the case of Alzheimer's dementia, these intellectual changes are often quite subtle in the beginning, but become debilitating as time passes. Our current understanding of the exact pattern of deficits seen with advancing stages of the disease is limited. However, there is no evidence that all cognitive skills deteriorate at the same rate in the afflicted patients, despite a clinical expectation for general decline. A recent study (10) reported that performance in attentional tasks deteriorated more quickly than performance on memory tasks over a 1-year period in a group of mildly impaired Alzheimer's patients. Research is needed to identify the pattern of cognitive fallout throughout the entire course of illness. Clinical experience suggests that it is likely that substantial individual differences will be seen. Many patients are capable of a wide repertoire of intelligent behavior despite obvious deficits.

## Natural History of Dementia: Changes with Time

Although the natural history of the Alzheimer type dementia is not yet well documented, the patient's capacity for self-care and ability to adapt to the physical and social environment deteriorates slowly and relentlessly. Recent data suggest that markers of immunodeficiency characteristic of Alzheimer's dementia predict the course of illness (11). Multi-infarct dementias are also progressive, but there appears to be a more exaggerated stepwise deterioration with time (12).

Clinically, large individual differences are observed in the rate of change during the course of dementia (13), and there does not appear to be a strong correlation between severity (i.e., degree of deficits) and duration of illness. These different patterns suggest the hypothesis that the disorder, primary neuronal degeneration of the Alzheimer type, like mental retardation, is not one disease, but a cluster of several disorders. A vigorous research effort to disaggregate dementia into its different forms will not only increase our knowledge of etiology and risk factors, but will lead to new methods of treatment and prevention.

## Need for Treatment and Management Strategies

Present opportunities for intervention with the demented patients and their families include drugs and medical intervention to maintain physical health, a variety of psychological therapies, and environmental interventions to change the physical characteristics of the home. Unfortunately, our intervention strategies are limited by our poor understanding of what is destroying the brain. Vigorous research is needed to understand how to arrest the progression of cell loss, to cure and, ultimately, to prevent dementing disorders.

The primary treatment objective for the patient suffering from a nonreversible dementia is optimization of function and quality of life for the patient and family. This is done through the management of medical, psychosocial, and family problems, as well as through cognitive enhancement and environmental alterations (13). Before discussing some of these available strategies, it is appropriate to emphasize some of the difficulties families face as well as to describe phases in the families' reactions. It is clear that the involvement and care of relatives as well as the availability of community resources and clinical services optimize the level of individual function and human dignity despite the inevitable degeneration of the brain.

Dementing illness affects 10–20% of the population over age 65. Although approximately 600,000 afflicted individuals are in nursing homes, the majority are in the community, and most families prefer to keep their relatives out of institutions as long as possible. As a result, care is often provided until the family's physical, emotional, and financial resources are exhausted (14–17).

## ISSUES IN THE MANAGEMENT OF THE FAMILY CARING FOR AN IMPAIRED RELATIVE

Families and caregivers are the major resource in the care and management of cognitively impaired older persons. Most older Americans have strong family bonds: 90% have seen one or more relatives during the previous week; 75% live within 30 minutes of their nearest child; and common living arrangements include living with a spouse, sibling, or other relatives (18, 19). When an older individual develops an impairment or disability, 80% of the support services are provided by families.

In an analysis of 280 admissions to a geriatric unit, Isaacs (20) observed that relatives' unwillingness to assist their older relative was not a factor contributing to the need for hospital admission. However, the condition most difficult for families to accept was the chronic care required with the presence of mental disorders. The willingness of relatives to accept responsibility for the care of the elderly has also been documented by Lowther and Williamson (21). In a review of 1,500 patients discharged from a geriatric unit, there were only 12 unreasonable refusals by relatives to provide home care.

The impact of dementing illness on family health can be severe, and as often as not, family members become patients themselves. The stress of caring for a cognitively impaired relative can result in serious personal distress as well as contribute to physical disorders (e.g., hypertension, heart attacks), psychiatric disorders (e.g., depression, alcohol and substance abuse), as well as maladaptive behaviors in family members, including children. Therefore, effective management of the patient requires not only a concern for the patient's health but appropriate concern for the health of the family members or caregivers.

## Difficulties that Families Face
## in Caring for Impaired Relatives

In an attempt to understand what happens in families caring for a relative with dementia, we need to review some of the problems these families face (Table 15.1). These problems group into several major areas:

- clinical, social, and economic factors;
- losses in the impaired family member;
- finding professional help;
- increased vulnerability of the family members;
- social isolation;
- interactions with the impaired family member; and
- long-term changes in the family.

The literature clearly shows that the psychiatric needs of the impaired aged and their families have not been adequately served and that the potential role of the family in caring for such patients has not been sufficiently supported. Many families report that little or no information is given to them by professionals, and therapeutic nihilism exists instead of clinical and community services. Lack of knowledge about dementia and lack of assessment, referral, and treatment centers in the community increase the vulnerability of the entire family. Although community resources are inadequate to meet families' home care needs, many families cannot afford whatever long-term health care services may be available (e.g., 24-hour nurse service). Consequently, some families will go without help, and others spend time and money without finding adequate help.

Too often, families report that they have spent a great deal of money and time to receive nothing. The patient may be given an inadequate label (senile, old) or a correct diagnosis (Alzheimer's disease), but families receive little practical information about how to help their relative. One professional may give them a dismal outlook ("She will be institutionalized in 3 months and dead in a year"); another may express uncertainty ("Let's wait a year and see what happens"). The end result of many families' experiences is hostility towards professionals. Some families feel that they will be the only ones who will take care of their relative. Others give up and live one day at a time. Alternatively, many families have formed self-help groups that meet and work together to solve their problems (22, 13, 23).

Relatives with an impaired adult in the family are often isolated

TABLE15.1 Difficulties That Families May Face in the Care of Relatives with Dementing Illness

**Medical, Social, and Economic Factors**
- Distribution of clinical resources
- Family structure
- Stigma and social vulnerability

**Losses in Demented Relative**
- Cognition
- Personality
- Health
- Family and social roles

**Finding Help and Experiences with Professionals**
- Absence of a comprehensive system of diagnosis, referral, and treatment
- Uncertainty
- Waste of time
- Desperation
- Hostility
- Unwillingness to seek or accept help

**Increased Vulnerability**
- Economic
- Health

**Social Isolation**
- Fatigue because of lack of help
- Poorer coping and less ability to gratify self and others
- Impaired relative is exposed to fewer normal and "outside" situations
- Family is seen as isolated, and this leads to further isolation
- Imposed vs. self-imposed isolation

**Interactions with Demented Adult**
- Personal care
- Family
- Activities
- Household
- Behavioral management
- Health

**Long-Term Changes in Family**
- Fatigue
- Isolation
- Marital problems (conflict and withdrawal)
- Family problems (conflict and withdrawal)
- Communication games
- Personal problems

from other members of the extended family—brothers, sisters, cousins, uncles, aunts. The result is that the spouse or the caregiver of a demented patient cannot receive support. Furthermore, families are usually characterized by a division of responsibilities, and the extent to which roles are inflexible has an important impact on the family. For example, if the husband or wife must work during the day or night, he or she may simply not be able to supervise the spouse adequately.

Many families are totally unprepared not only for the burden of 24-hour care but also for the negative reactions of friends and the greater community. Patients often have considerable insight into their problems, and report the withdrawal of friends as one of their most significant losses.

The behaviors of the demented patient are troublesome management problems. The family must deal with a range of behavior including agitation, aggression, disruptions, lack of motivation, and lack of self-care. Many of these problems in behavior can be effectively dealt with in the early and middle phases of the illness if the families are taught simple behavioral management plans. The progressive cognitive losses impose significant demands, and family members must find new ways of living with their impaired relative, often restructuring the physical environment of the home. Keeping the patient active and developing meaningful roles in the family often taxes the ingenuity and endurance of the caregivers.

Caring for an impaired relative not only affects the amount of work family members must do and their feelings about the present and future, but it also increases their economic vulnerability as they invest time and money looking and paying for professional help. They also become socially vulnerable as friends (including the patient's friends) drift away, social invitations decline, and leisure or work activities become impossible. The inevitable physical and emotional exhaustion becomes the basis for family conflict as well as for counterproductive ways of dealing with the impaired relative. In desperate attempts to find help, family caregivers become vulnerable to "miracle cures," as well as to anyone who offers them any information about dementing illness.

One of the major problems family members face in their search for help is uncertainty, even if they are able to get adequate diagnostic evaluation. Isolation in families caring for impaired relatives is caused not only by reactions of outsiders and experiences of professionals but also by the nature of the family structure, since many relatives are physically distant.

The results of the isolation may engender even more problems. Spouses or caregivers become fatigued because they cannot find or afford outside help. The more fatigued family members become, the less able they may be to cope with their impaired relative. Thus, as time goes on, the family may become a closed system in which the impaired family member is not exposed to outside settings that may still add to quality of life (e.g., sitting quietly by the ship canal or in the city park), and family members are perceived as eccentric, which often leads to more isolation.

What happens if problems facing the family continue for a long time? In most families, existing problems grow worse, new ones develop, the caregivers' health is often affected, and the quality of life for both patient and family deteriorates. Isolation may increase, marital problems may develop, caregivers become more drained, angry and nonproductive interaction occurs between the patient and family, and family routines become disorganized.

Fortunately, a great deal can be done to decrease family and patient isolation:

• working with patients and families to manage the behavioral manifestations of dementias,

● referring families to self-help groups from which they can obtain information about how others have coped effectively, and
● building family or community networks so that families can continue to
support, motivate, and reinforce each other.

A number of management strategies are possible to optimize health and
personal care as well as to increase activities and involvement in the
home (13, 24). The family must learn to interact with demented relatives
in a way that maximizes functional independence and health for all.
Further, the family members must also learn how to change their interaction as the dementia progresses. Just as the patient changes with the
course of the illness, so also does the family change.

## Development of a Geriatric and Family Services Clinic

An outpatient geriatric and family service clinic that provides comprehensive evaluation and treatment for cognitively and emotionally impaired older persons can also provide valuable counseling and support
for the family (8). The goal of such a clinic is to provide a comprehensive
evaluation for the patient, while offering the family counseling, support,
and advice (25).

The patient evaluation phase should consist of at least 3 or 4 visits,
including a home visit when feasible. On the first visit, the psychiatrist
conducts a diagnostic interview and observes the dynamics of the family
constellation. The social worker makes a home visit to assess family
stresses further and to gather information on the patient's physical and
psychosocial environment. A physical examination is conducted by an
internist or family physician with the primary goal of identifying and
treating reversible causes of dementing illness. An architect is a useful
consultant to assess the congruence between the individual's needs and
abilities and the actual living situation. The nurse and occupational therapist most frequently deal with an assessment of functional status.

Following the intake evaluations and home visit, staff conferences
are necessary to consolidate findings, develop a working diagnosis and
formulate recommendations in several specified areas:

● physical health of the patient;
● mental health of the patient;
● preparation for longer-term care of the patient in the home and/or
institutionalization;

●financial matters;
●community and clinical resources, including local self-help groups;
●structure of the patient's daily routine;
●food and nutrition;
●living situation and environmental alterations;
●stresses within the family caused by the patient's problems;
●physical and mental health of family members or caregivers; and
●the nature of the ongoing relationship between the clinic and the
  family as the dementia progresses.

## MANAGEMENT OF THE INDIVIDUAL
## WITH A DEMENTING DISORDER

Once the presumptive diagnosis of a nonreversible dementia of the
Alzheimer or multi-infarct type or a related disorder has been carefully
established (1, 2, 9, 26, 27), it is important to develop a regular schedule
for monitoring the adaptation of the patient and the family or caregivers.
Areas for patient evaluation should at least include the following:

●biomedical profile, including laboratory abnormalities;
●neurologic deficits;
●concomitant psychiatric disorders
●cognitive performance, including metacognition, the patients' insight
  and knowledge of their problems;
●functional abilities and disabilities; and
●psychosocial adaptation.

   A number of psychological therapies can be successfully implemented to manage the cognitively impaired patient (28). Current pharmacological therapies are effective in the treatment of concomitant psychiatric problems such as depression, anxiety, and paranoia, but a rational
effective drug for the treatment of the dementing process is currently
lacking (22). A number of drugs are being tested in cognitively impaired
patients, including cholinergic agents, with limited success (29, 30).
   Behavioral management techniques, including individual and group
psychotherapies, contingency therapies, family therapies, and environmental therapies, have been reviewed elsewhere (13, 28, 31, 32). The
remaining sections of this chapter review the basis for the use of cognitive enhancement or cognitive retraining techniques with cognitively
impaired patients (1, 33).
   A comprehensive evaluation of intellectual skills throughout the

course of dementia is important information to help the health care professional and family understand and manage the patient (Table 15.2). A wide range of abilities should be evaluated to establish the profile of deficits. These areas include:

- speed of simple and complex actions;
- the presence of aphasia or proficiency in the use of language;
- the ability to employ or respond to nonverbal cues;
- speed and accuracy in organizing, rehearsing, and retrieving learned information;
- the ability to focus and divide attention;
- the ability to remember and manipulate new information;
- the ability to read, write, and perform arithmetic tasks; and
- insight into the extent of cognitive dysfunction.

In conjunction with quality medical care and family support, cognitive remediation strategies based upon behavioral assessments may well be the best tools we now have to maximize the level of functioning of the patient with dementing illness.

Cognitively impaired individuals can continue to be active in a number of activities, including sports, shopping, and helping around the home, and they can play an active and valued role in the family, at least until the later stages of dementia. In addition to cognitive skills, several other factors must be evaluated in the evolution of management plans because of their effect on the adaptive style of the patient (Table 15.3). A careful, probing interview with the patient and caregivers during each follow-up visit should examine a range of environmental, family, psychosocial, and patient factors. For example, supportive psychotherapy with the demented patient can improve confidence and affect the patients' attitudes and beliefs regarding their limited control over their lifestyle.

TABLE 15.2 Areas of Cognitive Dysfunction
---
- Speed and motivation
- Language (expressive and receptive functions)
- Nonverbal communication
- General cognitive processes (coding, organizing, rehearsing, retrieving)
- Attentional systems (focused and divided attention)
- Memory systems (improvements in strategies, changes in executive functions, increases in knowledge base)
- Focal cognitive skills (reading, writing, mathematics, fluency)
- Metacognition

TABLE 15.3 Factors That Limit Cognitive Performance and Adaptation of Cognitively Impaired Individuals

**Disease Factors**
● Duration and severity of dementia
● Health

**Environmental Factors**
● Quality of clinical and community support systems
● Living situation and demands of environment (cognitive enhancing aspects of environment; ability to control and influence environment)
● Recent life events
● Family beliefs, attitudes, needs, and preferences
● Medications

**Patient Factors**
● Functional capacity
● Patient's beliefs, attitudes, needs, and preferences
● Life history (education, work and leisure experience, life roles)
● Affect (depression, anxiety, paranoia, anger and hostility)
● Repertoire of social skills (ability to relate to family and friends)

## Cognitive Assessment

The range of procedures useful to test both the healthy and the cognitively impaired aged is sharply limited. Although several clinical mental status examinations (34–36) provide gross measures of cognitive dysfunction, they do not clarify the types of cognitive processes that are impaired or the cognitive strengths that an individual may still retain. Their utility for diagnosis and assessment of change is limited (37).

A Cognitive Evaluation Battery composed of 15 major subtests has been developed to provide a profile of cognitive performance (Table 15.4) (38). These subtests group themselves into 4 major cognitive areas (Table 15.5):

●attentional systems,
●memory functions,
●focal cognitive skills, and
●clinical tests of mental status.

The battery was constructed to measure a series of discrete cognitive processes to evaluate the rate, quality, and accuracy of information processing in patients with a wide range of dementias. These tests provide an important assessment of the individual's strengths and weaknesses, as well as a basis for improved differential diagnosis and the assessment of

TABLE 15.4 Description of the Subtest in the Cognitive Evaluation Battery Developed for Evaluating a Range of Cognitive Functions in Older Persons, including Those with Dementing Illness (38).

1. **Orientation**
   Questions regarding biographical information

2. **Level of consciousness**
   Rate individual 0–2

3. **Speech**
   Rate individual 0–5

4. **Comprehension subtests**
   a. 3 simple questions, e.g., "Point to the floor"
   b. 3 yes/no questions, e.g., "Can a car go backwards?"
   c. 2 nonsense yes/no quesions, e.g., "If it is 100° and sunny outside, do I need to wear a raincoat?"
   d. 5 linguistic comprehension questions, e.g., Read a sentence, "CIRCLE ABOVE SQUARE," and decide whether a set of figures "————" is the "same" or "different"

5. **Memory Capacity**
   # digits forward;
   # digits backward

6. **Perceptual Store**
   Mean number of letters remembered from two 4 × 4 letter matrices presented for .5 second

7. **Selective Attention**
   Mean number of red letters remembered from six 4 × 4 letter matrices (alternating red and blue letters presented for .5 second)

8. **Semantic Visual Scanning**
   a. Sort 2 decks of 48 cards for a target "x" in a field of zeros
   b. Sort 2 decks of 48 cards for a target letter in a field of different letters

continued

change in performance. Cognitive skills (e.g., semantic vs. spatial, acoustic vs. visual, attention vs. memory skills) may not uniformly deteriorate in patients with dementia. Insight into the skills an individual retains during phases of illness can provide guidelines for cognitive retraining and also provide the family or caregivers with a realistic baseline for performance at home or in the institution.

## The Importance of Cognitive Assessment and Remediation

Ongoing cognitive evaluation provides an important focus on the changing abilities of the afflicted individual and guides changes in manage-

Table 15.4 continued

---

9. **Figural Visual Scanning (5 questions)**
   Identify which figure in a field of 5 is identical to a presented target figure

10. **Memory Search (6 sets of 8 trials)**
    Identify whether a set of numbers presented one at a time are identical to targets presented as a memory set

11. **Letter Matching**
    a. Compare 20 letter pairs for name identity, e.g., Aa
    b. Compare 20 letter pairs for physical identity, e.g., BB

12. **Episodic Memory**
    Report steps necessary to change a tire or bake a cake

13. **Selective Attention and Incidental Learning**
    Read short story orally, and then answer four questions about content

14. **Learning**
    a. Word list recall
    b. Record associations to 10 words (not included in score)
    c. Test immediate free recall, immediate cued recall, delayed free recall (10 min.) and delayed cue recall

15. **Focal Cognitive Skills**
    a. Writing, e.g., copy numbers (1–10), letters (5 Greek letters), and 3 designs, i.e., circle, square, and triangle
    b. Mathematics, e.g., mental arithmetic and simple written problems
    c. Oral reading and incidental learning
    d. Ideational fluency, e.g., name solids that are food and sweet

---

ment strategies. For example, in the early stages of dementia, if perceptual motor skills are relatively intact, limited driving to familiar locations may be permitted. When these abilities deteriorate significantly, other options should be explored to provide activities for the patient. For example, recreational activities such as cycling, which provides great pleasure to many people of all ages, should be encouraged if functional skills are present.

In general, physical exercise and activities should be structured for the patient and the family as part of a daily routine, even if it is as simple as running, walking, or gardening. Knowledge of the patient's strengths as well as weaknesses provides a basis for working with the family to find meaningful roles for the impaired relative throughout the course of the illness. Although memory and attentional dysfunctions often make the successful completion of household chores (e.g., cooking, cleaning, and shopping) impossible, individuals are often capable of successfully performing aspects of these tasks. Accurate evaluations can

TABLE 15.5  Major Areas of Cognitive Functions Evaluated by the Cognitive
Evaluation Battery (Number in Parentheses Identifies Subtest from Table 2)

**Memory Functions**
- Memory capacity (5)
- Perceptual memory (6)
- Retrieval from short-term memory (10)
- Retrieval from long-term memory (11)

**Attentional Performance**
- Selective attention (7)
- Semantic visual scanning (8a and b)
- Figural visual scanning (9)
- Oral reading with distraction (13)

**Focal Cognitive Skills**
- Writing (15a)
- Mathematics (15b)
- Reading (15c)
- Fluency (15d)

**Clinical Mental Status Tests**
- Orientation (1)
- Level of consciousness (2)
- Speech (3)
- Comprehension (4a–d)
- Episodic memory (12)
- Word learning (14a–c)

provide the framework to make recommendations about life and work
roles for the patient. An older impaired adult may not be capable of
doing the weekly shopping, but may derive satisfaction from running a
simple errand for the day (e.g., buying a loaf of bread or a quart of milk
for the evening meal). In general, the physical environment and life
roles should be structured to reward patients for successful performance
rather than to remind them of their disabilities. To go one step further,
research is needed to design cognitively enhancing environments for the
impaired aged—to implement physical and social alterations that motivate the individual, stimulate ordered behavior, and provide incentives
for using whatever capacities are intact or less impaired.

    Cognitive evaluation also provides a basis to establish the parame-
ters for management through psychotherapy, pharmacotherapy, and
cognitive enhancement. In early and middle stages of dementia, individualized and group training programs can be implemented to work
with less-impaired or intact cognitive functions to compensate as much
as possible for major cognitive deficits. These require a set of cognitive
shaping exercises so that easy and difficult tasks are ordered in a hierarchy (38).

## CONCLUSION

What do cognitively impaired aged patients and their families expect their lives to be like in the future? By and large, they expect that our relentless research, educational, and clinical efforts will continue to find a way to help them improve their quality of life. They expect to live fully until they die As Tennyson wrote in *Ulysses:*

> We are not now that strength which in old days
> Moved earth and heaven; that which we are, we are;
> One equal temper of heroic hearts,
> Made weak by time and fate, but strong in will
> To strive, to seek, to find, and not to yield.

## REFERENCES

1. Eisdorfer, C., Cohen, D. The cognitively impaired elderly: Differential diagnosis. In M. Storandt, I. Siegler, and M. F. Elias (eds.), *The Clinical Psychology of Aging*. New York: Plenum, 1978.
2. Eisdorfer, C., Cohen, D., Diagnostic criteria for primary neuronal degeneration of the Alzheimer type. *J. Fam. Prac.* 11:553–557, 1980.
3. Kay, D. W. K. The epidemiology of brain deficit in the aged: Problems in patient identification. In C. Eisdorfer and R. O. Friedel (eds.), *The Cognitively and Emotionally Impaired Elderly*. Chicago: Year Book Medical, 1977.
4. Gruenberg, E. M. Epidemiology of senile dementia. In, B. S. Schoenberg (ed.), *Advances in Neurology*, Vol. 19, New York: Raven, 1978.
5. Katzman, R. The prevalence and malignancy of Alzheimer's disease: A major killer. *Arch. Neurol.* 33:217–218, 1976.
6. (NIA) National Institute on Aging. Senility reconsidered. *JAMA* 244:259–263, 1980.
7. Eisdorfer, C., Cohen, D. and Kechich, W. Depression and anxiety in the cognitively impaired aged. In D. Klein (ed.), *Anxiety Reconceptualized*. New York: Raven, 1981.
8. Reifler, B., Eisdorfer, C. A clinic for impaired elderly and their families. *Amer. J. Psychiat.* 137:1399–1403, 1980.
9. Wells, C. E. Dementia (2nd ed.). Philadelphia: Davis Co., 1977.
10. Cohen, D., Eisdorfer, C. Longitudinal observation on cognition in patients with Alzheimer's dementia. Presented in Basel, Switzerland: Jan. 1980.
11. Cohen, D., Eisdorfer, C., Prinz, P., Leverenz, J., and Davis, M. Immunoglobulins, cognitive status, and duration of illness in Alzheimer's disease. *Neurobiol. Aging* 1:165–168, 1980.
12. Hachinski, V., Lassen, N. A., and Marshall, J. Multi-infarct dementia. *Lancet* 2:207–209, 1974.

13. Eisdorfer, C., Cohen, D. Management of the patient and family coping with dementing illness. *J. Fam. Prac.* 12:831–837, 1981.

14. Brody, E. M. Aging and the family personality: A developmental view. *Family Process* 13:23–37, 1974.

15. Brody, E. M. *Long-Term Care of Older People: A Practical Guide.* New York: Human Sciences Press, 1977.

16. Brody, E. M. The aging of the family. *Ann. Am. Acad.* 438:13–27, 1978.

17. Shanas, E. The family as a social support system in old age. *Gerontologist,* 19:169–174, 1979.

18. Shanas, E. Family and household characteristics of old people in the United States. In Hansen (ed.), *Age with a Future.* Copenhagen: Munksgaard, 1964.

19. Shanas, E., et al. *Old People in Three Industrial Societies.* New York: Atherton, 1968.

20. Isaacs, B. Geriatric patients: Do their families care? *Br. Med. J.* 4:282–285, 1971.

21. Lowther, C. P., Williams, J. Old people and their relatives. *Lancet,* 2:1459–1460, 1966.

22. Eisdorfer, C., Cohen, D., and Veith, R. *The Psychopathology of Aging.* Kalamazoo, Michigan: Scope, 1981.

23. Fengler, A. P., Goodrich, N. Wives of elderly disabled men: The hidden patients. *Gerontologist* 19:175–183, 1979.

24. Lezak, M. Living with the characterologically altered brain injured patient. *J. Clin. Psychiat.* 39:592–598, 1978.

25. Reitler, B., Larson, E., and Eisdorfer, C. Clinical strategies for the mentally ill elderly and their families. In A. Somers and D. Fabian (eds.) *The Geriatric Imperative: An Introduction to Gerontology and Clinical Geriatrics.* New York: Appleton-Century-Crofts, in press.

26. Katzman, R., Karasu, T. B. Differential diagnosis of dementia. In W. S. Fields (ed.), *Neurological and sensory disorders in the elderly.* New York: Stratton Intercon., 1975.

27. Wells, C. E. Chronic brain disease: An overview. *Am. J. Psychiatry* 135:1–12, 1978.

28. Eisdorfer, C., Cohen, D., and Preston, C. Behavioral and psychological therapies for the older patient with cognitive impairment. In M. Miller and G. Cohen (eds.), *The Clinical Aspects of Alzheimer's Disease and Senile Dementia.* New York: Raven, 1980.

29. Eisdorfer, C. Neurotransmitters and aging: Clinical correlations. In R. Adelman and V. Cristofalo (eds.), *Neural Regulatory Mechanisms During Aging.* New York: Alan R. Liss, 1980.

30. Reisberg, B., Ferris, S., and Gershon, S. Pharmacotherapy of senile dementia. In J. O. Cole and J. E. Barrett (eds.), *Psychopathology in the Aged.* New York: Raven, 1980.

31. Lawton, M. P. Psychosocial and environmental approaches to the care of

dementia patients. In J. O. Cole and J. E. Barrett (eds.), *Psychopathology in the Aged*. New York: Raven, 1980.

32. Rodin, J. Managing the stress of aging: The role of control and coping. In S. Levine and H. Ursin (eds.), *Coping and Health*. New York: Plenum, 1980.

33. Meichenbaum, D. Self-instructional strategy training: A cognitive prosthesis for the aged. *Hum. Dev.* 17:273–278, 1974.

34. Folstein, M. D., Folstein, S. E., and McHugh, P. R. Mini-mental status, a practical method for grading the cognitive state of patients for the clinician. *J. Psych. Res.* 12:189–198, 1975.

35. Blessed, G., Tomlinson, B. E., and Roth, M. The association between quantitative measures of dementia and of senile change in the cerebral gray matter of elderly subjects. *Brit. J. Psychiat.* 114:797–811, 1968.

36. Jacobs, J. W., Bernhard, M. R., Delgado, A., and Strain, J. J. Screening for organic mental syndrome in the medically ill. *Ann. Intern. Med.* 86:40–46, 1977.

37. Cohen, D., Dunner, D. The assessment of cognitive dysfunction in dementing illness. In J. O. Cole and J. E. Barrett (eds.), *Psychopathology in the Aged*.

38. Cohen, D., Eisdorfer, C. *The Cognitive Evaluation Battery*. New York: Springer, in press.

# CHAPTER 16

# The Diagnosis and Management of Depression in the Elderly Patient

Robert O. Friedel, M.D.

## INTRODUCTION

This chapter focuses on the major issues involved in the diagnosis and management of biological depressions in the elderly patient. The term biological depression is used here to refer to those depressive syndromes which are currently thought to be associated with a significant, persistent alteration in CNS chemistry and physiology, which do not respond to psychosocial interventions, but which often improve dramatically with somatic treatments. The most common biological depressions are endogenous unipolar and endogenous bipolar depressions with and without psychotic features.

The incidence of biological depressions appears to increase with age, peaking between the ages of 50 and 60 (1), and the relative frequency of the different types of biological depressions also appears to change with aging (2).

## DIFFERENTIAL DIAGNOSIS

Biological depressions in elderly patients are frequently overlooked by the practicing physician because the specific symptoms may be masked by somatic complaints and somatic illnesses, the side effects of drugs, symptoms of anxiety, and the "normal" complaints of aging. In addition, the symptoms of biological depressions may be produced by and confused with those of another common but less treatable disorder of aging, senile dementia, or other physical disorders such as myocardial infarction, gastrointestinal and neurological diseases, hypo- and hyperthyroidism, urinary tract disorders, pancreatic disease, and cancer (3). Finally, losses are a frequent occurrence in the life of the elderly, producing normal grief responses that may lead to either the underdiagnosis or overdiagnosis of depression. A high index of suspicion of depression when evaluating elderly patients with the above problems, and a knowledge of the specific symptoms of biological depressions to be described next, will enable the physician to develop a rational and successful approach to the detection and management of these common and highly treatable disorders of the elderly.

## TYPES OF BIOLOGICAL DEPRESSIONS IN THE ELDERLY AND THEIR TREATMENT

### Endogenous Unipolar Depression

This syndrome, the most common type of severe depression in the aged patient, is characterized by the following symptoms:

1. depressed mood with a significant impairment in ability to enjoy usual pleasures (anhedonia); the mood disturbance is often described as being qualitatively different from that experienced as a result of a significant loss,
2. decreased sleep, the patient awakening several hours earlier than usual and not being able to return to sleep,
3. decreased appetite with a significant weight loss,
4. marked increase or decrease in psychomotor activity,
5. unrealistic guilt.

This symptom pattern is commonly referred to as endogenous unipolar depression if the patient has no history of mania or hypomania, and if there is no family history of mania. Recent neuroendocrinological (4) and physiological (5) studies have confirmed the contention that endogenous depressions are associated with significant CNS biological changes and are distinct from "reactive," "neurotic," or "characterological" depressions. The confirmed finding that approximately two-thirds of patients with symptoms of endogenous depression (unipolar or bipolar, with and without psychotic features) demonstrate an abnormal response to dexamethasone now enables the physician to confirm his clinical diagnosis of this disorder in the laboratory (4). The dexamethasone suppression test (DST) is performed by having the patient take 1 mg of dexamethasone at 11:30 P.M. If an outpatient, the patient returns to have a blood sample drawn at 4:00 P.M. the next afternoon. Inpatients have an additional sample taken at 11:00 P.M. that evening. A plasma cortisol level above 5 μg/dl in either of these 2 samples indicates an abnormal response to the usual suppressive effects of dexamethasone on cortisol levels. If one excludes pregnant patients, patients who have Cushing's disease, anorexia nervosa, uncontrolled diabetes mellitus, a major physical illness, or temporal lobe epilepsy, and patients who are taking drugs inducing hepatic enzymes (see below), the test is 98% specific for endogenous depression. As the DST is approximately 65% sensitive in patients who have 2 blood samples drawn and analyzed (50% for 1 sample), the test will indicate only the presence of endogenous depression, *not* its absence. The DST is not altered in patients receiving psychotropic medications or other medications with the exception of phenytoin, barbiturates, and meprobamate as well as high doses of steroids or benzodiazepines (4).

The use of the DST in elderly patients suspected of having endogenous depression, including those with the other medical and behavioral problems noted above that may complicate the clinical presentation, will enhance the physician's certainty in making the correct diagnosis. Even in the absence of an abnormal DST, given the presence of most of the above clinical symptoms, it is worth proceeding with a therapeutic trial of tricyclic antidepressants (TCA), the treatment of choice for this disorder. Before doing so, however, the physician should conduct a thorough medical examination of the patient and perform routine blood and urine studies. In addition, an ECG should be done to rule out heart block, the major cardiac contraindication to the use of TCAs. The presence of orthostatic hypotension should also be determined, since this appears to be one of the best predictors of severe, TCA-induced orthostatic hypotension (6). This particular side effect occurs commonly in the elderly, and has been reported to be associated with dizziness or falling in approximately 40% of elderly outpatients treated with these drugs (7). Given the possible consequence of a fall in an elderly patient, this important side effect of TCA treatment must be minimized. Finally, prior to TCA treatment, patients should be removed from all nonessential drugs, especially steroids, L-dopa, Aldomet, guanethidine, reserpine, propranolol, hydralazine, and Tagomet, which may cause depression themselves.

Having done this, a TCA may then be selected and treatment initiated. Although it is clear that some patients with endogenous unipolar depression respond better to one TCA than another, there is no reliable way to predict such responses at the present time. Experienced clinicians, however, utilize a number of facts and clinical impressions about TCA response that aid in this choice. First, it appears that some TCAs have a tendency to cause greater sedation (e.g., amitriptyline or doxepin), and some TCAs have a tendency to cause less sedation (e.g., imipramine, desipramine, nortriptyline). Therefore, patients who are not sleeping well and are anxious or agitated may do better on one of the former drugs than the latter, which may increase "nervousness." Anticholinergic side effects of TCAs are more of a problem in the old than in the young because of the increased incidence of prostatic disease, glaucoma, chronic constipation, and a greater susceptibility to CNS anticholinergic toxicity. Consequently, TCAs with less anticholinergic potencies, such as doxepin in the sedating group, and desipramine and nortriptyline in the less-sedating group, are preferred. As previously noted, TCA-induced orthostatic hypotension in the elderly must be kept at a minimum. Doxepin and nortriptyline appear to be less problematic in this respect than the other members of their respective classes. Finally, TCAs are known to have a quinidine-like action on the heart. This enables the physician to use them in depressed patients who are also suffering from cardiac arrhythmias, even if they are being treated with quinidine, if the dosage of the latter drug is reduced appropriately. However, since TCAs all significantly increase cardiac conduction time, heart block of any degree is a major contraindication to their use (8).

The initial dose of a TCA given to an elderly patient should be less than that given to a young patient. For example, 25–50 mg/day, usually given 1–2 hours before bedtime, is a reasonable starting dosage range. Daily doses are then increased by 25–50 mg, no more frequently than once a week, until symptoms begin to clear, or side effects become problematic. Because the pharmacokinetic processes of drug absorption, distribution, metabolism, and excretion are often, but not always, altered in the aged patient (9), monitoring TCA plasma levels in this patient group permits greater individualization of treatment with improved response rate and decreased toxicity. To illustrate this point, in a recent evaluation of elderly patients treated with doxepin, apparent therapeutic plasma levels of doxepin plus desmethyldoxepin were achieved in some patients on a daily dose of 100 mg, while others required as much as 300 mg to reach the same drug plasma level (10). Table 16.1 lists the current best estimates of TCA therapeutic plasma levels derived from the current literature (11). It is important to realize that most of these data were obtained from studies using nongeriatric patient populations. Older patients might require somewhat lower or higher TCA plasma levels in order to achieve therapeutic responses,

TABLE 16.1 Tricyclic Antidepressant Plasma Levels
Associated with Maximal Therapeutic Response

| Drug | Plasma level (ng/ml) |
| --- | --- |
| Nortriptyline | 50–170 |
| Imipramine (+ desipramine) | > 200 |
| Desipramine | 40–160 |
| Amitriptyline (+ nortriptyline) | > 160 |
| Doxepin (+ desmethyldoxepin) | > 100 |

but these data can serve as guidelines for the physician treating the elderly depressed patient.

During the initial phases of TCA dosage adjustment, compliance can be enhanced, especially in outpatients, by alerting patients to the likely occurrence of certain side effects, such as drowsiness, dry mouth, etc., and their usual transient nature. If side effects do not subside within 3 days of the start of treatment or an increase of dosage, dosage reduction is often warranted, to be followed by a change to another TCA if improvement does not occur. It is also helpful to tell patients that they should not anticipate a reduction in their symptoms, with the exception of their sleep disturbance, sooner than 10–14 days after treatment is initiated. Patients often need to be encouraged to stay on their medications during this period when side effects seem to be the predominant "reward" for their efforts. TCA plasma levels will enable the physician to detect the noncompliant patient, who should then be gently questioned and encouraged to take the medication every day as directed.

Patients not responding to a TCA of one class (e.g., doxepin or amitriptyline) despite a therapeutic plasma level for 2 weeks duration, should be switched to a TCA of the other class (e.g., nortriptyline, desipramine, imipramine) and not to one of the same class, and the above process of dosage adjustment repeated. Patients not responding to thorough therapeutic trials on one TCA from each class require another form of therapy, some of which are mentioned below. Before doing so, however, the patient may be tried on a course of treatment with a new TCA recently approved by the FDA. Amoxapine (Asendin) appears to have an earlier onset of action than other TCAs currently used in this country and to have relatively minor anticholinergic and other side effects when given in the usual dosage range of 150–300 mg daily (12).

Although there are no clear research data on the subject, it is likely that TCA dosages may be reduced safely in elderly depressed patients after about 30 days of improvement. A common technique is to reduce daily dosage by about 25 mg, no more often than once a week, until approximately half the therapeutic dosage is reached or symptoms recur. The maintenance dosage is then given for an additional 3–4 months, and then reduced again by the above schedule until the patient is off the medication. It is estimated that 15% of patients may require long-term maintenance on TCAs in order to control symptoms. At this time, there are no known deleterious effects of such treatment, especially with doxepin (13, 14).

## Endogenous Bipolar Depression

This recurrent depressive syndrome is often characterized by the following symptoms:

1. marked depression of mood and anhedonia,
2. increased sleep,
3. increased appetite,
4. psychomotor retardation,
5. history of manic or hypomanic episode or family history of manic depressive disorder.

Although the age of onset of bipolar depression is typically in young adulthood, the disorder may first appear much later in life. Whenever it occurs, the illness is more effectively and safely treated with the combination of lithium carbonate and a tricyclic antidepressant. The use of lithium with a TCA protects the patient against the development of a manic episode produced by the TCA. Because they appear to act synergistically, a lower dose of both drugs may be used. A starting dose of 300 mg of lithium b.i.d. and 50 mg of a TCA per day is often sufficient. Response to this treatment is often more rapid than in unipolar depression, and the length of maintenance treatment may be substantially decreased (i.e., 2–4 weeks). Between attacks, the use of maintenance lithium alone should be considered. Older patients are more sensitive to lithium CNS toxicity than younger patients, even at relatively low blood levels. Therefore, any clouding of the sensorium of an elderly patient on lithium warrants a trial dosage reduction.

## Endogenous Depression with Psychosis

Either of the above-mentioned types of endogenous depression may present also with psychotic symptoms such as delusions of worthlessness, guilt, somatic illness, and/or auditory and visual hallucinations.

With the presence of any of these symptoms, the response to TCAs is markedly diminished. The treatment of choice for these patients then becomes unilateral electroconvulsive therapy (15) or the combination of a neuroleptic and a TCA (16).

These patients are very high suicide risks. In addition, most attempts at suicide in this age group are successful (17). Therefore, they, and all patients who have the diagnosis of depression, should be evaluated for suicidal potential.

## THE EVALUATION OF SUICIDAL POTENTIAL

Increased suicidal potential most likely coincides with the progression of patients through stages of thinking about suicide (ideation), frequent suicidal thoughts (rumination), considering methods of suicide (planning), and finally, actual attempts (action). Clearly, the further patients advance along this spectrum, the greater is the suicide risk. No specific recommendations can be made that will ensure such patients' safety and also keep hospitalization of depressed patients to a reasonable level. However, nonpsychiatrists are advised to request a psychiatric consult for a depressed patient who admits even to suicidal ideation. For those patients who have reached the planning stage, the situation has reached emergency proportions, and some action should be taken to safeguard the patient's life.

## SUMMARY

Biological depressions occur frequently in the elderly, and they are, unlike many life-threatening disorders that afflict this patient population, very treatable. These depressions are often masked by somatic complaints, other medical disorders, and the "normal" aging process or are confused with senile dementia or normal grieving. Different types of biological depression respond best to different somatic interventions including tricyclic antidepressants, lithium, neuroleptics, and electroconvulsive therapy. Suicidal potential should be evaluated in all elderly patients with symptoms of depression.

## REFERENCES

1. Post, F.: Diagnosis of depression in geriatric patients and treatment modalities appropriate for the population. In: Gallant, D. M. and Simpson, G.

M. (eds.), *Depression: Behavioral, Biochemical, Diagnostic and Treatment Concepts*. Spectrum, NY, 1976.

2. Winokur, G., Behar, D., Vanvalkenburg, C., and Lowry, M.: Is a familiar definition of depression both feasible and valid? J. Nerv. Ment. Dis. *166*: 764–768, 1978.

3. Lehmann, H. E.: Recognition and treatment of depression in geriatric patients. In: Ayd, F. J. (ed.), *Clinical Depressions: Diagnostic and Therapeutic Challenges*. Ayd Medical Communications, Baltimore, MD, 1980.

4. Carroll, B. J.: The dexamethasone suppression test for melancholia. Br. J. Psychiat. (in press).

5. Kupfer, D. J., Foster, F. G., Coble, P., McPartland, R. J. and Ulrich, R. F.: The application of EEG sleep for the differential diagnosis of affective disorders. Am. J. Psychiat. *135*(1):69–74, 1978.

6. Glassman, A. H., Giardina, E. U., Perel, J. M., Bigger, J. T., Kantor, S. J. and Davies, M.: Clinical characteristics of imipramine-induced orthostatic hypotension. Lancet *1*:468–472, 1979.

7. Blumenthal, M. D. and Davie, J. W.: Dizziness and falling in elderly psychiatric outpatients. Am. J. Psychiat. *137*:203–206, 1980.

8. Glassman, A. H. and Bigger, J. T., Jr.: Cardiovascular effects of therapeutic doses of tricyclic antidepressants. Am. J. Psychiat. (in press).

9. Friedel, R. O.: Pharmacokinetics in the geropsychiatric patient. In: Lipton, M. A., DiMascio, A., Killam, K. F. (eds.), *Psychopharmacology: A Generation of Progress*. Raven Press, NY, 1978.

10. Friedel, R. O.: The Pharmacotherapy of depression in the elderly: Pharmacokinetic considerations. In: Cole, J. O. and Barrett, J. E. (eds.), *Psychopathology in the Aged*. Raven Press, NY, 1980.

11. Silverman, J. J., Brennan, P. and Friedel, R. O.: Clinical significance of tricyclic antidepressant plasma levels. Psychosomatics *20*(11):736–746, 1979.

12. Ayd, F. J., Jr.: Amoxapine: A new tricyclic antidepressant. Int. Drug Ther. Newsletter *15*:33–38, 1980.

13. Ayd, F. J., Jr.: Guidelines for treating cardiac patients with tricyclic and tetracyclic antidepressants. Int. Drug Ther. Newsletter, *13*:9–12, 1978.

14. Ayd F. J., Jr.: Continuation and maintenance doxepin (Sinequan) therapy: Ten years' experience. Int. Drug Ther. Newsletter *14*:9–16, 1979.

15. Fink, M.: *Convulsive Therapy: Theory and Practice*. Raven Press, NY, 1979.

16. Minter, R. E. and Mandel, M. R.: The treatment of psychotic major depressive disorder with drugs and electroconvulsive therapy. J. Nerv. & Ment. Disorders. *167*:726–733, 1979.

17. Payne, E. C.: Depression and suicide. In: *Modern Perspectives in the Psychiatry of Old Age*, Howells, J. G. (ed.), Brunner-Mazel, NY, 1975.

# CHAPTER 17

# Schizophrenia in Old Age

## Charles M. Gaitz, M.D.

Often manifested early in life, schizophrenia is a mental disorder that may persist into the senium. Some persons, who have not had the disease earlier, may develop an illness similar to schizophrenia late in life. Whether or not the condition is the same for both periods of onset is of scientific interest, but this chapter directs attention to elderly persons who have had schizophrenic symptoms for many years.

## SYMPTOMATOLOGY

Friedel and Raskind (1) classified schizophreniform psychosis in elderly persons into five types:

1. patients with no cognitive impairment who develop acute schizophreniform illness with hallucinations and delusions,
2. patients with chronic progressive organic brain syndrome with memory loss, disorientation, and general intellectual impairment,
3. patients who have suffered from chronic schizophrenia since early adulthood,
4. patients with chronic brain syndrome who have also developed such schizophreniform symptoms as delusions and hallucinations, and
5. patients with chronic organic brain syndrome whose behavioral symptoms (agitation, irritability, assaultiveness) have become severe enough to cause distress to themselves or to those in their environment.

Perhaps a sixth type should be added. Some patients who have suffered from chronic schizophrenia since early adulthood may suffer dementing changes in the brain and present a combination of organic brain syndrome and schizophrenia rather than one or the other.

Post (2) offers a somewhat similar classification and describes three different forms of symptomatology in elderly persons. After studying a series of hospital patients, he concluded that there were paranoid states with a largely auditory hallucinosis, a second form with more widespread paranoid experiences, and third, a group of patients with clear schizophrenic symptoms about which there would be little disagreement. In the latter group, the symptoms were largely of a paranoid schizophrenic type; catatonic features and disruptions of formal thought were rare. The first two clinical syndromes tended to clear up when patients were moved from their homes to more sheltered surroundings, while patients who manifested "truly" schizophrenic symptoms rarely responded to social measures. In contrast to younger schizophrenics, elderly paraphrenics usually had had a good work record and did not show social decline. A family history of schizophrenia was far rarer in younger than in older schizophrenic patients. Long-standing deafness was strongly associated with late-onset schizophrenia. These patients tended to be socially withdrawn, leading an isolated existence as senile recluses. Few were married, and marriages were likely to occur late in life. Though some researchers concluded that the patients' abnormal personalities might be evidence of long-standing latent schizophrenic disorder that finally emerged because of the aggravated social deprivations of late life, deafness, or some cerebral aspects of the aging process, Post questions whether such conditions are related to gross brain changes. He also doubts that it is important to question whether such patients are schizophrenic or paraphrenic.

Raskin and Jarvik (3) noted that the factors attributed to the development of paranoid reactions at any age tend to be present more frequently in old age. These include social isolation, insecurity, and sensory deficits, particularly of vision and hearing. Some individuals may become overtly psychotic or develop late paraphrenia when senile degeneration or cerebral arteriosclerosis occurs; these patients may, in fact, have been borderline schizophrenic all of their lives. Raskin and Jarvik also discuss the often-expressed opinion that symptoms of depression, anxiety, and schizophrenia are frequently different in older as compared to younger persons, yet few data from empirical studies confirm this. To achieve more accuracy in diagnosing mental illness, it may ultimately be necessary to combine psychiatric rating scales, cognitive test measures, and such newer neurophysiological and vascular testing techniques as computed axial tomography and xenon inhalation.

## COURSE AND PROGNOSIS

Reviews of long-term studies reveal different opinions about the course and prognosis of schizophrenia. Bridge et al. (4) reviewed some of the long-term follow-up studies of schizophrenic patients into the involutional years. The researchers refer to the pessimistic views held by Kraepelin, Eugen Bleuler, and Arieti, who believed that remissions and exacerbations are acceptable as the natural history of the disorder, but that ultimately chronic schizophrenia leads to a terminal demented state. The latter idea is not confirmed in many other studies. As the Bridge group points out, some follow-up studies were of relatively short duration and often did not follow patients into old age. Their review of studies that did follow patients into middle and old age revealed, however, that the outlook was much more favorable than Kraepelin and Eugen Bleuler had believed. Manfred Bleuler (5), for example, reports that, on an average, schizophrenic persons show no further deterioration 5 years after onset of the illness, and he observed substantial symptomatic improvement of long-standing chronic psychosis, even among patients who were continuously hospitalized. Bridge et al. (4) report also on other studies that revealed reductions in paranoia, hyperactivity, phobias, and delusions and increases in sociability. There is at least indirect evidence for a "burn-out" associated with advancing years. Among implications for treatment, Bridge et al. call attention to several investigations that question the rationality of large-dose maintenance phenothiazine therapy across the life-span of the psychiatric patient.

Muller (6) reported on 101 schizophrenics who were 65 and older. Average duration of illness was 35 years and hospitalization 25 years. Evidence of a chronic brain syndrome was noted in about 10% of patients. When these patients were examined in 1959, senescence had not influenced the form of schizophrenia in half the cases. There were suggestive changes, such as disappearance of delusions and improved sociability. About 30 of the patients were reexamined about 10 years later. Many had been transferred to another facility where the ambiance was that of a nursing home for long-term patients. By then the average age of the patients was 80 years, and a number had evidence of dementia. For 23 of the 30 patients, the judgment was that there had been little change in schizophrenic symptomatology, but the aged patients had become more feeble, less vigilant, and less expressive. Modification of schizophrenia with age is not caused by an amnestic syndrome, Muller concluded, but takes place at the beginning of senescence in the sixties. Once this landmark has passed, advancing years, with or without organic mental deterioration, probably will not modify the schizophrenic illness.

Hold and Holt (7) conducted a 30-year follow-up study of 141 patients admitted to the Westborough State Hospital in Massachusetts. The dementia praecox group constituted 42% of the admissions and 37.5% of the discharges, 38% of recoveries, 36% of deaths, 33% of the surviving patients in the community, and 80% of surviving patients hospitalized more than 30 years. Perhaps to offer a note of optimism, Holt reports that 2 of the recovered patients left the hospital after 20 years and at time of follow-up were self-supporting and accepted as normal.

The possibilities and probabilities of cohort differences should not be overlooked in examining long-term studies. Beck (8) gives us an interesting report on patients who were admitted to the Prince Edward Island, Canada mental hospital during two 3-year periods, 1930–1932 and 1940–1942, with a 25- and a 35-year follow-up of first admissions. Patients over age 65 at time of first admission were excluded from the study. There seemed to be little difference in the long-term outcome of the types of cases first admitted for the two periods; at neither time were the newer somatic and pharmacologic therapies available when the patients were first hospitalized. Of 255 patients, 119 were patients who had not lived outside an institution for at least 3 consecutive years. This included 64% of the schizophrenic patients, 43% of those with affective disorders, and 16% of the alcoholic patients. Although about 36% of the schizophrenic patients had returned to the community for periods of more than 3 years, only about 12% seemed to have recovered or improved appreciably over the follow-up period. Thirty-five percent of those with affective disorders and 24% of those with alcoholism were believed to have improved. Although Beck does not report the age of the patients at time of follow-up, admission figures would lead one to conclude that the follow-up was of patients who are well into middle or perhaps old age. Data about economic productivity suggest that about 81% of the schizophrenic patients were either continually hospitalized or completely nonproductive while in the community. Those with affective illness and alcoholism fared somewhat better.

Stephens (9) examined long-term course and prognosis in schizophrenia by reviewing several reports of follow-up research and by his own study of 472 patients hospitalized at the Henry Phipps Psychiatric Clinic. Pointing out that there are relatively benign and malignant forms of the illnesses generally diagnosed as schizophrenia, Stephens reports that these extreme forms may be differentiated even though it cannot be determined with certainty whether they are discrete entities or points on a continuum. The subdivision of schizophrenia into paranoid, hebephrenic, catatonic, and simple has not proved useful, and Stephens emphasizes the need for a more revealing nomenclature. Narrowly defined schizophrenia still has a relatively poor outcome, he finds, whereas atypical schizophrenia has a much better prognosis for spontaneous remission, and for response to treatment by present-day methods. Possibly the syndrome variously labeled as reactive psychosis, nonprocess schizophrenia, schizophreniform psychosis, acute delusional psychosis, and acute schizoaffective psychosis should be considered a separate illness and not of the genus schizophrenia. Stephens's review of the effect of somatic therapies and drug treatment on long-term schizophrenia finds no evidence for better results in patients treated with insulin, Metrazol, or electroshock, but this may be related to the selection of patients. The short-term efficacy of antipsychotic drugs has been demonstrated, but differences are noted when attention is given to the type of schizophrenia being treated. It is perhaps too soon to evaluate fully the long-term effects of pharmacotherapy, but the evidence thus far suggests that careful diagnosis and classification is essential in evaluating the results of treatment. After noting the pessimism of some reports, Stephens concludes that only continuing research will resolve the questions concerning long-term drug efficacy. He also is impressed with the influence of social factors on the course of the illness, especially when duration of hospitalization is considered. No long-term studies deal with the effect of formal psychotherapy on the course of schizophrenia, but personal experience persuaded Stephens that psychotherapy may profoundly improve the course of schizophrenia in many patients.

## CLINICAL VIGNETTES

The following abstracts from case histories highlight some of the important aspects of treatment of these patients. With one exception, the histories are taken from the records of patients being treated at the Geriatric Services Outpatient clinic of the Texas Research Institute of Mental Sciences (TRIMS). Of 890 patients 65 years and older examined there between 1973 and 1978, 136 (15%) had a primary diagnosis of schizophrenia of some type. An undetermined but quite large proportion of these patients had manifestations of illness early in their lives. Although these patients do not usually receive as much attention as those with late-onset mental illness, clearly the management of patients with chronic schizophrenia is a major responsibility of personnel working in a geriatric psychiatric clinic.

The histories highlight two important aspects of management: the need for giving attention to social, psychological, and physical health problems and the need for constant monitoring of physical health status and drug effects. Ready accessibility of caregivers to patients and families is obviously beneficial.

> Mrs. L. is a 72-year-old woman who became ill at age 38 after separation from her husband. She imagined that men who were strangers were in love with her, and people were trying to keep them apart. Recurrent episodes of illness required three periods of hospitalization ranging from 2 to 4 years. She was diagnosed as having schizophrenia, chronic undifferentiated type. At age 56, 1 year after she had been in the hospital, she was referred to a clinic at TRIMS, where she received minimal supportive therapy and supervision of psychotropic medications. In 1975, when she was about 67, she was transferred to the TRIMS Geriatric Outpatient Clinic.
>
> She had been treated with trifluoperazine, chlorpromazine, and/or imipramine and maintained a good remission except for occasional crises and a recurrence of symptoms, when she required closer supervision. Sometimes she would not take her medications as prescribed, particularly at times when she needed them most. When her mother died, support offered by clinic personnel helped her adapt.
>
> After an attempt was made to discontinue psychotropic medications, Mrs. L.'s symptoms recurred, and she was again started on small doses of chlorpromazine. Mrs. L.'s daughter revealed that her mother, though on good behavior when she came to the clinic, actually needed close supervision in daily life. She lived alone, but had relatives to assist her. Formerly a bindery worker, she had been able to work only part-time lately because of an ulcerous dermatitis and respiratory infections. She continued taking chlorpromazine, 50 mg at bedtime. The clinic staff maintained close contact with Mrs. L. and her family, and together they encouraged Mrs. L. to take medications. Her condition fluctuated. A son-in-law complained that Mrs. L. was frequently irritable, and she seemed to be withdrawn. She had not worked for 2 years, but encouraging her to apply for work, perhaps part-time, seemed to lift her spirits. She became more interested in her appearance and generally seemed better, even though she did not find a job.

Mrs. L.'s history illustrates the importance of continuous supervision and close monitoring of psychotropic medications to determine adequacy of dosage. With minimal family support and support of the family by clinic staff, a chronically ill elderly person may remain in the community and perhaps even be able to work.

Mrs. F., a 70-year-old widow, had been in private psychiatric treatment for 36 years and had been delusional since about age 40. The onset of illness coincided with her hysterectomy. Mrs. F. believed that the operation was necessary because she had been poisoned. Her paranoid delusions varied; she spent hours washing herself and cleaning her home to get rid of contaminants, and she thought worms were coming out of her skin. Mrs. F. believed she had made one mistake in her life but nothing could be done about it until she got to heaven. Though her symptoms persisted, her husband refused to consider hospitalization. After his death, Mrs. F.'s two daughters continued to be very supportive. She has been treated for several severe physical disorders, including congestive heart failure, but presented no serious management problems, even when she was hospitalized. At one time she thought she had diabetes, but when her internist could not confirm it, she concluded he was unwilling to help her. She was very upset when the daughter with whom she lived took a 3-week vacation, but she got along quite well with the help of three teenaged grandchildren.

Mrs. F. has been seen infrequently by her psychiatrist, but phone contact has been maintained with her and her daughter. She has taken 15 mg of flurazepam as a bedtime sedative and 1 mg of haloperidol daily for several years. At the time of her last visit in August, 1980, she had clinical signs of parkinsonism for the first time. To determine if these were a side effect of haloperidol, the medication was discontinued and diazepam substituted. If the parkinsonian symptoms persist, she will need treatment for this condition. Her physical functional capacity has declined, and she has become more concerned about her physical health problems. She did not mention her delusions at the last interview, but when she was questioned, it was clear that she still had somatic and paranoid delusions.

Ongoing support by a psychiatrist can be very helpful to the patient and family. In Mrs. F.'s case the psychiatrist acted as case manager, assuring the patient's medical care when she needed it and offering support to family members.

Mr. D., 74, was referred to the TRIMS Geriatric Clinic in 1976 after a 2-month stay in a state mental hospital. He had a long history of psychiatric treatment, including a series of Veterans Administration hospitalizations from age 41–62 for schizophrenia, alcoholism, and borderline diabetes. Organic brain syndrome also had been diagnosed. Mr. D. had a fourth-grade education. When a brief mental status questionnaire was administered in 1976, it was difficult to determine whether his poor performance indicated dementia or reflected his limited education and social isolation. Mr. D. took Hydergine for several years before it was discontinued in 1979. Though organic brain syndrome had been diagnosed 12–15 years earlier, no evidence of advancing dementia appeared in the record.

After his last hospitalization, he did not believe he needed to be referred to TRIMS, was angry about having to give information about himself, and thought doctors had never helped him. An outreach worker made several home visits before Mr. D. would agree to come to the clinic. He was agitated and irritable at times, and was reported to awaken early, curse, and make noises that would disturb the relatives with whom he lived. These relatives worked, and his transportation to the clinic was a problem. Consequently, home visits by a field worker and phone contacts were used to monitor his progress. After several months he became more stable, and his behavior improved so that home visits were no longer necessary. He remained rather seclusive, and had occasional episodes of hostility. He was placed temporarily in a nursing home when the sister with whom he had been living became ill. When she improved, Mr. D. returned to their home. He was observed to be getting physically weaker. Mr. D. was maintained on haloperidol, and this was continued even after he had symptoms suggesting tardive dyskinesia. Another tranquilizer was substituted for a while, but Mr. D. became more agitated and hostile and was shifted back to haloperidol, which he preferred.

Clinic staff members, particularly outreach workers, may help retain patients in treatment and assist relatives, especially during crises. The history also illustrates a problem psychiatrists commonly face in deciding whether to continue prescribing a drug that has been helpful but may produce side effects; it is an example of the difficulties of diagnosing mental illness in old people, especially when there are hints that suggest organic brain syndrome.

Mr. D. lived in a nursing home when, at 76, he was referred to the TRIMS Geriatric Outpatient Clinic for treatment. He had spent about 45 years in state mental hospitals, diagnosed as having catatonic schizophrenia. On initial examination at TRIMS, his affect was flat, and he had little to say. His thought processes were fragmented, sometimes incoherent and irrelevant, and he talked as if he were living in the 1930s. Disorientation was suspected. Limited treatment goals at that time were to supervise his medications (25 mg of chlorpromazine twice a day), avoid psychiatric hospitalization, and help him maintain acceptable behavior in the nursing home. An outreach worker visited him there, and there were frequent contacts with clinic personnel. In 1975, the possibility of discontinuing chlorpromazine was considered. The nursing home personnel, however, were afraid of Mr. D., a large man, and were reluctant to discontinue his medication. He was described as disoriented and having a poor memory 5 years ago, but currently there seems to have been little progression of these symptoms. Mr. D. is relatively well adjusted to the nursing home. Records indicate that Mr. D. also has been treated for hypertension in a medical clinic. He had episodes of tachycardia and fainting spells, the latter possibly aggravated by chlorpromazine. His medication was changed to haloperidol, 0.5 mg twice a day, in September 1977, and he has continued taking this medication for the past 3 years.

Psychiatric clinic staff members must work with nursing home personnel, sometimes making compromises in treatment to accommodate the nursing home's needs, as one sometimes has to do with family members. The case also illustrates that physical health problems may arise and require attention. Constant supervision and close collaboration between internist and psychiatrist avoid problems such as drug-drug interactions and other effects of polypharmacy.

## General Guidelines for Treatment

Certain basic principles apply in treating patients with chronic schizophrenia regardless of age, but we apply these principles with a special awareness of the needs and characteristics of persons who are old. Our broad aims are to provide services that enable these persons to live in their communities in the least restrictive environments and to have opportunities for meaningful life experiences and self-fulfillment.

Psychopharmacologic treatment has been extremely helpful in caring for elderly schizophrenic patients, and it is probably the most important single factor in achieving these objectives. Drug therapy helps in mobilizing family and social supports. Psychiatrists' attitudes are also affected. Those who believe, correctly or not, that drugs effectively relieve the suffering of schizophrenic patients are understandably more optimistic, and this may well affect the outcome of interventions. But therapists must remember that drug therapy alone is not enough; a treatment plan must be comprehensive and mobilize all possible resources.

Elderly persons are likely to have a multiplicity of problems that can be categorized as social, psychological, and physical. Many problems are remediable, but they will be recognized and given attention only when a careful diagnostic evaluation has been done. Treatment often requires a multidisciplinary approach that is easier for the public than the private sector of health care. Private practitioners and those working in limited-manpower situations must provide or recruit a wide range of services. Insufficient attention to social factors, for example, may sabotage a carefully planned regimen for a medical problem. Physicians must look beyond the physical health aspects of care.

In all settings, caregivers must be accessible to patients and their families (10). Crises require active intervention and, perhaps more important, a continued expression of interest in the form of home visits and telephone contacts; regular, even if infrequent, office visits are useful. Patients and families who know that help is available make fewer demands than do those who are floundering, possibly overwhelmed by the demands made on them. Assurance that help is available when needed is a fundamental feature of treating patients for mental and/or physical chronic diseases.

Therapists who have little experience with elderly patients may not give enough thought to the likelihood that these patients often develop physical illnesses that must be treated concomitantly with the psychiatric disorder that was preeminent earlier in these patients' lives. Free-standing community mental health clinics must have arrangements for medical consultations and treatment. This must be done before the need arises; it is a corollary of the principle of comprehensive treatment.

If patients are in nursing homes, then nursing home personnel represent a surrogate family and should be included, as would family members. These collaborations yield a great deal of information and strength to the therapeutic alliance.

The importance of social and family support systems cannot be over-emphasized. Foster homes (11), day hospitals (12), day treatment centers (13), and board and care homes (14) are but a few examples of the kinds of placements that may be helpful to elderly schizophrenic patients. General hospitals and a variety of other community-based social and health agencies meet certain needs. Church groups and senior citizen recreation and nutrition centers provide opportunities for socialization (15).

## Treatment with Psychoactive Drugs

Ban (16), among others, has reviewed the "state of the art" of psychoactive drug treatment for schizophrenia. Research has suggested some specificity in selecting one phenothiazine over another in reducing schizophrenic disorganization, for example, in a withdrawn, suspicious patient, while another phenothiazine may be better for the withdrawn, periodically agitated patient. Response to one drug may be associated with cooperativeness, another with sociability, another with activity level, and still another with anxiety and tension—but there is no general agreement on this.

Ban's studies indicate that schizophrenic patients relapse when drug therapy is discontinued. Nevertheless, because of the increased likelihood of side effects, clinicians are encouraged to use discretion, to give patients drug holidays, and to reduce dosages whenever possible.

With reference specifically to the use of psychoactive drugs in elderly schizophrenic patients, several studies have given us some useful information. Prien et al. (17) surveyed 12 Veterans Administration hospitals, and found that 61% of 1,276 elderly psychiatric patients were receiving psychoactive drugs. Antipsychotic drugs had been prescribed for 70% of those with a diagnosis of schizophrenia, thioridazine and chlorpromazine being the most widely used. Drug dosage and the proportion of patients receiving them decreased with increasing age, so that patients over 75 were treated more conservatively than were patients 10 or 15 years younger, but the reduction in dosage and use may reflect more a change in drug tolerance than clinical condition.

Toxic effects may occur more frequently in older patients, and the risk of interaction between psychoactive drugs and those used to treat physical disorders increases. The Prien group noted that clinicians tend to prescribe familiar drugs, particularly thioridazine and chlorpromazine, which have been in use longer than most antipsychotic drugs. Thioridazine may be favored for geriatric patients because it produces fewer extrapyramidal reactions and involves less risk of falling or dizziness. These authors also conclude that combining two drugs and using smaller dosages rather than one drug in large dosage is not more effective and does not reduce side effects.

Branchey et al. (18) compared the efficacy and toxicity of a high-potency neuroleptic, fluphenazine hydrochloride, in 30 elderly chronic schizophrenic patients. Both drugs produced a similar degree of improvement, but their side effects differed. Fluphenazine caused slightly more extrapyramidal effects than thioridazine, though few occurred with use of either drug. Thioridazine caused weight gain, decreased blood pressure, and electrocardiographic changes. For these reasons, these investigators said, a high-potency neuroleptic agent seems to be the drug of choice for elderly schizophrenic patients.

Branchey et al. (19) also reported that the therapeutic effect of loxapine succinate is similar to that of other neuroleptic drugs in elderly chronic schizophrenic patients. That the degree of improvement was

only moderate was not surprising inasmuch as the subjects were treat-
ment-resistant patients. The maintenance dosage for older patients was
about half that used for younger patients.

Raskind et al. (20) compared the effects of 5 mg of fluphenazine
enanthate administered parenterally at 2 week intervals with those of 2
mg of haloperidol given orally, 3 times daily, for "crisis intervention"
treatment of elderly outpatients with late-onset paraphrenia. Fluphenazine was significantly superior, and this was attributed to improved
compliance with the prescribed regimen by patients receiving parenteral depot medication. At this low dosage, fluphenazine did not cause
adverse effects.

How long patients should continue taking drugs is an unsettled
issue. Imlah (21) reported on long-term follow-up studies of drugs for
schizophrenia. Because some patients improve and do not relapse after a
period of intensive treatment, some clinicians may decide to discontinue
psychotropic drugs. Yet it is the opinion of many psychiatrists that most
patients will relapse if drugs are withdrawn. Imlah discusses a number
of methodological issues regarding the evaluation of long-term studies,
among them uncertainty of whether or not patients have actually taken
the medications consistently and possible differences parenterally. Baseline data are often absent. There are virtually no control groups with
whom to compare patients who have been on long-term administration
of drugs. Imlah concludes with a conviction that severely ill schizophrenics with a seemingly poor prognosis have the most pressing need
for long-term treatment with neuroleptics. But questions of treatment of
the good-prognosis groups still remain. Because psychiatrists find it difficult to state prognoses, Imlah argues that all schizophrenic patients
should be treated continuously with drugs. Future long-term studies
may resolve the dilemma.

## DISCUSSION

There is a tendency to give little attention to mental illness as a persistent disorder from young adulthood into the senium. This has been
accentuated by the belief that mental disturbance in old people has an
organic substrate. Too often, our diagnoses and eventually our treatments are influenced by the age of the patient, so that "hardening of the
arteries" is used to explain a variety of symptoms. Misconceptions about
aging lead us to conclude that mental disorders of early life "go away,"
"burn out," or become insignificant when compared to the conse-

quences of physiologic and psychologic stresses experienced by elderly persons. The myth is that personality and psychotic disorders fade away as dementia takes over.

In reality, many illnesses persist into old age without shortening life. Paradoxically, older persons whose dependency needs have been frustrated in the past may find that changes associated with aging—such as changes in their physical health or society's demands on them—may actually facilitate achieving satisfaction of these needs.

Whether they are studying schizophrenia, affective disorders, psychosomatic conditions, bioavailability of drugs, psychosexual problems, or any of the other problems that deserve attention, researchers still tend to ignore age of subjects as an important parameter. And, too often, when pressed to consider age as a variable, they decide that subjects over age 45 are typical of the aged. It is unfortunate that studies of old people are so limited that we must rely on extrapolations from data obtained from younger persons. Studies involving long-term follow-up may include middle-aged subjects, but they may not include the clients we ordinarily associate with geriatric psychiatry.

One of the disorders that has an onset early in life and, in many instances, persists for many years is the condition once labeled dementia praecox, now called schizophrenia. This is not the place to review the history of this condition or to debate whether it is a disorder of a single or multiple etiologies. Continuous effort to define this condition, to describe various subtypes based on symptomatology, and to project from these classifications a prediction about treatment and outcome has met with little success. Until now, essays and research reports have been based on diagnostic criteria that are different from those of the recent edition of the American Psychiatric Association's *Diagnostic and Statistical Manual of Mental Disorders* (DSM-III) (22). The manual has specific criteria for the diagnosis of "schizophrenic disorder," and it points out the importance of differentiating this diagnosis from organic mental disorders, organic delusional schizophreniform disorders, atypical psychosis, pervasive developmental disorder, obsessive compulsive disorder, hypochondriasis, phobic disorder, factitious disorder, personality disorder, and mental retardation. Only time will tell whether the DSM-III categories represent an advance and a more useful approach for researchers and clinicians than have previous attempts to classify this sometimes ephemeral but always challenging condition (or conditions).

According to DSM-III, one essential criterion for the diagnosis of schizophrenic disorders is that of onset before age 45. This arbitrary approach has settled the question of whether "late paraphrenia," or paranoia with onset in late life, is a manifestation of schizophrenia. We no longer have to concern ourselves with this issue because DSM-III has told us that a schizophrenic disorder, by definition, has an onset before age 45! Such decisions, of course, do not alter the psychopathology or any other abnormalities associated with a disorder, but, logically, greater precision in classification may eventually lead to higher accuracy in diagnosis and a better understanding of the etiology, clinical course, and response to treatment.

It is also clear that evaluation of treatment, especially over a long period of time, is fraught with methodological problems, even when good baseline data are available. It is all but impossible, for example, to find a sample of patients whose histories could give us the natural history of schizophrenic disorders. Among patients who come to the attention of a psychiatrist, it is extremely rare to find one who has not had some kind of treatment that might affect the course of the illness.

Studies in the gerontologic literature have emphasized cohort differences that cannot be resolved in cross-section analysis of data and sometimes cannot be resolved even with longitudinal studies. That subjects are lost to follow-up may or may not be significant. Policy changes related to delivery of mental health services certainly affect the data, but in ways not fully understood. Because the impact of any single intervention is influenced by so many factors, only gross measurements can be used in long-term follow-up studies. One possible parameter is longevity, but why should we evaluate the impact of an intervention on survival when we are told that perhaps several hundred factors affect longevity? The effect of long-term institutionalization, or a particular treatment (e.g., psychotropic medications or insulin coma therapy), or a social variable (e.g., marital status) can be evaluated, but other factors have to be considered simultaneously. When the state of the art is such that we cannot adequately evaluate whether a treatment affects longevity, why should we place any reliance on variables such as plasma drug levels, length of hospitalization, need for repeated hospitalizations, and intensity of symptoms as affecting outcome? We know that these variables are in turn affected by many factors.

Methodological problems have brought studies of therapeutic results in dementia under severe criticism, while results of interventions that might affect the outcome or vary the course of schizophrenic disorders have been more widely accepted. But all outcome studies are subject to criticism. For example, serious researchers working with demented patients have acknowledged that instruments to measure change in behavior are inadequate, but the literature on chronic schizophrenia leads one to believe that, in this case as well, we are still searching for adequate evaluation methods.

## CONCLUSION

One must conclude that, under the best of circumstances, long-term studies of schizophrenic disorders have serious limitations. Under this rubric, we probably have a group of conditions that share many characteristics, but they have different etiologies and are influenced by many factors. How these factors operate is by no means clear. There is no question, however, that a significantly large number of old people, who have had a condition diagnosed as schizophrenia, come to the attention of psychiatrists and continue to require attention quite late in life. The situation would be simplified if, in fact, at some chronological age, say 65, all manifestations of these illnesses were no longer those of schizophrenia but rather of organic brain syndrome. Ridiculous as this approach is, it probably explains why psychiatric disorders that appeared earlier in life tend to be relegated to secondary importance when the patients are older. This approach has important therapeutic implications for aged persons. Too often, they are given diagnoses presumed to be associated with age; the assumption is that treatment is all but useless and the prognosis poor because of the patient's age.

The case histories given demonstrate that elderly persons who have had a diagnosis of schizophrenia deserve continued attention and treatment. The essential features of the treatment program are quite like those for elderly persons with any chronic disorder. A rational comprehensive approach, possibly using a multidisciplinary team, will help these patients attain a reasonable degree of happiness and contentment, and will offer comparable satisfaction to family members and therapists.

## REFERENCES

1. Friedel, R. O., Raskind, M. A.: Psychopharmacology of aging, in Special Review of Experimental Aging Research: Progress in Biology. Ed. by Elias, M. S., Eleftheriou, B. E., Elias, P. K. Bar Harbor, ME: EAR, 1976.
2. Post, F.: The functional psychoses, in Studies in Geriatric Psychiatry. Edited by Isaacs, A. D., Post, F. Chichester, John Wiley & Sons, 1978.
3. Raskin, A., Jarvik, L. F. (eds): Psychiatric Symptoms and Cognitive Loss in the Elderly. Washington, DC: Hemisphere 1979.
4. Bridge, T. P., Cannon, H. E., Wyatt, R. J.: Burned-out schizophrenia: Evidence for age effects on schizophrenia symptomatology. J Gerontol 33:835–839, 1978.
5. Bleuler, M.: The long-term course of the schizophrenic psychoses. Psychol Med 4:244–254, 1974.

6. Muller, C.: Schizophrenia in advanced senescence. Br J Psychiatry 118:347–348, 1971.

7. Holt, W. L., Holt, W. M.: Long-term prognosis in mental illness: A thirty-year followup of 141 mental patients. Am J Psychiatry 108:735–739, 1952.

8. Beck, M. N.: Twenty-five and thirty-five year follow up of first admissions to mental hospitals. Can J Psychiatry 13:219–229, 1968.

9. Stephens, J. H.: Long-term course and prognosis in schizophrenia. Seminars in Psychiatry 2(4):464–485, 1970.

10. Winston, A., Pardes, H., Papernik, D. S., Breslin, L.: Aftercare of psychiatric patients and its relation to rehospitalization. Hosp Community Psychiatry 28:118–121, 1968.

11. Linn, M. W., Caffey, E. M.: Foster Placement for the older psychiatric patient. J Gerontol 32:340–345, 1977.

12. Weldon, E., Clarkin, J., Hennessey, J. J., Frances, A.: Day hospital versus outpatient treatment: A controlled study. Psychiatric Quarterly 51(2):144–150, 1979.

13. Blume, R. M., Kalin, M., Sacks, J.: A collaborative day treatment program for chronic patients in adult homes. Hosp Community Psychiatry 30:40–42, 19 .

14. Van Putten, T., Spar, J. E.: The board-and-care home: Does it deserve a bad press? Hosp Community Psychiatry 30:461–464, 1979.

15. Goodstein, R. K.: The diagnosis and treatment of elderly patients: Some practical guidelines. Hosp Community Psychiatry 31:19–24, 1980.

16. Ban, T. A.: Psychopharmacology. Baltimore: Williams & Wilkins, 1969.

17. Prien, R. F., Harber, P. A., Caffey, E. M.: The use of psychoactive drugs in elderly patients with psychiatric disorders: Survey conducted in twelve Veterans Administration hospitals. J Am Geriatr Soc 23:104–112, 1975.

18. Branchey, M. H., Lee, J. H., Amin, R., Simpson, G. M.: High- and low-potency neuroleptics in elderly psychiatric patients. JAMA 239:1860–1862, 1978.

19. Branchey, M. H., Lee, J. H., Simpson, G. M., Elgart, B., Vicencio, A.: Loxapine succinate as a neuroleptic agent: Evaluation in two populations of elderly psychiatric patients. J Am Geriatr Soc 26:263–267, 1978.

20. Raskind, M., Alvarez, C., Herlin, S.: Fluphenazine enanthate in the outpatient treatment of late paraphrenia. J Am Geriatr Soc 27:459–463, 1979.

21. Imlah, N. W.: Long-term follow-up studies of drugs in schizophrenia. J Clin Pharmacol 3:411–415, 1976.

22. Diagnostic and Statistical Manual of Mental Disorders, Third Edition. Washington, DC: American Psychiatric Association, 1980.

# CHAPTER 18

# Psychotherapy in the Elderly

Sanford Finkel, M.D.

This chapter reviews four considerations in geriatric psychotherapy:

1. the frequency of the use of psychotherapy in the general private practice of psychiatry that includes elderly people,
2. some increasing interest on the part of professionals in doing psychotherapy with the elderly,
3. some special clinical elements of treatment and diagnosis, and
4. an individual case of long-term psychotherapy.

   In at least half the cases I see of elderly people in psychiatric distress, psychotherapy is an important part of treatment, whether as the primary therapy or as an adjunct. Among people who have recurrent affective disorders, unipolar or bipolar depression, psychotherapy is helpful in alleviating undue stress and anxiety and in reintegrating the patient into society. For many people who are depressed, the shame of avoiding friends, family, and responsibilities is a difficult obstacle to overcome. Most psychotherapy with older people is short term. In my practice, the average number of sessions is 8. It is not uncommon to see people 2 or 3 times a week for a few weeks. In long-term supportive psychotherapy, usually in conjunction with medication, people are seen every 3 or 4 weeks or sometimes as seldom as every 3–6 months. Long-term intensive psychotherapy requires that the patient be seen at least once a week for a year; I have found the need for this in elderly people to occur infrequently. Five percent of my practice (24 people over a 9-year period), required long-term intensive psychotherapy.

However, for this small group, psychotherapy is often the critical factor between living a productive and satisfying life and institutionalization.

More professionals are using psychotherapy with the elderly than before. Kastenbaum and others have described the reluctance of therapists to work with older people. I think that is changing. Just as many professionals are willing to work pharmacotherapeutically with older people, there is an increased interest in working psychotherapeutically as well. There are many advantages to working with older people. This is basically a good prognostic group, and the gratifications are immediate. You usually develop a sense of whether or not therapy will be helpful within 2 or 3 sessions. Alliances develop quickly, without a lengthy waiting period. For some types of clinical conditions, such as dementia or depression following physical illness, the psychiatrist can be particularly helpful using the combination of pharmacotherapy and individual psychotherapy. The psychiatrist with training and experience in working with physical illness, individual and family psychodynamics, and other psychosocial factors can be particularly helpful to the elderly patient and his family, and will often find himself in the role of a primary care physician, particularly for people who have a primary psychiatric problem with occasional medical complaints. Additionally, there are intellectual rewards in working with older adults, and certainly no other group of patients presents the psychiatrist with as great a challenge to his clinical acumen. Sorting out psychological, biological, and social factors is often difficult, particularly because a late-life illness can present atypically. We also have a unique opportunity to compare differing presentations of diseases from early life and late in life. We can learn about long-term coping mechanisms and try to determine what kinds are successful and unsuccessful. Furthermore, we can often best evaluate the natural history of an illness by observing it near the end of life.

Older people have interesting life histories. It has always been fascinating for me to talk with somebody who at age 11, a mere girl, would leave Russia and come to the United States by herself to live with a second cousin and then go right to work. Older people are very forthright and frank. If you ask a 35-year-old, "Why haven't you married?" you might get a response such as, "The right person hasn't come along." A 75-year-old will tell you frankly that she was very attached to her mother or that her father was such a great guy she didn't think she could improve on him. With elderly people, as compared to younger people, there is more opportunity—and it is more important—to share personal information. The real relationship is very satisfying, to both the patient and therapist. Discussions of food preferences, numbers of children, what the children are like, and hobbies form an important part of treatment.

Because of these special characteristics of older people, some particular kinds of questions should be asked during the diagnostic evaluation.

One question that is often omitted has to do with the aging of the patient's relatives. It's curious how often someone will come in at age 72 with some type of diffuse anxiety; in listening to the history, it turns out that at age 72 the mother died, or at age 72 the grandmother committed suicide. How did parents and grandparents function in the later years; how have siblings aged? Another special concern among the elderly is the issue of grandparenting: How a person sees his or her role as a grandparent, whether that has shifted, and how it has affected the role of the grandparents' own children. What kind of an experience has grandparenting been? In fact, many believe that a lack of interest in grandparenting is a sign of psychopathology and that recent changes in attitudes towards grandchildren, such as withdrawal, decreased intensity of affect, or rejection warrant further evaluation of a depression, dementia, or paranoia.

After diagnosis, it is important to consider how psychologically oriented psychotherapy in elderly people differs from similar procedures with younger people. In both groups, true functioning and enhanced self-acceptance and self-esteem are common aims. In younger people, more attention is likely to be focused on self-erected barriers, maladaptive defenses that cause psychological discomfort and prevent the realization of the person's work and interpersonal goals. In contrast, psychological work with the elderly often focuses on symbolic replacement of loss, often the loss of another person who was critical to the patient's psychological makeup and who provided a sense of stability. The therapist tries to replace the loss symbolically. There is no short answer about when to help with such problems; the empathic, tender-loving-care approach works for some people; for other people it is disastrous. For some people, sympathy may result in a worsening of the condition. For example, early on in my clinical practice, I saw a woman of 75 who had no psychiatric history and had a well-established history of good functioning in organizational work, but was universally disliked. People thought she was obnoxious, affected, bossy, and controlling, as her children related. The one person she didn't control was her husband, who was even more dominating than she; he would yell at her, making her cry and apologize. When her husband died, she threw herself into her activities all the more, and actually did well for a number of months, after which she started developing signs of depression, with delusional thoughts and loose associations. It looked as if she was becoming psychotically depressed, and she was referred for psychotherapy. Initially, I tried to empathize with her and talk about how difficult it must be for her to adjust to her husband's death, but she continued to get worse, until I adopted a tactic in which I became critical of her and somewhat directive. She became quite angry and upset at first, but she improved, became less depressed, and started functioning again. Her daughter came to me and said "My mother's delusional. She says that you yell at her all the time, and I know you wouldn't do anything like that." I said, "Of course."

Psychotherapeutic assistance for senility is often a very important and overlooked technique. It does not help with the dementia per se, but for people with dementia who have common depression or anxiety or paranoia, psychotherapy allows them to develop a relationship that can be vital. What determines whether or not psychotherapy is success-ful in later life probably is the same as what determines whether it is successful in early life: the ability to form an effective relationship. Indeed, there are people who cannot remember my name whom I see 3 and 4 times a week. I know, however, that they capture a sense of closeness and integration from the session.

I find the use of humor and sarcasm particularly useful in people who have chronic depressive and borderline personalities. For example, an elderly female patient was often enraged in the session. I always knew that she felt better when she laughed. Once she came in and said, "I hate your tie. If my husband wore that tie, I would take it off, and I'd strangle him with it." I answered, "If I were your husband, I'd let you do it gladly." Or she would come in and say, "I'm so angry with you, I'd like to crush your testicles and bite off your penis." I responded, "Your trouble is you don't know how to express anger."

"The Defeating of the Therapist" is also a useful technique. I am thinking of one very wealthy man in his mid-eighties who was very prominent in Chicago. He had incurred for the first time in his life a loss over which he had no control. A tyrant by nature, he became passive and very compliant. However, he also bought a gun and bullets, and his alarmed son asked me to see him. He was in a very passive state, feeling helpless; he had a disappointment, his life was over. I promptly hospital-ized him, which was the expedient thing to do. Shortly after we arrived at the hospital, he changed from a sycophantic, passive-client state to a demanding, tyrannical state. He wanted to go on pass whenever he did not like the food; he wanted to eat when he wanted to. He became quite angry and frustrated. He signed a 5-day release, and I threatened him with commitment, at which point I started getting calls from the offices of the attorney general, the mayor of the city, and the governor of the state. The man made a rather good recovery as he reestablished his common defenses and ordinary ways of coping.

Intensive psychotherapy is unusual in older people. In fact, I have never had an older person come to me over many months just to find out more about himself. However, the following case study is an example of successful long-term psychotherapy with a geriatric patient. The man had a stroke in November 1971, when he was 69. He had been the leading real estate salesman in his firm, and he was an exuberant, flamboyant gentleman. He had been loving to his family and friends, though vindictive to people he disliked. He had had one brief course of psychotherapy a few years earlier concerning his feelings about a son who divorced, and he thought that was successful. In his early sixties, he had both a cancer of the prostrate and a myocardial infarction, after which he had a tendency to be somatically preoccupied. Otherwise, he thrived on his fancy clothes, big cars, expensive vacations, card games, his work, his family, and his very active social life. The stroke changed all that. Not only was he unable to work, play cards, or drive, but he could no longer do arithmetic, and had extensive impairment in language and motor skills. Even his abilities to button his own clothes and to feed himself were impaired. He found after his hospitalization that his friends and acquaintances stayed away; they thought it too painful to see this powerful man diminished. He saw his previous psychiatrist, who placed him on minor tranquilizers, and over a period of 2 months his anxiety level diminished. He went to Florida for his annual vacation. While he was there, he became very paranoid and said his wife was stealing money from him. He actually physically lashed out at her for the only time in his life. This reaction occurring during vacation is not uncommon with older people. Family, friends, even the physician may advise the depressed older person to go on a trip to a favorite place in order to cheer up. When they get to the old environment that used to be so wonderful, seeing how much things have changed merely accentuates the losses, and manifests increased anxiety or paranoia.

The patient was hospitalized by his psychiatrist after he hit his wife. The mental status evaluation revealed that he was disoriented at the time. He could not do serial sevens, could not abstract proverbs. Despite a confused mental status, however, he said something quite interesting when asked about suicide: "I don't know if I have the courage. Maybe in this mess there may be still a life for me, maybe there is someone else who is even worse off, and maybe I'm just a fool enough to to lick this thing." During the first week of hospitalization, he felt optimistic, and showed symptomatic improvement. He was very charming, though in a very loose way. When it became clear to him that he was not going to be discharged immediately, he became quite angry, agitated, and confused, with increased somatic symptoms. He had to be transferred to a closed unit. He also discovered during that week that his psychiatrist was going on vacation; he threatened to sign out against medical advice. During the third week, consultation was sought with a senior psychiatrist who said the man was incapable of maintaining a psychotherapeutic relationship and that the prognosis was grave. During the fourth week, this psychiatrist went out of town and asked me to see the man for a 2-week period. He said that I probably would have to commit him because he was going to sign out against medical advice. The response was quite different, however. During the first few therapy sessions, he tried to bolster his own self-esteem by impressing me. His memory was impaired, his writing and reading were impaired, his speech was very poor. He was making a concerted effort thrice weekly in speech therapy. He would show me the work, brag to me about the progress he was making, and then started talking to me as if I were his grandson. He said at some point in time he would be better and we would go fishing and boating together, the kinds of things that he did with his grandson, whom he loved very much. The fourth time we met, I suggested we go to breakfast in the hospital cafeteria, something that we continued for the duration of his hospital stay. When we came back from that visit, he put his hand on my shoulder and looked in my eye and said, "Wouldn't it be a feather in your cap if you could cure me?" He did quite well over the following 2-week period; his memory improved. I said little during those first 2 weeks. Once I ventured what I thought was a helpful comment, on his need to accept certain limitations. He said, "I know I have a problem, I really have a problem accepting my own limitations." And then he reflected and said, "But you know that's the same problem that allows me to make my tremendous progress in speech therapy." He was right. When the other psychiatrist came back, the patient transferred to me, and I continued to see him. The wife had less confidence in me, since it was my first year in private practice. She had been told by several prominent persons that her husband was not going to make it. I had to work intensively with her because she had started an active mourning process and was beginning to get used to the idea that he would probably wind up in a nursing home or a state hospital. The work with her was important throughout this man's hospitalization. After I took over the case, this man needed concrete evidence of progress. I transferred him to an open unit where he was entitled to passes, and he continued to progress.

Now the course of therapy changed. I started an active life review. I have found it an exceptionally helpful technique for some older people. It lasted 21 sessions. At first the patient thought it was silly, until I told him that to understand the current chapter in his life I needed to know more about the previous chapters, to make a more complete story for both of us. As he started becoming better acquainted with some of the feelings from the past, he began recognizing himself again. What had happened to this man, which happens to many older people with a series of dramatic losses, is a lost sense of identity, a break from the sense of himself in the past. In the process of the life review, there is a reorganization and a reestablishment of the sense of who an individual is.

By the eighth or ninth week of his stay, the patient had become quite active and popular in our geriatric group at Michael Reese Hospital. We started talking about discharge at that time. The wife's anxiety recurred. I reduced the number of sessions from 5 a week to 4. The combined pressures made him more anxious. Whenever this man became anxious or somewhat depressed, his cognitive functioning temporarily diminished. However, as discharge approached, my role changed again from a listener who was dazzled by him to an active participant in a life process. I took advantage of the power that he had given to me, and became very directive and reassuring. I promised him that we would struggle through together. At times I would see his face start to change from a frown to determination.

When he was discharged, the first visit was at his house, by my request, which was the only time that I was there. He saw to it that his wife made my favorite food for breakfast. In many ways our problems were just beginning; after his discharge from the hospital he had no work, his friends stayed away, he could not play cards, his self-esteem was badly damaged, he was envious of healthy people, and very jealous of his wife. He was angry about the dependency on his wife, and at the same time his speech therapy was being cut back because his language skills were improving. I left town for 2 weeks during the second month after discharge, which was during the seventeenth and eighteenth weeks of his treatment. Upon my return, he was planning to go to California for a son's wedding. This was his first time away since the Florida episode, and he was quite anxious. He recalled that his father had died of a strangulated hernia while visiting *his* daughter. Nevertheless, the patient did very well. When he came back, he chose to reduce the frequency of our visits to twice a week. During this phase, I functioned in a different role again. He really was controlling the therapy and telling me what to do, although I was the confidant and on occasion gave him feedback on his plans. He started to draw and to paint, which he had never done before (his daughter was an artist). Then, exactly 1 year to the day after his initial hospitalization, when his speech therapist was away, his only other child, a daughter, decided to move out of the city.

He became suicidal again, and was rehospitalized for a 9-day period. He was very resilient, however; he recovered, and over the next few months began working again. In the fourteenth month after the stroke, he consumated his first real estate deal, something that no one thought he would ever be able to do again. He cut down his therapy further, and by the sixteenth month, we were meeting on an every-other-week basis. By the eighteenth month he began driving again. He loved his art lessons. He was becoming increasingly independent. He had always been accompanied by his wife, whom I usually saw for a few minutes during the course of the sessions, but now he started to come alone. By December, the twenty-second month, he had an operation for a strangulated hernia, but he survived. After that, his social contacts improved. He started playing bridge and gin again, and our therapy stopped altogether. I saw him once in June 1974, and for 4 sessions in November 1975. He came back at that time feeling kind of sad, and again there was some impairment of cognitive functioning. By this time, however, his language skills had returned completely. I placed him on Hydergine. He wrote me a letter saying he was fine. He discontinued the medicine in 1976, and although I never saw him again, I sent him a birthday card every year, which he acknowledged in writing. He wrote to me from his vacations and I to him. When he saw my name in local papers, he would write a letter. Our relationship continued.

Besides being a very personally rewarding experience, this story provides an example of preventive psychiatry. It was unnecessary to see this man as long as he felt well. Small written contact sufficed. In February 1980, he died suddenly of a heart attack at the age of 77, the night before he was to receive a plaque and car as the award for being the number-one real estate salesman in his firm. He had made it back to the top. When I saw his wife a few months after his death, she told me he had been fine, in every way, as a husband and as a friend. All his friends had come back, he had played cards again, he had insisted on going back to Florida to the same place they had gone before. They had had a wonderful time. That was his way. He had accepted back people who had rejected him, and had seemed to enjoy every aspect of life. I learned a good deal from this patient about the value of long-term psychotherapy with the elderly, and relate the case as a useful example of the possibility of good prognosis in people who may not be considered good candidates for this modality.

# CHAPTER 19

# Alcoholism and the Elderly: An Overview

Joan C. Martin, PH.D.
Ann P. Streissguth, PH.D.

Although there have been hundreds of studies conducted on alcoholism and drinking problems among the elderly, no clear picture of the nature or extent of the problem has emerged. The populations surveyed, and the tests and other measures which have been administered have all been too diverse to warrant firm conclusions. Most authors, however, agree that alcohol consumption is a significant problem among the elderly.

Questions which remain unanswered include: What percentage of old people are alcoholics or problem drinkers? Who are they demographically? What are the special factors associated with aging which may predispose the elderly toward alcohol abuse? What special problems does alcoholism pose for the elderly person? What are risk factors in the onset of alcoholism among the elderly who have not previously been alcoholics? What are the neurological, behavioral, economic, and legal consequences of alcohol abuse among the elderly? And finally, what can be done to prevent or intervene in alcoholism and drinking problems in aging populations? This chapter will address these issues.

## PREVALENCE OF ALCOHOLISM AND DRINKING PROBLEMS IN AGING POPULATIONS

The extent of the alcohol problems among the elderly is not known. However, data on age-related factors in alcoholism, alcohol problems, and drinking patterns have been reported in several cross-sectional population surveys as well as in a variety of special populations such as hospitalized or nursing home patients. These studies have been reviewed in terms of possible risk factors which might be related to increased prevalence of drinking in the elderly, male/female differences, and factors associated with abstention. Tables 19.1 and 19.2 present a summarization of studies reviewed that estimated prevalence of alcohol problems and/or drinking patterns.

## Surveys and Cross-sectional Studies.

Studies in this section are those which were conducted on representative national samples, or samples defined by a geographic boundary. Investigators have typically focused on either broadly defined alcohol problems (including alcoholism, problem drinking and alcohol abuse) or on patterns of drinking, in which heavy drinking is defined by the amount consumed rather than the consequences to the drinker.

*Studies of Alcohol Abuse.*    Bailey et al. (1965) conducted an epidemiological survey on rates of alcoholism in 8,082 persons 20 years old and over residing in the Washington Heights Health District of New York City. Alcoholism was defined as a positive response to questions about health and monetary problems, job difficulties, family arguments or marriage dissolution, trouble with neighbors or the police, and violence. A total of 132 alcoholics were identified, which resulted in a prevalence rate of 19 per 1,000, with the male to female ratio being three to one.

The most vulnerable subgroups in the population were widowers and divorced and separated persons of both sexes. Blacks had a higher rate than Caucasians, and the rate of alcoholism was inversely related to education.

Age trends in studies of this type are of considerable interest. As Table 19.2 indicates, the rate of alcoholism in the 65–74-year-olds is comparable to peak rates in the middle years. Furthermore, although there is a decline in the rate after age 75, the rate in these very elderly persons is still comparable to the rate in the early twenties.

For women, the peak rate of alcoholism was in the 45–54 year range, while for men, the peak rate was in the 65–74 age group. Haberman and Baden (1974) noted that this latter finding was related to the number of elderly widowers who acknowledged a drinking problem. Widows, on the other hand, had a very low rate of alcoholism, which may be related to the difference in the number of role changes between the sexes at older ages, or to concealment of alcohol problems among

TABLE 19.1 Studies of the prevalence of heavy or problem drinking: Surveys and Cross-sectional Studies

| Author | Sample Characteristics | Alcohol Problems | |
|---|---|---|---|
| Bailey, Haberman & Alksne, 1965 | 8,082 persons ≥ 20 years old living in Washington Heights, NYC, (1960–61) | 19/1,000 overall rate of alcoholism men to women: 3.6:1.0<br>55–64: 17/1,000<br>65–74: 22/1,000<br>75+ : 12/1,000 | |
| Bollerup, 1975 | 588 70-year-olds living in Copenhagen suburbs (1966–1968) | 9.6/1,000 = Alcoholic<br>13.2/1,000 = Men<br>6.2/1,000 = Women | |
| Cahalan & Cissin, 1968 | 2,746 ≥ 20 years old, living in households; national sample, (1964–1965) | 10% Men (≥ 60 yrs.)<br>16% Men (50–59 yrs.)<br>3% Women (50–59 yrs.)<br>1% Women (≥ 60 yrs.) | "heavy–escape drinkers" |
| Cahalan, 1970 | 4,105 persons > 21 years old residing in households; national sample, (1964–65, 1967) | Men:<br>Age 50–59: 13%<br>Age 60–69: 12%<br>Over 70: 1%<br>Women:<br>Age 50–59: 2%<br>Age 60–69: 1%<br>Over 70: ½% | "problem drinkers" |
| Cahalan & Room, 1974 | 1,561 men aged 21–59 residing in house holds; national sample, 1967 & 1969. | Men: Age 50–59<br>Heavy intake: 6%<br>Binge drinkers: 2%<br>Problem drinkers: 11% | |
| Encel, Kotowicz & Resler, 1972 | Random sample of 820 persons > 15 years old in Sydney, Australia, (1968–69). | Heavy drinkers (daily drinking and/or 3–5 drinks/occasion) in persons > 60 years old:<br>45% for men<br>6% for women | |
| Johnson, 1974 (Chafetz, 1974) | 169 noninstitutionalized elderly (≥ 65 years) in Manhattan's East Side (< 1974). | 24% Regular drinkers<br>Men: 39%<br>Women: 20% | |

TABLE 19.2  Rates of Probable
Alcoholics per 1,000 Persons Aged
20 Years and Over in Age-Selected
Subgroups, Washington Heights
Master Sample Survey, 1960-61*

| Age, Years | Rates |
|---|---|
| 20–24 | 13 |
| 25–34 | 22 |
| 35–44 | 16 |
| 45–54 | 23 |
| 55–64 | 17 |
| 65–74 | 22 |
| 75 and over | 12 |

*Taken from Bailey et al. (1965), p. 27.

women of this age. As Table 19.2 indicates, alcohol problems are remarkably high during the retirement-crisis years. The lower rate observed in persons 75 years and over may be due to the many family and occupation-related criteria by which alcoholism was defined in this study. Such criteria may not be relevant to older persons who are already retired, widowed, or socially isolated. It is quite possible that this study underestimates the extent of alochol problems in elderly persons.

Cahalan (1970) devised a "problem drinking" score which included questions on intoxications, binge drinking, psychological dependence, and a variety of problem consequences of drinking. It was administered to a national sample. High scores on these drinking problems were tabulated against age and sex. For men, drinking problems peaked at 25% during the twenties and tapered off gradually with increasing age, but remained fairly high (12%) through the sixties. For women, peak problem drinking years were in middle age, with a rate of 1% in the sixties. The absence of questions on bereavement, loneliness, retirement, loss of status, and so forth may be one factor influencing the lower rates of reported problem drinking in older persons.

The higher proportion of problem drinkers cited by Cahalan (1970) compared to Bailey et al. (1965) may be a reflection of a more representative sample and a broader categorization of drinking problems and behaviors. These two surveys are the only ones reviewed which screened a large nonclinical sample of men and women across age groups who were living in the community, which used self-report (rather than physicians' diagnoses) to identify cases, and which focused on alcohol problems (rather than drinking patterns). Such studies are particularly important because they permit a broad comparative look at age-related trends in alcohol problems.

Cahalan and Room (1974) reported on alcohol problems in men sampled in a national survey, but unfortunately did not include men over age 60. The percentage of nondrinkers increased markedly with age and the proportion of "drinking problems" decreased. Binge drinking also decreased with age but "heavy intake" remained fairly constant across age groups. Among the 50–59-year-olds, "heavy intake" was over three times as high for men who lived with neither wife nor child, a pattern not found with younger men. In the older groups, "high consequences" of heavy drinking was negatively associated with social class, whereas heavy drinking per se remained fairly constant across the social classes.

No studies were reviewed which surveyed the extent of alcohol abuse specifically in an elderly population residing in a particular geographic region. However, Bollerup (1975) reported on the prevalence of mental illness among 588 70-year-olds all living within a circumscribed area in nine Copenhagen suburbs. Alcoholism in the absence of other diagnoses was diagnosed in 9.6 per 1,000 persons (13.2 per 1,000 for men and 6.2 per 1,000 for women). The criteria for alcoholism or demographic sample characteristics were not available in the English-language version of this study.

*Studies of Drinking Patterns.*    Important data on drinking habits in the elderly can be derived from the nationwide random sample of 2,746 households conducted by Cahalan and Cissin (1968) which provided breakdowns by age, sex, and socioeconomic status (SES). These data appear to provide the most complete picture of how drinking patterns vary across different age groups, although the focus of this national study was on drinking *habits* rather than alcoholism per se. The two categories of drinkers assessed were "heavy" drinking and "escape" drinking. "Heavy" drinking was not rigorously defined, but generally meant consuming five or more drinks at a sitting with some regularity. As Table 19.3 indicates, eighteen percent of the drinkers were "heavy" drinkers, including 28% of the men and 8% of the women. For men, the rate of heavy drinking was fairly constant from age 21 through 59, but dropped to 20% after age 60. For women, the highest rate (12%) occurred in the 40–49 range, with a marked decline to 2% occurring after age 50. The prevalence of "heavy" drinking declined with increasing age within each sex and SES group.

Cahalan and Cissin defined "escape" drinkers as persons who assigned some importance to at least two of the five "escape" reasons for drinking. These included: for relaxation, to forget everything, to forget one's worries, to overcome a bad mood, to overcome tension and ner-

TABLE 19.3 Drinkers, Heavy Drinkers and Heavy-Escape Drinkers, by Sex and Age[a]

| | Total Sample N[b] | % | Drinkers[c] N | Heavy Drinkers[c] % | Heavy-Escape Drinkers[c] % |
|---|---|---|---|---|---|
| Total Sample | 2,746 | 68 | 1,848 | 18 | 9 |
| Men | 1,177 | 77 | 909 | 28 | 13 |
| Women | 1,569 | 60 | 939 | 8 | 5 |
| **Men:** | | | | | |
| Age 21–29 | 216 | 84 | 179 | 28 | 12 |
| 30–39 | 243 | 86 | 211 | 30 | 15 |
| 40–49 | 264 | 79 | 209 | 31 | 14 |
| 50–59 | 197 | 73 | 145 | 29 | 16 |
| 60+ | 257 | 65 | 165 | 20 | 10 |
| **Women:** | | | | | |
| Age 21–29 | 256 | 70 | 181 | 9 | 6 |
| 30–39 | 345 | 72 | 252 | 9 | 7 |
| 40–49 | 333 | 65 | 218 | 12 | 6 |
| 50–59 | 265 | 50 | 132 | 3 | 3 |
| 60+ | 367 | 44 | 154 | 2 | 1 |
| No age given | 3 | | 2 | | |

[a]From Cahalan & Cissin, 1968, p. 137.
[b]Percentages are based on weighted sample, N = numbers of interviews in each group. Classifications defined in text.
[c]Base: Total drinkers.

vousness, and to escape problems. "Escape" drinking occurred with a frequency of 32% for men and 26% for women drinkers, while 9% of the drinkers were both "heavy" drinkers and "escape" drinkers. The prevalence of "heavy-escape" drinking in men rose steadily from age 21, with the highest rate (16%) in men aged 50–59. In elderly men, the rate dropped to 10% which was probably correlated with earlier death found in alcohol abusers. For women, the rate of "heavy-escape" drinking was constant from age 21–49, but dropped below 3% with advancing age.

In a study which focused specifically on drinking habits in the elderly, Johnson (1974) (as reported in Chafetz, 1974) assessed drinking patterns in 169 persons aged 65 and above who lived on the upper east side of Manhattan. Most of them were from lower socioeconomic groups, living alone or in small households. Regular drinkers comprised 24% of the total elderly sample: 39% of the men and 20% of the women. "Regular" drinking was preponderant among the highly active people in good health, with abstinence more common among the less active.

Encel et al. (1972) have reported on drinking patterns in Sydney,

Australia. They hypothesized that acceptable heavy drinking sets the stage for alcoholism, and concluded that it was therefore important to study drinking habits. They interviewed a random sample of 820 representative persons over 15 years old, and defined heavy drinking quite inclusively (daily drinking and/or 3–5 drinks per occasion). The findings are comparable to those of Cahalan and Cissin (1968), although the rates of heavy drinking are understandably much higher: (1) a sharp increase in abstainers and infrequent drinkers occurred at age 60 and over for both men and women; (2) the proportion of heavy drinkers in persons over 60 years was 45% for men and 6% for women; (3) men drank considerably more than women at each age; and (4) the primary change in drinking in the elderly was in terms of quantity consumed rather than the frequency of consumption. Encel et al. conclude that since heavy drinking is a normative behavior for the adult population in Sydney, heavy drinking by men was socially accepted and encouraged, and that such drinking customs provided a social context highly conducive to the development of alcoholism in susceptible persons.

Russell et al. (1978) reported data from a large representative sample of the U.S. population. The rate of "heavier drinking" (one ounce or more of absolute alcohol per day) was 23% in men 50–64 and 15% in men 65 years and over. In women, comparative figures for the two ages were 7% and 4% respectively. Since these are higher percentages of heavier drinking than those reported by Cahalan and Cissin (1968) and the Harris poll 1972–74, they could reflect an increase in heavier drinking among the elderly over the past 10–15 years.

These survey findings are frequently cited to indicate that alcohol abuse declines with age and is therefore not a particular problem among the aged. However, it would seem that several considerations are important in interpreting these data:

1. With declining physiological competence, smaller quantities of ingested alcohol may have an effect that is comparable to lower doses in younger imbibers. Wallgren and Barry (1970) have described the slower clearance of alcohol in the elderly due to a generally slowed metabolism.
2. Even though the absolute percentage of "heavy-escape" drinking in the elderly may be less than in younger men, a prevalence of 10% is still indicative of an important problem.
3. The apparent higher prevalence of heavy drinking among the lower classes suggests that certain environmental factors which relate to drinking in the elderly could be isolated.
4. Sampling procedures involving household surveys may well preclude transient, homeless or institutionalized persons, as well as elderly

persons in residential care, thus biasing the sample against finding alcoholism.

5. Cross-sectional studies can never be free of social/cultural/economic factors that could influence one cohort and not another. Longitudinal studies which can examine individual and environmental factors which change over time need to be performed in addition.

## Studies on Specialized Populations

Many prevalence studies of drinking habits and alcohol problems in the elderly have been conducted on specialized populations and are therefore of more limited generalizability than local or national surveys. One group of studies has examined drinking habits in specific groups of persons identified by their occupation or insurance membership, and thus may be particularly unrepresentative of the elderly population. Another group of studies, even more unrepresentative, focused on alcohol problems in various types of hospitalized patients, including the elderly. Table 19.4 presents a summarization of studies reviewed that estimated the prevalence of heavy drinking and/or alcohol problems in special populations.

*Surveys of Noninstitutionalized Persons.*    Klattsky et al. (1977) reported decreased alcohol use with increasing age among each sex and race for 91,659 persons receiving care at Kaiser-Permanente Medical Center, Oakland, California. The peak age for heavy drinking for white males was 50–59. Although the proportion dropped to 2.3% at age 70–79, the percentage of heavy drinkers in the 70–79-year-old range was equivalent to that reported for 20–29-year-olds. The peak drinking years were earlier (30–39 years) for black males, with 4.2% still heavy drinkers at age 60–69. The peak drinking years were also earlier for white and black females, and drinking dropped to almost nothing by 70–79 years. These figures were somewhat lower than those reported by Cahalan and Cissin (1968), perhaps reflecting the more specific nature of the Klattsky sample.

Siassi et al. (1973) used a household survey technique to assess drinking in a sample of 937 workers who were members of the United Auto Workers. Only a little more than half of the men and one-quarter of the women reported using alcohol at all. However, 65% of the male drinkers 60 years old or older were "heavy" drinkers and 10% of this group were "heavy-escape" drinkers. Among women drinkers 60 years old or older, 40% were classified as "heavy" drinkers. These high proportions were no doubt related to the rather minimal criteria for a "heavy" drinker (6 or more drinks per week).

Several studies have surveyed residents of residential hotels or homes for the aged in an effort to discover what proportion of the residents have or have had drinking problems.

Table 19.4 Studies of the prevalence of heavy or problem drinking. Studies in Special Populations

| Author | Sample Characteristics | Alcohol Problems | | |
|---|---|---|---|---|
| Baker, et al, 1974 (cited in Chafetz, 1974) | 98 persons ($\bar{x}$ age 77 years) living in nursing homes or homes for elderly in Boston. Retrospective interview re practices before institutionalization (<1974). | Regular drinkers: 30% | | |
| Daniel, 1972 | 693 geriatric admissions to psychiatric ward, Queensland, Australia (65–90 years old) (1965, 1970). | 6% of sample 4% of men 2% of women | Clinical alcoholism and alcoholic psychosis | |
| Funkhauser, 1977/78 | 47 V.A. admissions to medical/surgical ward over 55 years old (1977). | 55.3% alcoholic (by self-report on most) | | |
| Gaitz & Bahr, 1971 | 100 consecutive psychiatric admissions 60 years and older (<1970). | 44% alcoholic (36% primary alcoholic diagnosis) | | |
| Harrington & Price, 1962 | 1,000 V.A. domiciliary patients, (1959). | 22.3% medical dx. of alcoholism | | |
| Klattsky, et al. 1977. | 91,659 Kaiser-Permanente members in Oakland, California (1964-1968). | 5.2% white men 50-59 years 4.2% black men 60-69 years 2.3% white men 70-79 years 1.1% white women 50-59 years 0.5% white women 60-69 years 0.1% white women 70-79 years | | ≥6 drinks per day |
| McCusker et al., 1971 | 118 new admissions to medical wards at Harlem Hospital, New York City, 1969. | Rated alcohol abuse based on research interview: Men: 63% Women: 35% Men: 50% Women: 0% | 50-69 years ≥70 years | |

250

| | | |
|---|---|---|
| Pascarelli & Fischer, 1974 | 86 persons >60 years old living in a residential hotel on Manhattan's West Side (mostly poor; 57% women) (<1974). | 21% diagnosed alcoholic |
| Rosin & Glatt, 1971 | 103 patients with alcohol problems and over 65 years of age who were referred for geriatric or psychiatric care in England (1963-1970) | Women to Men: 3:2 ⅔: longstanding problem drinkers ⅓ were previously not problem drinkers but effects of aging increased their drinking. |
| Russell, et al, 1978 | Representative U.S. persons surveyed (HANES data) (1971-1973) | Percentage drinking one or more ounces absolute alcohol per day. Age: 50-64 Men: 23% Women: 7% Age: 65+ Men: 15% Women: 4% |
| Schuckit, Miller & Hahlbahm, 1975 | 50 consecutive elderly male admissions to medical surgical wards (1974). | 8% alcoholic |
| Schuckit & Miller, 1976 | 113 elderly acute medical ward admissions at V.A.Hospital, (1974-1975). | 18% alcoholic |
| Schuckit, 1976 | 327 elderly acute medical/surgical ward patients, at V.A.Hospital (1974-1975). | 5% alcoholic (alcoholism was 2nd most frequent psychiatric diagnosis). |

Table 19.4 continued

| Author | Sample Characteristics | Alcohol Problems |
|---|---|---|
| Siassi et al., 1973 | Probability sample of 8,000 UAW workers, interview sample: 937 respondents, 1966-1971 | Heavy drinkers (≥6 drinks/week) in persons >60 years old (% of drinkers) 65% of men 40% of women |
| Simon, Epstein & Reynolds, 1968 | 543 geriatric first admissions, resident of California one year, > 60 years old, no hx of arrests or psychiatric hospitalization < 60 years old. | 23% = alcohol diagnosis 7% became alcoholic > 60 years 16% became alcoholic < 60 years + 5% very heavy drinkers |
| Zimberg, 1969 | 17 admissions to geriatric psychiatry out-patient program in Harlem: NYC, 1966-1967 | 12% diagnosed alcoholic |
| Zimberg, 1971 | 24 patients receiving psychiatric consulta-tion as part of a medical home care program Harlem, NYC, < 1971 | 13% diagnosed alcoholic |
| Zimberg, 1974 | 87 geriatric admissions to surburban Rock-land County Community Health Center, New York | 17% alcohol abuse problems |

In a 1973 study of 86 persons over 60 years of age, mostly poor, living in a residential hotel on Manhattan's West Side, Pascarelli and Fischer (1975) found that 21% of the women were alcoholic. Their average age was 69 years. Furthermore, alcohol abuse was compounded by fairly high levels of psychoactive or mood-altering drugs. Darvon was taken regularly by 23% of the sample, Librium by 12% and Valium by 7%, with 19% receiving multiple prescriptions. On the basis of these findings, Pascarelli and Fischer conclude that "drug dependence and alcoholism among the elderly are major problems." Most abuse occurred in the categories of the depressants, including alcohol, and the opiates. Fewer problems with stimulants and hallucinogens were reported in this sample.

Garrett and Bahr (1973), who studied homeless and transient persons seeking help at New York City shelters, reported that 24% of the men and 10% of the women were over age 65. Half of the men and one-third of the women in the sample were heavy drinkers, but no attempt was made to study the extent to which drinking problems might have been particularly related to homelessness in the elderly.

*Studies of Hospitalized Persons.* Another type of study evaluated admissions to medical, geriatric, or psychiatric wards in terms of frequency of diagnosis as alcoholics or problem drinkers. Findings from these studies are highly variable, probably due to discrepancies in the method used for identifying a "case."

Wechsler et al. (1972) studied blood alcohol levels in 6,266 admissions to a Boston hospital emergency room, and found that over 7% of the men and 3% of the women over age 65 had high blood alcohol levels. Unfortunately, the more interesting question from our standpoint, namely, what percentage of all persons with elevated blood alcohol levels was over 65 years old, was not asked.

Daniel (1972) published a 5-year study of 693 geriatric admissions to an Australian psychiatric ward. It was implied that physicians established the diagnosis, and that 6% of the admitted patients had a primary diagnosis of chronic alcoholism or alcohol psychosis. The ratio of men to women was a little over 2 to 1. Compared to other diagnostic categories, alcoholics were admitted at an earlier age, primarily in the 65–69-year range, with no admissions beyond age 79.

Gaitz and Baer (1971) studied 100 consecutive psychiatric admissions, 60 years and older, and found that 44% were alcoholic, including 36% with a primary diagnosis of alcoholism. Over half of the alcoholics also had organic brain syndrome.

McCusker et al. (1971) studied new admissions to the medical wards of Harlem Hospital Center in New York City. Fifty-six percent of males over 70 and 63% aged 50–69 were considered alcoholic. Alcoholism was defined as intoxications once or twice weekly and/or significant social, occupational, or physical impairment related to alcohol consumption. Thirty-five percent of the women in the 50–59 age group, but none over age 70, were also considered alcoholic. These figures are among the highest frequency of alcoholism reported in any of the specialized populations studied. Whether these results are characteristic of a predominantely black, lower class population, is not known. Zimberg (1969, 1971) found other evidence of alcoholism as a major problem in this community. Twelve percent of the patients seen in the first year of operation of the geriatric psychiatry outpatient program had an alcoholism problem, and 13% of the patients receiving psychiatric consultation through a medical home care program were alcoholic. In more recent studies conducted in Suburban Rockland County Community Health Center in New York, 5.3% of the admissions in 1972 were over 65 years of age, and 17% of these 87 patients had alcohol abuse problems on admission (Zimberg, 1974). So the problem is clearly not confined to minorities or the poor.

U.S. veterans obtaining care through Veterans Administration hospitals have frequently been studied for alcoholism. Caution is required in the generalization of these findings to the population as a whole.

Harrington and Price (1962) studied 1,000 veterans who were living in a domiciliary care setting, and therefore represented the patients least able to maintain themselves in independent care. Twenty-three percent of this sample was diagnosed alcoholic.

Fifty-five percent of patients over age 55 admitted to a medical and surgical unit of a V.A. hospital in Seattle were diagnosed as alcoholic on a self-report questionnaire (Funkhauser, 1977–78). These rates are considerably higher than those reported in other studies, but the sample size was small.

Schuckit and Miller (1976) found that 18% of consecutive admissions to an acute medical ward at a V.A. hospital were diagnosed as alcoholic. All patients were male and over 65. Alcoholism was diagnosed from an interview and included any of the following criteria: (1) job layoff, firing, or inability to carry out work activities; (2) a marital separation or divorce; (3) two or more nontraffic arrests; or (4) report by a physician that alcohol had actually harmed health. Twenty-five percent of the alcoholics had a secondary diagnosis of organic brain syndrome.

Schuckit (1977) has also evaluated the rate of psychiatric disorders in relation to medical diagnosis, using the same diagnostic and intake procedures described earlier (Schuckit and Miller, 1976). Alcoholism was the second most frequent psychiatric diagnosis among the 327 elderly medical V.A. patients, surpassed only by atherosclerotic dementia. Patients with heart disease had an increased level of alcohol intake and a greater history of minor alcohol problems. Since Gould et al. (1971) have reported that one cocktail will decrease cardiac index and stroke index in vulnerable individuals, it is again apparent that the critical levels of alcohol intake in the elderly may be lower than in their younger counterparts.

The question of unrecognized alcohol problems among the elderly is an important issue, not only in obtaining accurate research data but also in generating help and care for elderly alcohol abusers. Schuckit et al. (1975), in a study of 50 elderly acute medical and surgical ward patients, found that 24% had major mental disorders that were unrecognized by the admitting physicians. Half of these with unrecognized problems had either alcoholism or depression. Missed alcoholic diagnosis could lead to severe withdrawal on the ward, or dangerous drug-alcohol interaction when patients resume drinking after discharge.

## Longitudinal Studies of Aging and Alcoholism

Very few studies have followed a group of middle-aged individuals over their lives to determine to what extent alcohol abuse becomes related to life crises such as bereavement, retirement, isolation, and physical disability. Such studies are urgently needed for a full comprehension of the dynamics of alcohol abuse in the elderly. One important longitudinal study which followed college students for 20 years into their middle years (Fillmore 1974) is discussed later in this chapter in the section "Characteristics of Elderly Alcohol Abusers."

In general, longitudinal studies of alcohol problems in the elderly have followed specific demographic groups of alcoholics and reported on later health, social, and/or drinking variables. Hyman (1973) has reported on a 15-year study of white male alcoholism treatment center clients. The follow-up located 87% of the original sample who were 30–54 years at intake. Those not located were assumed to be worse off socially, economically and medically based upon their condition at the time of initial treatment.

Among the 54 subjects located for follow-up, the mortality rate was 38%, over 2½ times that of the general population. Heart attack, cancer, acute alcoholism, cirrhosis, and suicide were the primary causes of death. Twenty-six subjects or families were interviewed. Marital break-ups and/or serious alcohol-related health problems characterized many of the subjects. A total of 63% of the original sample were either dead, clearly mentally deteriorated, or had had recent and serious manifestations of problem drinking. Considering that the median age at follow-up was around 56, this seems an exceptionally poor outcome for a group of men who were still middle-aged.

Simon et al. (1968) examined an alcoholic subsample of geriatric first admissions to a mental hospital. The sample was predominantly from the lower socioeconomic classes. Twenty-three percent had an alcoholic diagnosis and an additional 5% were very heavy drinkers. The alcoholics were somewhat younger and had a higher proportion of males than the 72% who were not alcoholics. Although alcoholics had lived alone more frequently prior to admission and had a higher proportion of broken marriages, they did not differ from the nonalcoholic groups in terms of measures of social interaction and isolation or in measures of cognitive and social function. Compared to the nonalcoholic patients, the alcoholics were lower on measures of physical self-maintenance at the time of the crisis which precipitated hospitalization. As might have been expected, the alcoholics with chronic brain syndrome (CBS) were the lowest of all groups on this measure.

Although the authors state that 7% of the entire sample became alcoholic *after* age 60, there were no data on precipitating factors, or whether the alcoholism was a result of cognitive deterioration. It would also be of considerable interest to know to what extent alcoholism before age 60 was related to a subsequent diagnosis of alcohol-related brain disease. Alcoholic patients with CBS had a mortality rate of 32% within 2 years. Alcoholic patients without CBS (who were 5 years younger than the nonalcoholics), had a mortality rate of 20% two years post discharge, compared with 10% for the nonalcoholics. Alcoholism, with or without CBS, clearly puts the elderly patient at a higher risk.

This interesting study demonstrates two major weaknesses in the sparse literature on alcoholism among the elderly: (1) the data are presented almost exclusively in a descriptive fashion without appropriate statistical tests of significance between comparison groups; (2) the data are not tabulated in a manner that contributes important new hypotheses about the unique problems of this alcoholism in the elderly. It is clear, however, that alcoholism among geriatric mental patients is a greater problem than might be anticipated based upon the commonly held assumption that because alcoholism rates decline with age the magnitude of the problem in the elderly is less significant.

# Male/Female Factors in Alcohol Problems of the Elderly

Survey studies typically locate a very small proportion of elderly women who are heavy drinkers, compared with elderly men (Cahalan, et al., 1968; Klattsky, et al. 1977; Bailey, et al., 1965). These figures may be an underestimation of the magnitude of alcohol abuse in elderly women for several reasons. Alcohol-use scales have been validated on male intake criteria. For women, it might be more appropriate to use a lower level for "heavy" usage since body size is considerably less in women. Furthermore, indicators of alcoholism such as work problems, police arrests, etc., may be more appropriate for elderly men than elderly women since the latter group is less likely to have had such experiences.

Garrett and Bahr (1973) in their study of homeless men and women seeking shelter, report data that are relevant to this point. Women were just as likely as men to *perceive* themselves as heavy drinkers, even though the actual amount reportedly consumed by the women was lower. Women in this study were also much more likely to be solitary drinkers compared to men.

Rosin and Glatt (1971), on the other hand, found more women than men in the alcoholic sample of elderly psychiatric patients in England. Two other British studies were cited, in which elderly women with alcohol problems also outnumbered the men, at a ratio of 2 to 1. This was attributed to the larger number of female survivors in the older age ranges in Britain.

McCusker et al. (1971) reported the male to female ratio of alcohol abuse among general medical ward admissions at Harlem Hospital was almost two to one. These data were interpreted as indicating that alcoholism is no longer primarily a male disorder. However, since one-half of the alcoholic women were also heads of households and 91% of the sample was black, these data may actually represent the incidence of alcoholism in a black inner-city population, rather than being representative of the larger group of elderly women.

Schuckit et al. (1978) compared consecutive admissions to two alcohol treatment centers by age and sex. Twenty-four percent of the sample were older men and 16% were older women but differences in the centers precluded direct comparison of these percentages. Sixty percent of the women were living alone at the time they sought treatment, from either having been widowed (37%), or divorced or separated (23%). In contrast, only 32% of the elderly alcoholic men lived alone. There were also some interesting similarities between the elderly alcoholics from each sample. The mean age of 59 years was the same for males and females; the elderly alcoholics of both sexes had no more years of alcohol problems than younger alcoholics, and both elderly male and female alcoholics had had more stable lives than younger alcoholics. The elderly alcoholics of both sexes seemed to be persons who had developed alcohol problems in middle to late life (Type II or late-onset alcoholism to be described in the next section).

Studies on middle and upper class alcoholics, particularly women, are sparse. Even such thorough recent reviews of women alcoholics as Greenblatt and Schuckit (1976) and Beckman (1975) reported no studies that focused specifically on alcoholism in elderly women.

Curlee (1969) reported that middle class, middle-aged women were much more likely than their male counterparts to perceive an external situation as the precipitating factor in the onset of alcoholism. In a study of 200 consecutive male and female admissions to a private alcoholism treatment center, retirement was the most commonly stated precipitating factor (6 out of 100 of the men), while 20% of the women related the onset of excessive drinking to problems associated with the middle-aged identity crisis (sometimes referred to as the "empty nest" syndrome). Similar studies need to be carried out on situational crises facing older women, such as widowhood, husbands' retirement, and so on.

## Studies of Abstention Behavior in the Elderly

Very few of the studies on drinking problems in the elderly have dealt with the equally interesting question of abstentious behavior in the elderly. Although most surveys indicated a higher proportion of abstinence among the elderly, it is not clear whether this represents generational differences sampled by the cross-sectional studies, or actual changes in drinking habits that accompany aging. Factors related to abstinence in the elderly would be of interest to investigate.

Perhaps the most interesting of such reports is the work of Westermeyer (1972) who has reported on drinking and abstaining behavior in a Chippewa community in Minnesota. A sudden and abrupt onset of abstention apparently characterized some elderly Indians who inexplicably stopped drinking one day and did not resume again. Westermeyer reported that these persons became "fed up" with their own drinking and the problems it caused them. He postulated that understanding how this process occurred within the atmosphere of "Indian" drinking with long binges, specified social and individual behaviors, and heavy alcohol intake might be of considerable use. However, the motivational factors which may have precipitated such abstinence are not discussed.

Chafetz (1974) also discussed the issue of abstentious behavior in the elderly, by citing the work of Johnson (1974) on elderly abstainers who at one time had been drinkers. Sixty-one percent of the men and 29% of the women who had formerly been drinkers were abstainers at the time of the study. Half had stopped because it made them ill or was considered detrimental to health. There was, however, no actual difference in the proportion of abstainers to drinkers who reported good health. One hypothesis was that the fear of the emotionally disinhibitory effects of alcohol and the desire to avoid these may have been a predominant reason for drinkers to become abstainers in old age. One-third of the nondrinkers stated that one of the reasons for not drinking was the behaviors that drinking caused.

The studies reviewed thus far have reported divergent prevalence rates for alcohol problems among the elderly. Many factors are involved in these studies, which could contribute to the reported differences. Sample characteristics, definition of "elderly," and diagnosis of alcoholism or the methods for assessing drinking may be three of the most important variables.

Whereas survey studies of drinking habits demonstrate that the prevalence of problem drinking is lower among the elderly, studies of special populations indicated that alcoholism among the elderly is a significant and often unrecognized problem. Unfortunately, no longitudinal studies were found which dealt with the important question of what unique factors associated with aging might increase the risk of alcohol abuse in the elderly.

## CHARACTERISTICS OF ELDERLY ALCOHOL ABUSERS

Most studies agree that elderly alcohol abusers cannot be defined along a single dimension. Two types of data will be reviewed here: reports that differentiate elderly alcohol abusers according to the age of onset of alcohol problems, and studies that describe unique aspects of alcohol abuse in the elderly.

### Early vs. Late Onset of Alcohol Problems

Many authors writing about problems of the elderly agree that there are basically two types of elderly alcoholics. These types are classified according to age of onset of alcoholism: Type I, or early-onset alcoholics, are those with a long history of alcohol abuse who continue to drink excessively into their later years. Type II, or late-onset alcoholics, are those who react to the stresses of aging by excessive drinking (Droller, 1964; Glatt and Rosin, 1964; Rosin and Glatt, 1971; Pascarelli, 1974; Pascarelli and Fischer, 1974; Zimberg, 1974, 1978; Glatt, 1978 and Schuckit and Pastor, 1978). Such studies indicate that the relative proportion of the two types is two-thirds Type I and one-third Type II. Psychopathology is seen as the most important underlying factor in early-onset alcoholics, while social factors precipitate late-onset alcoholism (Glatt and Rosin, 1964).

The Type I, or early-onset alcoholic, has been described as a person with remarkable physical resistance to have survived the long-term effects of alcohol, but most have one or more consequences, such as cirrhosis of the liver, of heavy drinking (Pascarelli, 1974). Early-onset alcoholics have a history of greater social and occupational problems (Schuckit and Pastor, 1978) but may not be drinking as heavily in their old age due to decreased tolerance, poorer financial circumstances, limited social circles, or hampered physical mobility (Glatt, 1978).

The Type II, or late-onset alcoholics, are perhaps of greater interest to the field of geriatrics, because they have responded to the stresses of aging by drinking excessively, while as younger persons they were typically only moderate or infrequent drinkers (Glatt and Rosin, 1964). Precipitating events for the late-onset alcoholics include bereavement, retirement, and increased social isolation (Glatt and Rosin, 1964; Zimberg, 1974; Pascarelli and Fischer, 1974).

In some of the earliest descriptions of late-onset alcoholics, Droller, 1964, has presented case reports on seven patients, aged 63–80. Six of these patients were women and five of those were widows. Only two began drinking in their 30s and 40s but five of the seven "took to alcohol after increasing isolation, grief, and the other erosions of life inseparable from old age."

However, both Droller and Glatt agree that the prognosis is good for the late-onset alcoholics because of their better basic personality structures. In a follow-up study of alcoholic patients in England, Glatt (1961) found that the prognosis in the 41–70 age group was significantly better than in the 21–42 year olds.

Bahr (1969), in an early study of Skid Row habitués, distinguished between early and late onset of alcoholism in elderly male alcoholics. In early-onset alcoholics, the drinking functioned as a "primary causal influence" in the subsequent lifestyle, while in late-onset alcoholics, the drinking followed as a response to a personal crisis or physical decline. The hypothesis was confirmed that men who began to drink heavily in their 20s and 30s were less affiliated with families and jobs, had lower occupational status, and belonged to fewer voluntary organizations than later-onset drinkers. The behavior patterns of the two groups tended to converge as they reached the 50s, although in one sample studied, the convergence was never complete.

In another empirical study, Rosin and Glatt (1971) classified the precipitating causes of drinking problems in 103 elderly alcoholics. "Primary" factors (particularly inveterate drinking and personality factors associated with long-standing pathological drinking), were primarily characteristic of Type I, or early-onset alcoholics, while precipitating causes classified as "Reactive" (bereavement, retirement, and infirmity) were primarily characteristic of Type II alcoholics. They hypothesized that late-onset alcoholics could be taught to function with lowered alcohol intake since they had been social drinkers for much of their lives, but believed that additional social support systems to replace their loss and coping mechanisms would have to be implemented as well. Certainly the prognosis for late-onset alcoholism augers better in terms of treatment possibilities and eventual return to an independent mode of functioning. Such individuals appear to be healthier, better integrated, and more capable of being absorbed again into a social milieu than do the early-onset alcoholics. Early alcoholics, on the other hand, may be a more marginal group in that their drinking problems have resulted from physical, mental, or social deficiencies within themselves.

Tarter et al. (1977) found that hyperactivity and/or minimal brain dysfunction in childhood was often associated with early-onset alcoholism, as well as a family history of excessive alcohol intake. Foulds and Hassall, 1969, in an early study in Great Britain, found that male alcoholics who had become excessive drinkers by age 30 had more frequent job changes, more police convictions and prison sentences, more suicide attempts, and more divorces and separations as compared with males who became chronic drinkers after age 30.

One of the most important longitudinal studies in this area has unfortunately only carried the subjects through middle age at last report. Fillmore (1974), who examined the drinking habits of middle-aged men and women who had been first studied as college students, used pathway analysis as a model to predict problem drinking in later life. While frequency of drinking in young adulthood had little effect on later problem drinking, young male and female problem drinkers continued to be problem drinkers in middle age. Furthermore, the quantity that young women drank was related to problem drinking later in life. These may be the forerunners of Type I or early-onset alcohol abusers. An additional group of young abstainers had become problem drinkers by middle age (10% of the young male abstainers and 7% of the young female abstainers). These may represent the first appearance of Type II or late-onset alcohol abusers. It will be interesting to see the next 20-year follow-up, when the individuals will be in their early sixties. This sample is of particular interest in that it began with a homogeneous, white, upper middle class, well-educated group of young persons, thus enabling assessment of the consequences of alcohol problems in terms of social, economic and occupational variables.

The demographic evidence that there are proportionately fewer alcoholics in the elderly than would have been expected from the numbers at younger ages has led to the hypothesis by Drew (1968) that alcoholism is a self-limiting illness which corrects itself with advancing age. Zimberg (1974) stated that although this indeed may be true, the extent of alcoholism in the elderly has been underestimated and remains a serious problem. Zimberg's extensive work on the prevalence of alcoholism in Harlem would support this contention. In one of his studies 63% of the males and 35% of the females admitted to the medical ward were alcoholics.

Nevertheless, there is some evidence in support of Drew's hypothesis. Schuckit (1976) described the cessation of drinking in men in the seventh decade as "maturing out." This abstinence syndrome correlated with early onset of heavy drinking. Schuckit suggests that many individuals who begin heavy drinking at an earlier age may not survive unless abstinence ensues.

The genetic theory of alcoholism, which presupposes an inherited propensity for drinking or at least a predisposition for alcohol abuse, would encompass the early-onset more readily than the late-onset alcohol abuser. Ericksson (1974) cited the well-known Scandinavian twin studies which demonstrated concordance in drinking habits for monozygotic rather than dizygotic twins. The correlation of early childhood hyperactivity and later alcoholism would also be indicative of a familial concordance for alcoholism. Thus, in evaluating alcoholism in the elderly, it would seem important to differentiate between the early- and the late-onset alcoholic. Treatment implications and prognosis appear to both be related to these factors.

## Unique Aspects of Alcohol Abuse in the Elderly

Rathbone-McCuan and Bland (1974) suggested that geriatric problem drinkers and alcoholics be added to Brody and Brody's (1974) list of subgroups of the elderly population which are at particularly high risk. They cited a Rutgers study which estimated that 7.5% of the population over age 55 were problem drinkers. That the number is this large is surprising in view of the fact that U.S. (Knupfer and Room, 1974; Cahalan and Cissin, 1968) and Australian studies (Encel et al., 1972) have shown that drinking declines with age, although in the Australian study the drop was less precipitous. An Irish study, however, found no age-related drop in alcohol consumption (Blaney and Radford, 1973).

*Demography.*   Schuckit (1976) found that older alcoholics as compared with younger alcoholics are more often white, have lower separation and divorce rates, and have fewer social problems. According to Schuckit and Pastor (1978), elderly Veterans Administration alcoholics compared with medical and surgical patients of the same age were more likely to live alone (33% vs. 25%), less likely to be married (40% vs. 65%), and less likely to have been living in the same house for 5 years or more (25% vs. 50%). In addition, alcoholics over 60 are more likely to be Caucasian than younger alcoholics (90% vs. 70%). All of the above studies describe hospital or treatment center populations and are probably not representative of the general population.

*Drinking Patterns.*   Older alcoholics are more likely to drink daily than a younger group and to drink less per occasion (Schuckit and Pastor, 1978). They are also less likely to use illicit drugs than their younger counterparts. They correspond in drinking pattern to the Ashley et al. (1976) description of "continuous" rather than intermittent alcoholics, and to Jellinek's (1960) "delta" alcoholic, who is described as a steady, inveterate, sustained, or nonperiodic drinker. Russell, et al. (1978) commented that the decrease in body water which is concomitant with old age results in higher blood alcohol levels in this population, since alcohol is almost entirely distributed in water.

*Precipitating Factors.*   Elderly persons who become alcoholic in the absence of a prior history of alcoholism appear to be more influenced by various precipitating conditions that often accompany aging. Such factors include retirement, bereavement, loneliness, illness, and loss of social, family, and economic resources. Unfortunately, with the exception of a few studies already mentioned (e.g., Rosin and Glatt, 1971; Fillmore, 1974) there has been little examination of the unique factors associated with aging that help precipitate the onset of alcoholic problems in the elderly.

## LONG-TERM CONSEQUENCES
## OF SUSTAINED DRINKING
## IN THE ELDERLY

### Morbidity and Early Mortality

Numerous studies have replicated the finding that alcoholics die 10–15 years sooner than the general population. Costello (1974) in a retrospective study found the fatality rate in 400 alcoholic clients in a rehabilitation center was far in excess of the general population, with an increase in deaths due to violence, suicide, cirrhosis of the liver, and some increase in cardiovascular disease. Blum and Braunstein (1967) have reviewed the literature earlier and confirmed the correlation between excessive drinking and suicide, homicide and accidental death. In the most recent literature review, Brody and Mills (1978) concluded that alcoholics die 10–12 years prematurely due to many causes including cirrhosis, pancreatitis, heart disease, cancer of the upper gastrointestinal tract, accidents, and suicide.

Haberman and Baden (1974) reported on a study of postmortem findings in a sample of 1,000 sudden traumatic or medically unattended deaths in a major city. Thirty-seven percent of all alcohol decedents died as a result of accidents, homicide, narcotics, or suicide. Thirty-two percent of these had blood alcohol concentrations of 0.10% or higher, which indicated alcohol impairment immediately prior to death. Twenty-one percent of those identified as alcoholics were sixty years old or older at the time of death.

A paper by Waller (1974) documented factors related to injury in the aged. A study he performed on 150 emergency room patients aged 60 or older found that 13% reported alcohol use prior to the injury for which they were being treated. McCusker et al. (1971), in a study of 118 admissions to general medical wards at Harlem Hospital, reported higher rates of pneumonia, bronchitis, cirrhosis, seizure disorders, gastritis, and pancreatitis in patients who were alcoholic compared to nonalcoholic admissions. All ten cases of seizure disorders were also alcoholic.

According to data from the Division of Vital Statistics cited by the Metropolitan Life Insurance Company (Anon., 1974), the mortality rates from alcoholic disorders vary according to age, peaking among white males at 32.1 per 100,000 at ages 60–69, and at 65.0 per 100,000 for black males in the same age group. For white women, the peak rate is 28.0 per 100,000 at ages 40–49.

Malin et al. (1978) have reported on the high rate of deaths due to cirrhosis of the liver in women of all races who were over 75 years old, with the highest rate in Native Americans (45 per 100,000), followed by Caucasians (20 per 100,000), and Blacks (14 per 100,000).

Another related consequence of alcoholism in the elderly is early institutionalization. In a study of 1,000 male domiciliary inpatients, Harrington and Price (1962) compared those with a history of alcoholism with those who had not had an alcoholic diagnosis. The alcoholic patient entered the domiciliary at a significantly earlier age and significantly more alcoholics (23%) had had no income at the time of admission to domiciliary care. Furthermore, in terms of diagnosis, significantly more alcoholics than expected had personality disorders and chronic brain syndrome.

Wiik-Larsen and Enger (1978) point out that a relatively high number of persons die unintentionally of alcohol intoxication. In Oslo in 1975, there were 35 such deaths listed. The majority of them occurred outside of the hospital, and all were listed officially as "accidental." The peak age for death by intoxication in men was 50–60 years while for women it was 40–50 years.

## Suicide

The aged comprise 9% of the population but commit 25% of the reported suicides. The suicide rate in Caucasians over age 65 is four times the national average for males and twice the national average for females (Resnik and Cantor, 1970). The suicide rate not only increases with age, but there is some evidence that alcoholics may be particularly at risk. Ripley (1973) has reported age-related trends in approximately 400 completed suicides in Seattle and Edinburgh. The peak years for suicide were ages 50–64 for Seattle men and for Edinburgh women. Seventy-six percent of the men who committed suicide had had drinking problems. Robins, et al. (1959) and Dorpat et al. (1968) both reported high rates of chronic alcoholism among completed suicides, 23% and 30% respectively.

Factors precipitating suicide are often those associated with aging and alcoholism. Physical illness was the most common precipitating factor in both the Dorpat and Ripley studies of completed suicide, while Tuckman and Youngman (1968) reported that persons living alone, including the widowed and divorced, were at greatest risk for successful suicide. To this list can be added the unemployed and retired (Patterson et al., 1974). Loss of loved ones, loneliness, declining faculties, feelings of hopelessness and inability to cope are compounded in the elderly alcoholic. Schuckit and Pastor (1978) also found that older alcoholics had an increased suicide rate compared with elderly medical and surgical patients (5% vs. 1%). The extent of alcoholics' feelings of hopelessness and the accuracy of their perceptions is indicated in a study of prior communications in completed suicides. Seventy-seven percent of the chronic alcoholics who had committed suicide had communicated their intent to family and friends prior to the act. However, of all diagnostic groups, the suicidal communications of the alcoholic were the least likely to have been believed by relatives and friends.

## Neural Damage

*Korsakoff's Psychosis.*    Korsakoff's psychosis, the chronic phase of the Wernicke-Korsakoff syndrome, is an organic brain disease characterized by the retrograde and anterograde amnesia with relative sparing of other intellectual functions (McEntee and Mair, 1978). These investigators found evidence that the memory impairment may be due to damage to ascending noradrenergic pathways resulting from diencephalic and brainstem lesions associated with the disease. Korsakoff patients have been experimentally found to be deficient in short-term memory particularly in the verbal area, but have more or less normal memory for auditory, visual, or tactile stimuli. Since severe intoxication may result in an amnesiac (blackout) episode during which short-term memory is impaired, it was hypothesized by Goodwin et al. (1975) that a group of alcoholics who suffer frequent blackouts might resemble Korsakoff patients in exhibiting poorer verbal than nonverbal recall. Unfortunately, 11 of 12 of their frequent blackout patients failed to have one during the test period and this interesting hypothesis could not be adequately tested.

Jones et al. (1975) found that Korsakoff syndrome alcoholics were severely impaired in their ability to determine whether common odors were the same or different in a paired comparisons test. Alcoholics per se did not differ from controls on this task. It was hypothesized that olfactory information processing may have been compromised due to disease-related damage to the dorsal medial and ventrical medial thalamic nuclei, which are olfactory pathways to cortex. Another study in that laboratory by Cermak et al. (1971) found Korsakoff patients, compared to alcoholic and normal patients, to be significantly impaired in short-term verbal recall. Recognition short-term memory was similarly impaired, as was long-term memory for associated word pairs. Neither degree of stimulus difficulty nor amount of material was shown to be a factor. Since the Korsakoff patients performed relatively better on the recognition task, it was hypothesized that their memory deficit was primarily a problem of retrieval rather than storage of short-term memories and of transferral of information from short-term to long-term memory. To date no such impairments have been demonstrated for alcoholic patients without Korsakoff's syndrome (Butters et al., 1977). Older alcoholics who have been recently intoxicated performed similarly to Korsakoff patients on short-term tasks, but their performance approached that of younger alcoholics after a month's abstinence. The Korsakoff patients exhibited no such improvement (Cermak and Ryback, 1976). The mechanism for this effect is not known.

Plutchnik and DiScipio (1974) have noted the similarity in behavioral patterns between alcoholics with Korsakoff's syndrome and nonalcoholic geriatric patients with evidence of organic brain syndrome. They cite this as evidence against the hypothesis that there exists a constellation of behaviors which uniquely characterize the alcoholic, that a lifetime of heavy drinking results in probable neurologic involvement, and that the two groups of patients may have a common underlying metabolic or nutritional disorder. Apropos of this, the acute phase of Korsakoff's psychosis, Wernicke's syndrome, has long been associated with the specific thiamine deficiency occurring in nutritionally depleted chronic alcoholics. The section on nutrition in the elderly goes into more detail.

*Organic Brain Syndrome* (OBS).    A study by Epstein and Simon (1967) found that 29% of organic brain syndrome patients who were over age 60 were excessive drinkers. Half of these were late-onset problem drinkers. This syndrome is reserved for generalized cognitive deficits accruing from structural neural damage to the brain. A subset of the Wechsler Adult Intelligence Scale (WAIS) has been found to be effective in selecting out OBS patients. Overall and Gorham (1972) analyzed profile patterns to separate "mental aging" from "organicity," with which it is often confounded.

A study was then performed on 158 hospitalized alcoholic patients who ranged in age from 25–64 (Williams et al. 1973). Alcoholic patients differed from WAIS normative scores on both mental aging and organicity with a significant acceleration in mental aging and organicity in the alcoholic patients. A suggestion of greater organic involvement after age 35 in the alcoholic group was also found. This suggestion of premature aging in alcoholics was substantiated by Korboot and Naylor (1972), who examined 26 males with a mean age of 56 who had been diagnosed as alcohol dementias by two psychiatrists. The implication of dementia is of an irreversible intellectual decline as opposed to the relatively static

Korsakoff condition. The demented alcoholics' maximum rate of information acceptance was significantly below the rate for two groups of normal elderly subjects between the ages of 60–69 and 70–79, but very close to normals who were 80–89 years of age. The alcoholic subjects then, appeared to be prematurely aged, possibly due to a nonfocal neuronal loss.

Tarter (1975) examined the evidence for three hypotheses which have been advanced to describe neuropsychological deficits exhibited by chronic alcoholics: (1) alcoholics have diffused generalized cerebral impairment; (2) alcoholics are differentially impaired in the right hemisphere; and (3) neurological disruption is primarily in the anterior-basal regions of brain. Tarter concluded that neither psychiatric symptomatology, psychological test profiles, nor neuropathological/neurological evidence can be found for the hypothesis of nonfocal brain damage. Evidence for the right versus left hemispheric damage is considered to be provocative and worthy of further study, since alcoholics have been found to be impaired on many, but not all, tasks involving spatial perception. The greatest support was found for anterior-basal neurological deficit. Psychological test performance of cognitive flexibility, spatial concepts, perceptual field orientation, task persistence, and several others all suggest structural lesions in anterior-basal regions in chronic alcoholics. Autopsied chronic alcoholic brains have been found to exhibit frontal cerebral atrophy and disruption of tracts connecting frontal to limbic and diencephalic regions. This suggests that alcoholics exhibit a pattern of disorders similar to that manifested by the more deteriorated Korsakoff patients who have been shown to suffer from the same disruption.

## Premature Aging

The hypothesis that excessive drinking results in some form of "premature aging" has been suggested and tested in regard to sensory-motor, perceptual, and cognitive functions by Blusenwicz et al. (1977). Unfortunately, no elderly alcoholics were tested, but young alcoholics were deficient on tasks involving short-term memory as were the elderly normal group who had a mean age of 71. Gaitz and Baer (1971) who administered a test battery and the mental status scale to 100 consecutive elderly psychiatric hospital admissions found that only when alcoholism was compounded by organic brain syndrome were there elevations in mental status scores, particularly in the areas of inappropriate or bizarre behavior, confusion, speech disorganization, and disorientation or memory loss. Since the nonalcoholic with organic brain syndrome exhibited scores which were equally elevated, it was concluded that the organic brain syndrome accounted for the results. The hypothesis that excessive alcohol use results in early aging was supported since the alcoholic/OBS patients were significantly younger than the OBS/nonalcoholic patients.

Parker and Noble (1977) administered a battery of four test of cognitive function to 102 male, middle-aged, social drinkers (1.42 oz. per session of absolute alcohol). There was no correlation found between the amount of alcohol consumed over the subject's lifetime and cognitive scores; however, correlations were found between the amount of alcohol consumed *per session* and impaired performance. Significant performance decrements were in the areas of abstraction, adaptive abilities, and conceptualization. Although this provocative study was performed in middle-aged males, one would expect the accrued deficits to be greater in older individuals.

Kleinknecht and Goldstein (1972) reviewed the literature of neuropsychological deficits associated with alcoholism and found that age is not well controlled or accounted for in such studies of alcoholics. The ages of subjects tend to cover the range from young adulthood to old (but not extreme old) age, with standard deviations being seldom reported. Sample size in each age range tends to be small as well. Since there is a well-known decline in abilities with age as measured by psychological and perceptual tests, it is crucial that normal decline be separated from the effects of alcoholism. One area of normal decline is in the area of abstract reasoning culminating in organic brain syndrome, and the second is in the area of speed tasks and complex perceptual motor abilities. Standard I.Q. tests did not discriminate alcoholics from the normal population, with the possible exception of some of the WAIS subtests. The hypothesis that excess alcohol intake results in cognitive and perceptual impairments resembling extreme old age is supported by the above data. Excessive alcohol intake represents a potential excessive economic, social, and personal loss in a shortened effective life span.

## Antisocial Behaviors

Schuckit et al. (1970) found that male alcoholics who began drinking heavily before age 20 (early-onset) had significantly more antisocial behaviors than did alcoholics who did not become alcoholics until after age 30. Specifically, the early-onset group had had more severe school problems, repeated marital separations, arrests while drinking, arrests for

fighting, poor work history, sexual promiscuity, and drug experimenta-
tion. A study of disciplinary problems in a veteran's home in which 58%
of the sample was aged 60 or older (Apfeldorf et al. 1972) found two
groups of individuals who had records of offenses resulting in disciplinary action: diagnosed alcoholics without overtly hostile behavior patterns, and individuals with expressed hostility who had drinking problems in addition. It was not determined if the latter group were likely to
become alcoholics, but self-report scales seemed to indicate that the two
groups perceived themselves differently.

Hoffman and Nelson (1971) administered the MMPI, Edwards Personal Preference Scale and the Shipley-Hartford Intelligence Scale to a
group of 148 alcoholics divided into three age and three intelligence
levels. Age accounted for more of the variance than did alcoholism or
intelligence, with the more intelligent and younger alcoholics scoring
closer to the normal (nonalcoholic) population. Older alcoholics showed
a significant decrease in abstract reasoning as well as decreases in Domi-
nance, Change, and Psychopathic Deviance, and increases in Defer-
ence, Order, Nurturance, and Endurance. Higher intelligence removed
most of these differences.

## Nutritional Deficiencies

Nutritional deficiencies as a result of poor eating habits in the elderly
are compounded by alcohol abuse, since there is an increased need for
nutrients to repair alcohol-induced tissue damage. Barboriak, et al.
(1978) examined a domiciliary V.A. population in which free meals are
provided to residents, thus eliminating the problem of reduced food
intake in alcoholics who spend their money instead for liquor. Even
though all food was provided for these 51 males whose mean age was
59½ years, their caloric intake was reduced below the recommended
2,400 Kcal/day. In addition, vitamin intake was reduced, which could
compound the malabsorption of thiamine and pyridoxine found in alcoholics. Serum albumin levels and plasma triglyceride levels were lower
in the drinkers and perhaps augered the onset of nutritional deficits.

Alcohol abuse is associated with an increased excretion of nutrients
such as zinc and magnesium. Russell et al. (1978) point out that some
nutrients are less efficiently utilized in the presence of excess ethanol,
and that years of heavy alcohol use can damage the liver, gastrointestinal
tract, and pancreas, which then results in impairments in the digestion,

absorption, and metabolism of nutrients. Alcohol abuse and poor nutrition interact, particularly in the elderly person whose physical and financial resources may already be limited.

## TREATMENT OF ALCOHOL ABUSE IN THE ELDERLY

### Diagnosis

Diagnosis of alcohol abuse in the elderly is a difficult procedure and elderly patients with such problems are frequently missed by the examining physician (Zimberg, 1974; Droller, 1964; Glatt and Rosin, 1964). McCusker et al. (1971) found that only 55% of alcoholic patients were identified on admission by the house staff and 45% on discharge. Failure to properly diagnose alcohol abuse resulted in few requests for psychiatric consultations for alcoholism and failure to make appropriate referrals to the alcoholism clinic of the hospital upon discharge. In general, prevalence studies employing self-report or special interview procedures reveal higher rates of alcoholism than those relying on physician diagnosis alone.

According to Zimberg (1978) a number of factors make alcoholism in the elderly less obvious than in younger patients.

1. Older alcoholics consume less alcohol.
2. Alcohol abuse in the elderly often leads to social rather than acute physical problems.
3. The acute physical distress associated with alcoholism is seen less in the elderly and leads to their greater reluctance to utilize alcoholism treatment programs.

Several authors (Zimberg, 1974; Rosen and Glatt, 1971) cite denial on the part of the elderly patient and especially his family as another important factor. Droller (1964) reported that his elderly patients' physicians often did not realize what was happening to these individuals as they developed symptoms of alcoholism late in life. Thus, the diagnosis of alcoholism becomes particularly difficult in late-onset alcoholics.

Self-report scales for alcoholism detection have generally not been specifically used in elderly populations, but Apfeldorf and Hunley (1975) reported that two alcoholism scales from MMPI (the McAndrew and the Holmes Scales) detected not only domiciled alcoholics, but nonalcoholics with records of offenses which indicated that they had drinking problems. They concluded that these scales may be of value in detecting elderly patients who have drinking problems but are not flagrantly alcoholic.

Most survey data assess the frequency and quantity of alcohol consumption but age-related studies of blood alcohol levels would add another dimension. Russell, et al. (1978) stated that a given dose of alcohol is associated with higher blood alcohol levels in the elderly, due to the general decrease in body water associated with aging. Longitudinal studies of individual changes in drinking habits associated with aging, as well as individual changes in blood alcohol, would bear further investigation. Vestal et al. (1975) have demonstrated age differences in peak blood alcohol levels following a standard alcohol dose.

## Treatment

Droller (1964) has prescribed a specific treatment procedure for elderly alcoholics involving rehydration with a glucose-saline solution and vitamin $B_{12}$, immediate withdrawal from all alcohol, dietary intervention to attain a 2,500 calorie diet, and protein supplementation when indicated. Barbiturates or sedatives were also utilized on a short-term basis. Once physically and mentally restored, he encourages his elderly alcoholics to live in some form of community rather than returning to their own homes. Social contacts are of primary importance.

Zimberg, (1969, 1971, 1974, 1978) views alcoholism as a signal that the patient is unable to cope with loneliness, depression, hopelessness, and other stresses of aging. For these late-onset (Type II) alcoholics, he recommends a therapeutic regimen combining antidepressant medication with resocialization. He believes that neither drug therapy, referral to alcohol treatment programs or detoxification is required by many of these elderly alcoholics (Zimberg, 1978), and recommends that the treatment of the elderly alcoholic is best carried out through facilities serving the aged rather than through alcohol treatment agencies. He remains optimistic about the effectiveness of intervention strategies for both early and late-onset elderly alcoholics.

While some authors share Zimberg's view that community treatment and social intervention are important in the treatment of the elderly alcoholic (Subley, 1974; Droller, 1964; Glatt and Rosin, 1964) others, such as Mayfield (1974), focus entirely on treatment and management of alcohol withdrawal. The unexpected appearance of alcohol withdrawal symptoms among hospitalized patients is often overlooked and thus may be inappropriately treated. He cautions against vigorous hydration in view of the work by Beard and Knott (1968), which indicated that overhydration rather than dehydration is a more constant concomitant of chronic alcohol intake. Thus, it is not clear that there is accord in the alcohol literature about the best approach to treating the elderly alcoholic; the treatment may be as diverse as the problem.

## Therapeutic Use of Alcohol in Geriatric Settings

Leake and Silverman (1967) summarized earlier authors who cite the beneficial effects of alcohol for the elderly. Alcohol, in moderate amounts, is reported to increase the flow of gastric secretions, stimulate the gastrointestinal tract, alleviate the pain and discomfort from angina attacks, and help in maintaining healthy circulation. In 1973, Turner, in an editorial comment in JAMA, cited recent controlled studies in this area and also concluded that in many geriatric patients favorable physical and psychological effects accompanied the therapeutic use of mild alcoholic beverages.

The studies in this area are fraught with methodological problems. Only one article (Johnson, 1974) dealt with the issue of whether moderate alcohol use was beneficial for those among the elderly who consume it normally. Most of the empirical studies in this area have administered alcohol to patients and measured staff ratings of socialization (Carroll, 1978) or attempted to evaluate the influence of the "pub" setting on the behavior of elderly patients (Chien, 1971; Chien et al., 1973). In general, these studies concluded that the primary effect results from the alcohol, but that the congenial pub atmosphere may enhance the alcohol effect. Another common problem is that of bias since the ward staff, who know the treatment conditions of the patients are the primary raters or recorders of outcome variables. However, one study (Mishihara, et al., 1975) utilized "blind" examiners and a comparison group, and reported several favorable effects related to moderate alcohol use (including improved morale, sleep, and ratings of vigor, intactness, orientation, and relationships). The primary focus of these studies has been an assessment of short-term favorable effects, with the longest alcohol administration phase evaluated being 18 weeks (Mishihara, et al., 1975).

There is little information on the effects of long-term alcohol administration, either on general behavior, health, or subsequent alcohol consumption. The concern most frequently expressed by critics of alcohol treatment for the elderly (e.g., Zimberg, 1974; Droller, 1964), that is, that it will become addictive, does not appear to have been addressed by the empirical studies in general. Furthermore, with the exception of one study which compared data from physical exams and ECGs from experimental vs. control groups (Mishihara et al., 1975), studies in this area seem in general to have been primarily concerned with social and behavioral variables rather than physiological or health-related outcomes.

Long-term studies of the potentially adverse effects on subsequent alcohol use and abuse do not appear to have been carried out. Furthermore, most of the empirical studies have been conducted in inpatient geriatric settings. There are obvious difficulties in generalizing such studies to elderly persons living in a community setting.

The demarcation between moderate alcohol use with possibly favorable outcomes and alcohol abuse (and its obvious disadvantages) is no more clear in the field of geriatrics than it is for the field of alcohol studies in general.

Criticism of alcohol treatment for the elderly appears to come from practitioners such as Zimberg (1974) and Droller (1964) who deal more intensively with the numerous problems arising from alcohol abuse in the elderly.

## SUMMARY

Although several dozen articles have been written addressing the topic of alcohol use and abuse in the elderly, there has been no systematic attack on the problem's extent, or ultimate cost to society of alcoholism in individuals over age 65. The majority of studies have been cross-sectional in design, which is a limitation, although it is easy to understand why such studies are performed, since they are considerably less expensive. The methods by which alcohol use is assessed are probably not relevant to the elderly since they have been standardized on young males. In addition, the effective amounts consumed are underestimated, since older individuals are lighter in body weight and less of their mass is composed of water. Therefore it takes less alcohol to have an effect. Few studies have been performed specifically on older individuals who are still residing in the community rather than in nursing homes or V.A. hospitals, and there is very little information on women over the age of 65, since most of the studies have examined drinking in males.

The population in the U.S. is aging; birth rate is continuing to drop and health care has been improved. By the year 2000, 20% of all individuals will be over 65 compared with 4% in 1900. Furthermore, alcohol use in younger men and particularly in younger women is increasing markedly. The extent to which excessive alcohol use compounds the normal problems of aging must be clarified. Now is the time to begin long-term prospective studies on the physical and mental health of this population and to standardize tests and methodology in this area. The cost to society of neglecting drinking problems in the elderly will be considerable in the future.

# REFERENCES

Anon., Alcoholism in the United States. *Stat. Bull. Metrop Life Ins. Co.*, 2–5, July, 1974.

Apfeldorf, M., Hunley, P. J. & Cooper, G. D.: Disciplinary problems in a home for older veterans: Some psychological aspects in relation to drinking behavior. *Gerontologist*, 12:143–147, 1972.

Apfeldorf, M. & Hunley, P. J. Application of MMPI alcoholism scales to older alcoholics and problem drinkers. *J. Stud. Alc.*, 36:645–652, 1975.

Ashley, M. J., Olin, J. S., le Riché, W. H., Kornaczewski, A., Schmidt, W. & Rankin, J. G.: "Continuous" and "Intermittent" alcoholics: A comparison of demographic, sociological, and physical disease characteristics in relation to the pattern of drinking. *Addict. Dis.*, 2:515–532, 1976.

Bahr, H. M.: Lifetime affiliation patterns of early- and late-onset heavy drinkers on Skid Row. *Quart. J. Stud. Alc.*, 30:645–656, 1969.

Bailey, M. B., Haberman, P. W. & Alksne, H. The epidemiology of alcoholism in an urban residential area. *Quart. J. Stud. Alc.*, 26:19–40, 1965.

Barboriak, J. L., Rooney, C. B., Leitschuk, T. H. & Anderson, A. J. Alcohol and nutrient intake of elderly men. *J. Amer. Diet. Assn.*, 72:493–495, 1978.

Beckman, L. J. Women Alcoholics: A review of social and psychological studies. *J. Stud. Alc.*, 36:797–824, 1975.

Blaney, R. & Radford, I. S.: The prevalence of alcoholism in an Irish town. *Quart. J. Stud. Alc.*, 34:1255–1269, 1973.

Blum, R. H. & Braunstein, L.: Mind-altering drugs and dangerous behavior. In: *U.S. President's Commission on Law Enforcement and Administration of Justice Task Force Report: Drunkenness*. Washington, D.C.: Government Printing Office, 1967.

Blusewicz, M. T., Dustman, R. E., Schenkenberg, T. & Beck, E. C.: Neuropsychological correlates of chronic alcoholism and aging. *J. Nerv. Ment. Dis.*, 165:348–354, 1977.

Bollerup, T. R. Prevalence of mental illness among 70-year olds domiciled in nine Copenhagen suburbs. *Acta. Psychiat. Scand.*, 51:327–339, 1975.

Brody, J. A. & Mills, G. S. On Considering alcohol as a risk factor in specific diseases. *Amer. J. Epidemiol.*, 107:462–466, 1978.

Butters, N., Cermak, L. S., Montgomery, K. & Adinolfi, A.: Some comparisons of the memory and visuoperceptive dificits of chronic alcoholics and patients with Korsakoff's disease. *Alc. Clin. Exp. Res.*, *1*:73–80, 1977.

Cahalan, D. Problem Drinkers: San Francisco. *Jassey-Bass, Inc.*, 1970.

Cahalan, D. & Cissin, I. H.: American drinking practices: Summary of findings from a national probability sample. I. Extent of drinking by population subgroups. *Quart. J. Stud. Alc.*, *29*:130–151, 1968.

Cahalan, D. & Room R. *Problem Drinking Among American Men*. Monog. No. 7, New Brunswick, N.J.: Rutgers Center for Alcohol Studies, 1974.

Carroll, P. J. The social hour for geropsychiatric patients. *J. Amer. Geriat. Soc.*, *26*:32–35, 1978.

Cermak, L. S., Butters, N. & Goodglass, H.: The extent of memory loss in Korsakoff patients. *Neuropsychologia*, *9*:307–315, 1971.

Cermak, L. S. & Ryback, R. S.: Recovery of verbal short-term memory in alcoholics. *J. Stud. Alc.*, *37*:46–52, 1976.

Chafetz, M. E. Alcohol and older persons. In: *Alcohol & Health*. Department of Health, Education and Welfare. Washington, D.C.: Government Printing Office, 1974, Chapter II.

Chien, C.-P. Psychiatric treatment for geriatric patients: "Pub" or drug? *Amer. J. Psychiat.*, *127–128*, 1070–1075, 1971.

Chien, C.-P. Stotsky, B. A. & Cole, J. O. Psychiatric treatment for nursing home patients: Drug, alcohol and milieu. *Amer. J. Psychol.*, *130*:543–548, 1973.

Costello, R. M. Mortality in an alcoholic cohort. *Int. J. Addict.*, *9*:355–363, 1974.

Curlee, J. Alcoholism and the "empty nest." *Bull. Menn. Clin.*, *33*:165–171, 1969.

Daniel, R. A. Five-year study of 693 psychogeriatric admissions in Queensland, *Geriatrics*, *27*:132–155, 1972.

Dorpat, T. L., Anderson, W. F. & Ripley, H. S. The relationship of physical illness to suicide. In: *Suicidal Behaviors*, H. L. P. Resnick (ed.), Boston: Little, Brown & Co., 1968, Chapter 15.

Drew, L. R. H. Alcoholism as a self-limiting disease. *Quart. J. Stud. Alc.*, *29*:956–967, 1968.

Droller, H. Some aspects of alcoholism in the elderly. *Lancet*, *2*:137–139, 1964.

Encel, S., Kotowicz, K. C. & Resler, H. E. Drinking pattern in Sydney, Australia. *Quart, J. Stud. Alc.*, *Suppl.* *6*:1–27, 1972.

Epstein, L. J. & Simon, A. Organic brain syndrome in the elderly. *Geriatrics*, *52*: 145–150, 1967.

Eriksson, K. Genetic aspects of alcohol drinking behaviour. *Int. J. Neurol.*, *9*:125–133, 1974.

Fillmore, K. M. Drinking and problem drinking in early adulthood and middle age: An exploratory 20-year follow-up study. *Quart. J. Stud. Alc.*, *35*:819–840, 1974.

Funkhouser, M. J. Identifying alcohol problems among elderly hospital patients. *Alc. Health & Res. World*, 27–37, Winter, 1977/78.

Gaitz, C. M. & Bear, P. E. Characteristics of elderly patients with alcoholism. *Arch. Gen. Psychiat.*, *24*:372–378, 1971.

Garrett, G. R. & Bahr, H. M. Women on Skid row. *Quart. J. Stud. Alc.*, *34*:1228–1243, 1973.

Glatt, M. M. Experiences with elderly alcoholics in England. *Alc.: Clin. & Exp. Res.*, *2*:23–26, 1978.

Glatt, M. M. & Rosin, A. J. Aspects of alcoholism in the elderly. *Lancet*, *2*:472–473, 1964. (Letter to Editor).

Goodwin, D. W., Hill, S. Y. & Hopper, S. Alcoholic blackouts and Korsakoff's syndrome. *Adv. Exp. Med. Biol.*, *59*:585–593, 1975.

Gould, I., Zahir, M., DeMartino, A., & Gomprecht, R. Cardiac effects of a cocktail. *JAMA*, *218*:1799–1802, 1971.

Greenblatt, M. & Schuckit, M., (Ed's.). *Alcoholism Problems in Women*. New York: Grume & Stratton, 1976.

Haberman, P. W. & Baden, M. M. Alcoholism and violent death. *Quart. J. Stud. Alc.*, *35*:221–231, 1974.

Harrington, J. G. & Price, A. C. Alcoholism in a geriatric setting. *J. Amer. Geriat. Soc.*, *10*:197–211, 1962.

Hoffman, H. & Nelson, P. C. Personality characteristics of alcoholics in relation to age and intelligence. *Psychol. Repts.*, *29*:143–146, 1971.

Hyman, M. M. Alcoholics 15 years later. In: *Alcoholism and Problem Drinking Among Older Persons*, E. P. Williams, B. Carruth, & M. M. Hyman, (eds.). New Brunswick: Rutgers University Press, 1973.

Jellinek, E. M. *The Disease Concept of Alcoholism*. New Haven, Connecticut: Hillhouse Press, 1960.

Johnson, L. A. Use of alcohol by persons 65 years and over, upper east side of Manhattan. *Final report to NIAAA/ADAMHA under contract HSM-43-73-38-NIA*. Washington, D.C.: Government Printing Office, January, 1974.

Jones, B. P., Moskowitz, H. R. & Butters, N. Olfactory discrimination in alcoholic Korsakoff patients. *Neuropsychologia*, *13*:173–179, 1975.

Klattsky, A. L., Friedman, G. D., Siegelaub, A. B., Gerard, M. J. Alcohol consumption among white, black, or oriental men and women: Kaiser-Permanente multiphasic health examination data. *Amer. J. Epidemiol.*, *105*:311–323, 1977.

Kleinknecht, R. A. & Goldstein, S. G. Neuropsychological deficits associated with alcoholism. *Quart. J. Stud. Alc.*, *33*:999–1019, 1972.

Knupfer, G. & Room, R. Age, sex and social class as factors in amount of drinking in a metropolitan community. *Social Prob.*, *12*:240, 1964.

Korboot, P. & Naylor, G. F. K. Patterns of WAIS and MIA in alcoholic dementia. *Austral. J. Psychol.*, *24*:227–234, 1972.

Leake, C. D. & Silverman, M. The clinical use of wine in geriatrics. *Geriatrics*, *22*:175–180, 1967.

Malin, H. J., Munch, N. E. & Archer, L. D. *A National Surveillance System for*

*Alcohol and Alcohol Abuse*. Presented at 32nd Internat. Cong. Alc. & Drug. Dep., Warsaw, Poland: Sept. 3–8, 1978.

Mayfield, D. G. Alcohol problems in the aging patient. In: *Drug Issues in Geropsychiatry*, Fann, W. E. & Maddox, G. L. (eds.), New York, Williams & Wilkins, 1974, pp. 35–40.

McEntee, W. J. & Mair, R. G. Memory impairment in Korsakoff's psychosis: A correlation with brain noradrenergic activity. *Science, 202*:905–907, 1978.

McCusker J., Cherubin, C. E. & Zimberg, S. Prevalence of alcoholism in general municipal hospital population. *N.Y. State J. Med.,* 71:751–754, 1971.

Mishara, B. L., Kastenbaum, R., Baker, F., & Patterson, R. D. Alcohol effects in old age: An experimental investigation. *Soc. Sci. & Med.*, 9:535–547, 1975.

Overall, J. E. & Gorham, D. R. Organicity versus old age in objective and projective test performance. *J. Consult. Clin. Psychol.*, 39:98–105, 1972.

Parker, E. A. & Noble, E. P. Drinking practices and cognitive functioning. In: *Alcohol Intoxication and Withdrawal*. M. M. Gross (ed), New York: Plenum Press, 1977. pp 377–388.

Pascarelli, E. F. Drug dependence: An age-old problem compounded by old age. *Geriatrics, 29*:109–115, 1974.

Pascarelli, E. F. & Fischer, W. Drug dependence in the elderly. *Int'l. J. Aging & Hum. Develop.*, 5:347–356, 1974.

Patterson, R. D., Abrahams, R. & Baker, F. Preventing self-destructive behavior. *Geriatrics, 29*:115–121, 1974.

Plutchik, R. & DiScipio, W. J. Personality patterns in chronic alcoholism (Korsakoff's syndrome), chronic schizophrenia, and geriatric patients with chronic brain syndrome. *J. Amer. Geriat. Soc.*, 22:514–516, 1974.

Rathbone-McCuan, E. & Bland, J. *Diagnostic and Referral Considerations for Geriatric Alcoholic and Aging Problem Drinker*. Presented at the 27th Ann. Mtg. Gerontological Soc., Portland, Ore: Oct. 28-Nov. 1, 1974.

Resnik, H. L. P. & Cantor, J. M. Suicide and aging. *J. Amer. Geriat. Soc.*, 18:152–158, 1970.

Ripley, H. S. Suicidal behavior in Edinburgh and Seattle. *Am. J. Psychiat.*, 130:995–1001, 1973.

Robins, E., Gassner, S., Kayes, J., Wilkinson, R. H. & Murphy, G. E. The communication of suicidal intent: A study of 134 consecutive cases of successful (completed) suicide. *Med. J.*, 12:724–733, Feb. 1959.

Rosin, A. J. & Glatt, M. M. Alcohol excess in the elderly. *Quart. J. Stud Alc.*, 32:53–39, 1971.

Russell, M., Welte, J. W., Hattwick, M. A. W. & Hadden, W. *Estimation of Alcohol Consumption from HANES Questions*. Presented at the Society for Epidem. Res. 11th Ann. Mtg., Iowa City, Iowa, June 14–16, 1978.

Schuckit, M. A. *An Overview of Alcohol and Drug Abuse Problems in the Elderly*. Testimony before the Subcommittee on Alcoholism and Narcotics and Subcommittee on Aging of the Senate Committee on Labor and Public Welfare. Washington, D.C.,: Congressional Record, June 7, 1976.

Schuckit, M. A. The high rate of psychiatric disorders in elderly cardiac patients. *Angiology*, 28:235–247, 1977.

Schuckit, M. A. & Miller, P. L. Alcoholism in elderly men: A survey of a general medical ward. *Ann. N.Y. Acad. Sci.*, 273:558–571, 1976.

Schuckit, M. A., Miller, P. L. & Hahlabohm, D. Unrecognized psychiatric illness in elderly medical-surgical patients. *Gerontology*, 30:655–659, 1975.

Schuckit, M. A., Morrissey, E. R. & O'Leary, M. R. Alcohol problems in elderly men and women. *Addict. Dis.*, 3:405–416, 1978.

Schuckit, M. A. & Pastor, Jr., P. A. Alcohol-related psychopathology in the aged. University of Washington., *Alc. Drug Abuse Inst. Tech. Rept.*, 10:78, 1978.

Schuckit, M. A. & Pastor, Jr., P. A. The elderly as a unique population: Alcoholism. *Alc. Clin. Exp. Res.*, 2:31–38, 1978.

Schuckit, M. A., Rimmer, J., Reich, T. & Winokur, G. Alcoholism: Antisocial traits in male alcoholics. *Brit. J. Psychiat.*, 117:575–576, 1970.

Siassi, I., Crocetti, G., & Spiro, H. R. Drinking patterns and alcoholism in a blue-collar population. *Quart. J. Stud. Alc.*, 34:917–926, 1973.

Simon, A., Epstein, L. J. & Reynolds, L. Alcoholism in the geriatric mentally ill. *Geriatrics*, 23:125–131, 1968.

Subley, P. *A Community Based Program for the Chemically Dependent Elderly*. Presented at the No. Am. Cong. Alc. & Drug Prob., San Francisco, December 1974.

Tarter, R. E. Brain damage associated with chronic alcoholism. *Dis. Nerv. Syst.*, 36:185–187, 1975.

Tarter, R. E., McBride, H., Buopane, N. & Schneider, D. U. Differentiation of alcoholics: Childhood history of minimal brain dysfunction, family history, and drinking pattern. *Arch. Gen. Psychiat.*, 34:761–768, 1977.

Tuckman, J. & Youngman, W. F. Assessment of suicide risk in attempted suicides. In: *Suicidal Behaviors: Diagnosis and Management*, Resnik, H. L. P. (ed.), Little Brown & Co. Boston: 1968.

Turner, T. B. Beer and wine for geriatric patients. *JAMA*, 226:779–780, 1973.

Vestal, R. E., Norris, A. H., Tobin, J. D., Cohen, B. H., Shock, N. W., & Andres, R. Antipyrine metabolism in man: Influence of age, alcohol, caffeine, and smoking. *Clin. Pharmcol. & Ther.*, 18:425–432, 1975.

Waller, J. A. Injury in aged. *N.Y. State J. Med.*, 74: 2200–2208, 1974.

Wallgren, H. & Barry, H. *Actions of Alcohol*, vol. I. *Biochemical, physiological, & Psychological aspects*. New York: Elsevier, 1970.

Wechler, H., Thum, D., Demone, H. W. & Dwinnell, J. Social characteristics & blood alcohol level. *Quart. J. Stud. Alc.*, 33:132–147, 1972.

Westermeyer, J. Options regarding alcohol use among the Chippewa. *Amer. J. Orthopsychiat.*, 42:398–403, 1972.

Wiik-Larsen, E. & Enger, E. Drug and alcohol induced deaths within and outside hospitals in Oslo due to acute self-induced intoxication. *Tidsskr. Nor. Laegeforen (Norw)*, F-8:371–373, 1978.

Williams, J. D., Ray, C. G. & Overall, J. E. Mental aging and organicity in an
   alcoholic population. *J. Consult. Clin. Psychol.*, *41*:392–396, 1973.
Zimberg, S. Outpatient geriatric psychiatry in an urban ghetto with nonprofes-
   sional workers. *Amer. J. Psychiat.*, *125*:1697–1702, 1969.
Zimberg, S. The psychiatrist and medical home care: Geriatric psychiatry in the
   Harlem community. *Amer. J. Psychiat.*, *127*:102–106, 1971.
Zimberg, S. The elderly alcoholic. *Gerontologist, 14*:221–224, 1974.
Zimberg, S. Diagnosis and treatment of the elderly alcoholic. *Alc.: Clin. & Exp.
   Res.*, *2*:27–29, 1978.

# Index

# Index

Substance abuse, 196
Substantia nigra, 71, 73
Succinylcholine, 100, 102
Sudden death, 23, 113
Suicide, 98, 139, 216, 236, 238, 255,
    264, 265
"Sundowner's syndrome," 92, 148,
    149
Suspiciousness, 184, 189
Sympathetic activation, 55
Sympathetic hyperactivity, 54, 65
Sympathetic nervous system, 52
Sympathetic tonus, 52, 54, 55

Tachycardia, 99, 226
Tagomet, 212
Tardive dyskinesia, 19, 155, 225
Temazepam, 38, 39
Tension, 228, 246
Testosterone, 97
Tetracyclic antidepressants, 119, 122,
    149
Thiamine, 167, 270
Thiazide diuretics, 151
Thioridazine, 9, 15, 17, 22, 23, 90,
    149, 150, 171, 228
Thiothixene, 23, 24, 190
Tinnitus, 70
Torticollis opisthotonos, 18
Toxic confusional state, 20
Tranylcypromine, 5, 6, 151
Trauma, 194
Tremor, 18, 76, 141, 149
Triazolam, 35, 64, 91
Tricyclic antidepressants, 1, 2, 6, 21,
    23, 24, 97, 105, 112–122, 147,

150–153, 165, 169, 170, 212–
    216
Trifluoperazine, 150, 223
Triglyceride, 270
Trihexyphenidyl, 150, 155
Tryptamine, 2, 3

Unilateral ECT, 101
Unipolar depression, 215, 234
Urinary obstruction, 170

Vascular dementia, 194
Vasoactive medications, 127, 128, 133
Vasodilators, 133
Vasolantin, 131
Ventricular arrhythmias, 117, 121,
    122, 151, 152
Violence, 243, 264
Vitamin $B_{12}$, 270, 272
Vitamin E, 131

Weight gain, 22, 229
Weight loss, 98, 211
Wernicke-Korsakoff syndrome, 266,
    267
Widowhood, 258
Withdrawal, 75, 76, 78, 85, 90, 236,
    255
Work history, 257, 270
Worthlessness, 98, 215

Xanthinol niacinate, 131
Xenon inhalation, 219

Zinc, 270